of the hair and scalp

Handbook of diseases of the hair and scalp

Rodney D. Sinclair MB BS FACD

Senior Lecturer
Department of Dermatology
St Vincent's Hospital
Melbourne
Australia

Cedric C. Banfield MSc MBBS MRCP(UK)

Stoke Mandeville Hospital
Dermatology Department
Aylesbury
UK

Rodney P.R. Dawber MA FRCP

Consultant Dermatologist
Department of Dermatology
The Churchill Hospital
Oxford
UK

b

**Blackwell
Science**

© 1999 by
Blackwell Science Ltd
Editorial Offices:
Osney Mead, Oxford OX2 0EL
25 John Street, London WC1N 2BL
23 Ainslie Place, Edinburgh EH3 6AJ
350 Main Street, Malden
    MA 02148 5018, USA
54 University Street, Carlton
    Victoria 3053, Australia
10, rue Casimir Delavigne
    75006 Paris, France

Other Editorial Offices:
Blackwell Wissenschafts-Verlag GmbH
Kurfürstendamm 57
10707 Berlin, Germany

Blackwell Science KK
MG Kodenmacho Building
7–10 Kodenmacho Nihombashi
Chuo-ku, Tokyo 104, Japan

The right of the Authors to be
identified as the Authors of this Work
has been asserted in accordance
with the Copyright, Designs and
Patents Act 1988.

First published 1999

Set by Excel Typesetters Co., Hong Kong
Printed and bound in Italy
by Rotolito Lombarda SpA, Milan

A catalogue record for this title
is available from the British Library

ISBN 0-86542-928-6

Library of Congress
Cataloging-in-publication Data

Sinclair, Rodney D.
    Handbook of diseases of the hair and
    scalp /
    Rodney D. Sinclair, Cedric Banfield,
    Rodney P.R. Dawber.
        p.   cm.
    Companion v. to: Diseases of the hair
        and scalp /
        edited by Rodney Dawber.
        3rd ed. 1997.
    ISBN 0-86542-928-6
        1. Hair—Diseases—Handbooks,
    manuals, etc.
        2. Scalp—Diseases—Handbooks,
    manuals, etc.
    I. Banfield, Cedric. II. Dawber, R. P. R.
    (Rodney P. R.) III. Diseases of the hair
    and scalp. IV. Title.
        [DNLM: 1. Hair Diseases handbooks.
    2. Hair Diseases atlases.
    3. Scalp Dermatoses handbooks.
    4. Scalp Dermatoses atlases.
    WR 39 S616h 1999]
    RL151.S586   1999
    616.5'46—dc21
    DNLM/DLC
    for Library of Congress   98-29004
                                        CIP

For further information on
Blackwell Science, visit our website:
www.blackwell-science.com

The Blackwell Science logo is a
trade mark of Blackwell Science Ltd,
registered at the United Kingdom
Trade Marks Registry

DISTRIBUTORS
Marston Book Services Ltd
PO Box 269
Abingdon, Oxon OX14 4YN
(Orders: Tel: 01235 465500
            Fax: 01235 465555)

USA
Blackwell Science, Inc.
Commerce Place
350 Main Street
Malden, MA 02148 5018
(Orders: Tel: 800 759 6102
                    781 388 8250
            Fax: 781 388 8255)

Canada
Login Brothers Book Company
324 Saulteaux Crescent
Winnipeg, Manitoba, R3J 3T2
(Orders: Tel: 204 837-2987)

Australia
Blackwell Science Pty Ltd
54 University Street
Carlton, Victoria 3053
(Orders: Tel: 3 9347 0300
            Fax: 3 9347 5001)

1-04 PPC 99-W-6258-PB

Contents

Introduction

This book has been written as a companion to the parent text, *Diseases of the Hair and Scalp* edited by Rodney Dawber. The aim of this book is to act first as a text-atlas that can be used by the clinician to confirm a diagnosis and then as a source of concise, management orientated information for that condition.

The book is organized into sections based on the chief symptom complained of by the patient and further divided into chapters based on the pathological process. A description of the histology of those conditions where a biopsy is useful in establishing or confirming the diagnosis is included.

This book deals with a comprehensive range of hair and scalp disorders faced by physicians. For those conditions where a treatment is available, that treatment is discussed. While for those conditions without effective treatment the emphasis is on being able to communicate sufficient information to the patient so that they understand the nature of the condition and the likely natural history.

The text that accompanies the photos is not referenced; however, if references or more detailed information on a particular topic are required then the reader is referred to the parent text.

While individually many of the diseases described in this book are rare, there are a sufficient number of these rare conditions for most clinicians to encounter one or more of them in the course of clinical practice. There is a role for a well illustrated book dealing concisely with a broad range of conditions that affect the hair and scalp and this book is aimed to slot in between standard dermatology texts that emphasize the more common disorders and the expensive tomes that are designed for dermatologists with a specific interest in these diseases and for hair research workers. Additionally endocrinologists, paediatricians and dermatopathologists who encounter hair disorders may find this text of interest.

Rodney D. Sinclair
Cedric Banfield
Rodney P.R. Dawber

Acknowledgements

We would like to thank all the Australian, British and international dermatologists who have allowed us to reproduce their photographs in this book. We also thank those dermatologists who have referred their patients to us as well as Dorovitch Trezise Pathology and the medical illustration departments at St. Vincent's and the Alfred Hospitals in Melbourne and the John Radcliffe Hospital in Oxford for their help and expertise.

We also thank Julian Barth, David de Berker, David Fenton, Chris Gummer, Andrew Messenger and Nick Simpson who coauthored the parent textbook on which this handbook is based.

Finally, we dedicate this book to our wives and partners Ellen Williamson, Ann Banfield and Maggie Dawber in appreciation of their considerable support.

Rodney D. Sinclair
Cedric Banfield
Rodney P.R. Dawber

Section A
Hair biology

Chapter 1

Hair structure and function

1.1 Hair biology

Hair is a defining characteristic of mammals. Evolution has robbed humans of the fine pelage seen on our simian ancestors, but vestigial hair remains on the scalp, axillary, beard and perineal areas. The importance of hair to humans is obvious, not only to those who deal with diseases of the hair and scalp, but also to those who profit from it in the hairdressing and hair cosmetic industries.

The human skin supports approximately five million hair follicles, of which only one hundred thousand are on the scalp. Most of these follicles produce vellus hairs that are cosmetically insignificant. Many never produce hairs long enough to protrude from the follicular ostium. The majority of hairs on the scalp are terminal hairs that uncut may grow up to a metre long. Hair can be red, blond, brown or black and straight, wavy or curly. These natural variations are an important part of our identity that can be manipulated according to the dictates of fashion or society.

Each hair arises from a follicle consisting of epidermis that has invaginated the dermis to form a sleeve-like structure. The base of the follicle is intimately associated with the dermal papilla, and hair is the product of interaction and communication between dermis and epidermis. The hair shaft consists of keratinocytes that are compacted and cemented together. The final product is remarkably strong and resistant to the extremes of nature (Fig. 1.1).

Types of hair

The type of hair produced by an individual follicle can change with age or under the influence of hormones. The three, main recognized types of hair are listed below.
1 Lanugo hair is formed and shed during the seventh or eighth month *in utero*. It consists of fine, soft, nonpigmented hair that has no central medulla.
2 Vellus hair is the fine, unmedullated hair found on glabrous skin that is usually shorter than 2 cm and non-pigmented (Fig. 1.2)
3 Terminal hair is the coarse pigmented, long hair found on the scalp, eyebrows and eyelashes prior to puberty and additionally in the pubic, axillary, chest and beard areas of adults.

Intermediate or indeterminate forms of hair also exist on the scalp of infants at 3 months and last until the age of 2 years. They are coarser than lanugo hair and sparsely pigmented, however, they do not have a well-defined medulla like that found in terminal hair. Similar hair also appears on adult scalps in the context of androgenetic alopecia, a process that results in miniaturization of terminal hairs and ultimate reversion into vellus hairs (Fig. 1.3).

1.2 Hair anatomy

The sites of attachment of the arrector pili muscle and the sebaceous gland act as anatomical boundaries separating the hair follicle into three parts:
1 the bulb, which extends from the base of the follicle to the insertion of the arrector pili muscle;
2 the isthmus, which extends from the insertion of the arrector pili muscle to the sebaceous duct;
3 the infundibulum, which runs from the entrance of the sebaceous duct to the follicular ostium (Fig. 1.4).

Each terminal hair consists of either two or three elements depending on whether it is of sufficient size and calibre to develop a central core or medulla. If present, this central medulla, which arises from hair matrix cells, may occur intermittently along the hair. It is encased by the hair cortex, which forms the major part of the hair shaft and contributes most to

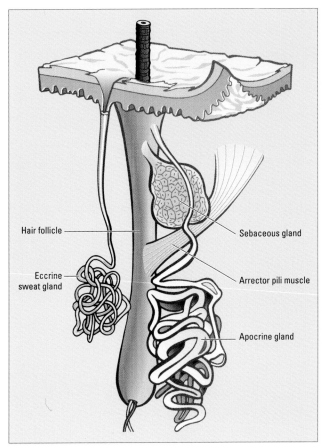

Fig. 1.1 Pilosebaceous apparatus arises from the epidermis and invaginates into the dermis.

the colour and the mechanical properties of hair. The cortex is in turn encircled by the hair cuticle, a shield that protects the hair cortex and is responsible for the lustre and texture of hair.

The medulla exists as a framework of spongy keratin supporting thin shells of amorphous material bounding air spaces of variable size. It is best seen on light microscopy of hair where, because of refraction of light, the air

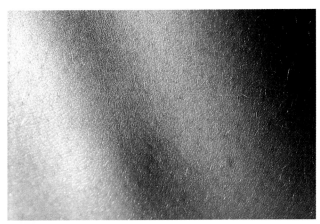

Fig. 1.2 Vellus hairs.

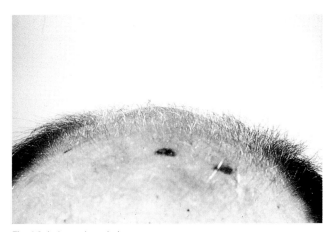

Fig. 1.3 Indeterminate hairs.

spaces appear dark (Fig. 1.5). In animals the central air canal of hair provides an insulating effect crucial to thermoregulation. However, in humans the medulla is a vestigial structure.

The cortex consists of closely packed spindle cells containing cytoplasmic filaments that run parallel to the long axis of hair (Fig. 1.6). These filaments are hard alpha keratin fibres that appear different to the tonofibrils found in epidermal keratinocytes. Each cell is separated by a narrow gap containing proteinaceous material that cements the cells together and contributes to the incredible strength of the hair shaft. Melanocytes are found only in the hair matrix at the base of the cortex and produce melanin granules that intersperse throughout the cortex.

The cuticle consists of a single layer of cells that overlap in a similar way to roof tiles, with the free margin pointing towards the tip of the hair (Fig. 1.7). These cells are the first part of the emerging hair to harden by undergoing keratinization, and determine the shape of the emerging hair (Fig. 1.8). If the cuticle is damaged the cortex will quickly degenerate, resulting in broken hairs and split ends. The strength of the cuticle comes from the strong high sulphur protein present in the outer part of each cuticular cell. Absence of this protein, which occurs in trichothiodystrophy produces weakened, fragile hairs that break off close to the root.

The inner root sheath is one of the two root sheaths that surround the hair shaft. It is also produced by the hair matrix and comprises three distinct layers of cells (Fig. 1.4). The single-cell layer of Henle is outermost, the double cell layer of Huxley is central and the innermost inner root sheath cuticle consists of a single layer of overlapping cells akin to roof tiles, but in contrast to the hair cuticle, the free margin of these cells points downwards allowing the two cuticles to interlock. The two cuticles are so completely integrated that the interlocking cells appear as a single cell layer on light microscopy. The inner root sheath forms trichohyaline granules (which are more eosinophilic than keratohyaline granules) and keratinizes before the hair shaft does and so is an important scaffold for the developing hair and it determines the ultimate shape of the hair shaft. The hair that ultimately emerges from

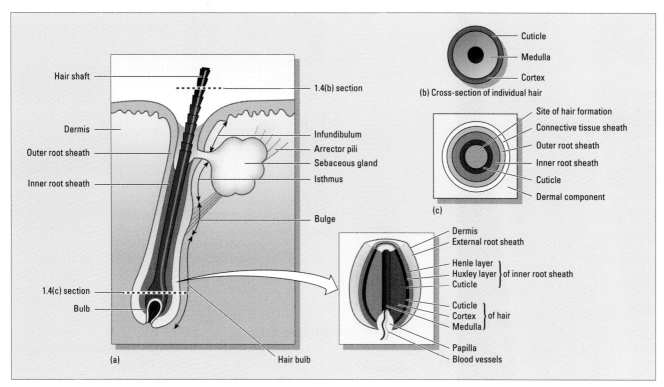

Fig. 1.4 (a) A mature hair in vertical section. Arrowed lines show levels of transverse section shown in parts (b) and (c). (b) Cross-section of individual hair. (c) Cross-section of hair follicle.

the follicle is devoid of its inner root sheath. This disintegrates at the isthmus and the residue is discharged into the pilosebaceous canal.

The outer root sheath is also known as the tricholemma (Greek: coating or sac around the hair). Its upper part surrounding the follicular ostium merges imperceptibly with the adjacent epidermis. In the dermis the outer root sheath is thickest at the isthmus and narrowest at the bulb where it is only one or two cells thick. The outer layer is a germinative layer resting on a basement membrane that is continuous with basal epidermis. Differentiation occurs centrally towards the inner root sheath with the cells enlarging, flattening and becoming vacuolated. The exact fate of the cells adjacent to the inner root sheath is not known but it is presumed they keratinize without the formation of keratohyaline granules and are shed into the pilosebaceous canal along with cells of the inner root sheath. The vitreous or glassy membrane lies external to the basement membrane of the outer

root sheath and is a noncellular connective tissue sheath enveloping the follicle.

The arrector pili muscle arises from of the outer root sheath at the junction between the bulb and isthmus. It inserts

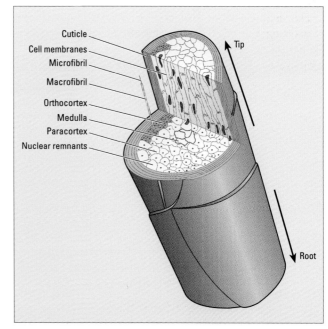

Fig. 1.6 Ultrastructure of a hair shaft.

Fig. 1.5 Terminal hair showing continuous central medulla.

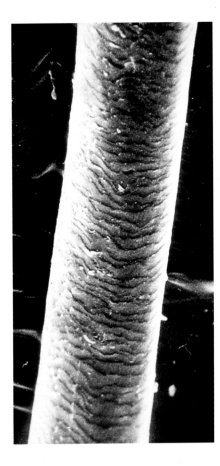

Fig. 1.7 Normal hair, root end, with unweathered, closely opposed, overlapping cuticular scales.

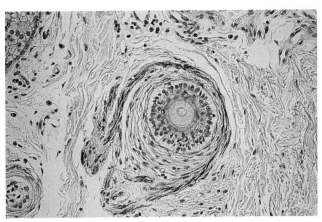

Fig. 1.9 High magnification of a vellus hair follicle in transverse section showing circumferential insertion of the arrector pili muscle (desmin, peroxidase 3-amino-9-ethylcarbazole stain). (Reproduced with permission from Narisawa, Y., Kohda, H. *British Journal of Dermatology* (1993) **129**, 138–9.)

predominantly into a bulge on the posterior wall, but some fibres insert circumferentially (Fig. 1.9). This bulge contains a group of germinative cells that can be identified histochemically. With the onset of anagen, bulge cells proliferate and repopulate the transient portion of the follicle that involutes with catagen. The cells within the bulge are the immortal stem cells of the hair follicle, and destruction of the bulge will permanently destroy the follicle.

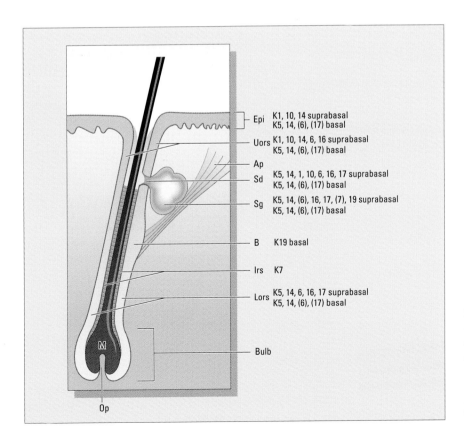

Fig. 1.8 The structure and expression of epithelial keratins in the hair follicle. Epi, epidermis; Uors, upper outer root sheath; Sd, sebaceous duct; Sg, sebaceous gland; Ap, arrector pili muscle; B, bulge stem cell region; Irs, inner root sheath; Lors, lower outer root sheath; M, matrix; Dp, dermal papilla. (After C. Wilson.)

Cells of the outer root sheath express different keratin markers (Fig. 1.7) to the cells of the medulla, cortex, cuticle and inner root sheath which all express similar keratins. This reflects the common origin of these latter hair components from specialized matrix, while the outer root sheath derives from adjacent epidermis.

The dermal papilla consists of an oval mass of spindle cells resting in a local environment rich in mucopolysaccharides. The papilla is surrounded by hair matrix epithelium from which it is separated by a thick basement membrane except where it sits on a dermal fibroelastic plate called the Arao-Perkins body. The papilla receives a rich neurovascular supply. It plays a vital role in stimulating embryological follicle formation and regulating the hair cycle. There is a close relationship between the mitotic activity of the dermal papilla fibroblasts and the hair matrix keratinocytes and the size of the dermal papilla correlates closely with the size of the hair follicle.

The vascular supply surrounding the hair follicle arises from the subdermal arterial plexus. It is richest at the bulb and the insertion of the sebaceous duct. It too involutes during hair dormancy (late catagen) and regenerates early in anagen.

Sensory nerves and neural end organs (predominantly Pinkus corpuscles) encase the entire length of the hair follicle like a glove (Fig. 1.10), however, nerve axons do not penetrate the outer root sheath. All hairs are innervated, usually by several myelinated nerve fibres. While hairs may act as subtle organs of touch, the physiological and pathological significance of this innervation requires further investigation. Additional efferent autonomic nerve fibres supply the arrector pili muscles, and stimulation produces the sensation of goose bumps.

1.3 Hair embryology

The full quota of hair follicles is present at birth, and no new follicles develop thereafter. Secondary sexual hair is the result of an androgen triggered switch to the production of terminal hairs rather than vellus hairs in pre-existing follicles.

Hair follicles develop as epidermal down growths that invaginate the dermis and subcutaneous fat and enclose at their base a small stud of highly specialized dermis known as the dermal papilla. The site of these down growths is probably determined by the location of these papillae in the dermis. Follicles exist as pilosebaceous units that also give rise to the sebaceous glands, arrector pili muscles and in certain areas the apocrine glands.

In the ninth week of embryonic development, rudiments of hair follicles appear on the eyebrows, upper lip and chin; sites in which vibrissae (whiskers) are present in other mammals. At 16 weeks hair is developing within these follicles while the development of other follicles is gradually extending cephalocaudally.

The first sign of hair follicle development is the focal crowding of basal cell nuclei in the fetal epidermis to form

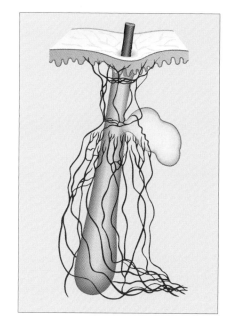

Fig. 1.10 Nerve endings in the hairy skin. The hair follicles innervated by free endings of circular fibres and expanded tips of the palisade fibres. (After Montagna.)

what is called the primitive hair germ (Fig. 1.11). These appear on the skin surface in groups of three at fixed intervals of between 274 and 350 µm. The hair germs enlarge asymmetrically and grow obliquely downwards into the dermis to form a solid column of cells known as the hair peg. The lower end of the enlarging hair peg becomes bulbous and encloses a group of mesodermal cells destined to become the papilla.

At the same time two or three swellings develop on the posterior wall of the hair peg. The upper bulge is the germ of the apocrine gland. It is uncertain whether apocrine glands only develop in the axilla, groin, external ear canal, eyelid and breasts or if they initially develop in all follicles, only to later involute other than in these selected sites.

The middle swelling is the germ of the sebaceous gland, while the lower swelling becomes the site of attachment of the arrector pili muscle. This lower swelling persists as the hair bulge and is a source of follicular stem cells crucial to the regeneration of anagen hairs during the hair cycle. The arrector pili muscle was previously assumed to attach only to the bulge on the posterior wall of the hair follicle, but recently it has been shown to attach circumferentially.

The cells immediately surrounding the dermal papilla constitute the hair matrix, comprising undifferentiated proliferating cells that produce the hair medulla, cortex and cuticle as well as the inner root sheath. The outer root sheath of the hair is derived from epidermis, while the mesodermal cells surrounding the bulb give rise to the connective tissue sheath.

1.4 The hair cycle

In man hair follicles show intermittent activity. Thus each hair grows to a maximum length, is retained for a period of time without further growth and is eventually shed and

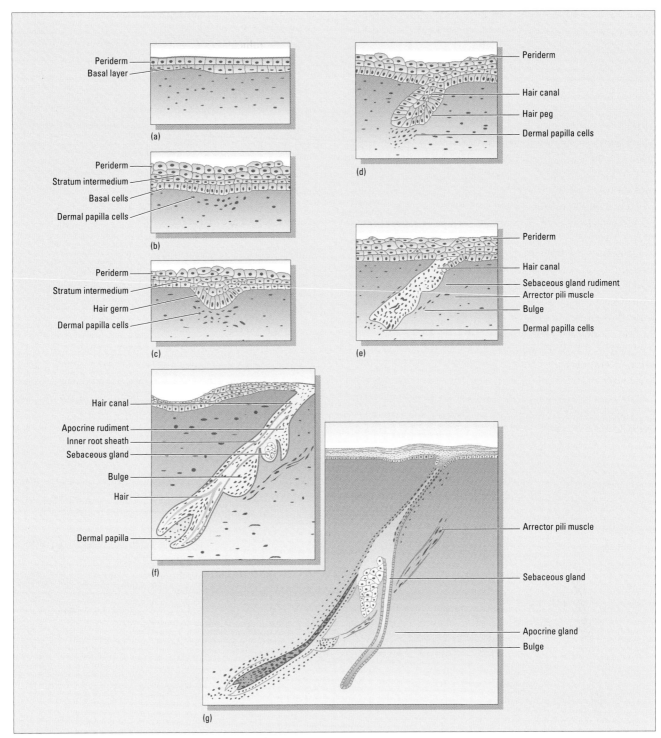

Fig. 1.11 Development of the hair follicle. (a) Section of skin of a foetus at about 4 weeks. The periderm is clearly seen, and a basal or generative layer appears in occasional areas. (b) Skin at about 11 weeks. The epidermis is made up of basal cells, cuboidal in shape, and cells of the stratum intermedium are beginning to appear above them. The periderm consists of two or three cell layers. Dermal papilla cells are beginning to aggregate below the presumptive hair follicle. This is the primitive hair germ. (c) Hair germ stage. Basal cells are now columnar and starting to grow downwards. (d) Hair peg stage. Cells of the so-called hair canal form a solid strand. (e) Bulbous hair peg. Note solid hair canal, sebaceous gland rudiment and bulge for attachment of the developing arrector pili muscle. This is the presumptive location of hair stem cells. (f) Later stage showing apocrine rudiment, sebaceous gland, now partly differentiated, and bulge. The dermal papilla has been enclosed and hair is starting to form, with an inner root sheath. (g) Complete pilosebaceous unit of axillary skin from a 26-week-old fetus. The sebaceous gland is well differentiated and the apocrine gland is canalized. (Courtesy of the late Professor F.J.G. Ebling.)

replaced (Fig. 1.12). The duration of activity varies greatly from region to region and subtle variation also occurs with age and between males and females.

Anagen is the period of active growth and in a vellus follicle lasts between 6 and 12 weeks. In terminal hairs anagen lasts 4–14 weeks on the moustache, 6–12 weeks on the arms, 19–26 weeks on the leg and 2–5 years on the vertex of the scalp.

Anagen can be subdivided into six stages that to some extent recapitulate the embryological development of the hair follicle. The first five are collectively known as proanagen and are characterized by progressively higher levels of the new hair tip within the follicle. Anagen 6, also known as metanagen, is defined by the emergence of the hair above the skin surface.

Catagen is the transitional phase that follows anagen and usually lasts 2 weeks. It is not clear what triggers induce the spontaneous cessation of mitosis, rapid terminal differentiation of keratinocytes and apoptosis within the regressing hair bulb that all occur in catagen. Changes in the vasculature appear to be secondary events. With the onset of catagen, melanin production ceases and melanocytes resorb their dendrites. Keratinization of the hair and inner root sheath continues and the result is a nonpigmented expansion at the base of the hair in the shape of a club.

Telogen is the resting phase of the hair cycle. The club hair with its nonpigmented bulb is held in a sac and is retained in the follicle until the development of the next anagen hair is well established. Telogen usually lasts 3 months on the scalp before the follicle spontaneously re-enters anagen, however a premature anagen can be triggered by plucking the resting club hair.

Hair stem cells in the bulge begin to proliferate at the end of telogen and daughter cells differentiate into the new anagen bulb (anagen 1). The new bulb grows downwards, encloses the dermal papilla (anagen 2) and anagen is once again under way. Finally the new anagen hair pushes the old club hair out just before it emerges from the follicular ostium.

In animals the hair cycle is synchronized such that the entire pelage grows continuously through winter. When summer comes growth abruptly ceases and a cephalocaudal malt ensues. This synchronized growth pattern also occurs in human hair *in utero*. Hairs first appear on the scalp at 20 weeks gestation and then grow over the rest of the body cephalocaudally. Initially all hairs are in anagen. At 26 weeks the scalp hairs enter catagen and then telogen in a progressive wave from the frontal to the parietal region over a period of seven days (Fig. 1.13). These telogen hairs are mostly shed *in utero*. Occipital hairs, however, remain in anagen until about 38 weeks and then they too enter catagen. Meanwhile the frontal and parietal hairs have re-entered anagen and formed the second pelage. When these hairs subsequently enter catagen the second wave forms.

At full term there are two consecutive waves of hair, each of

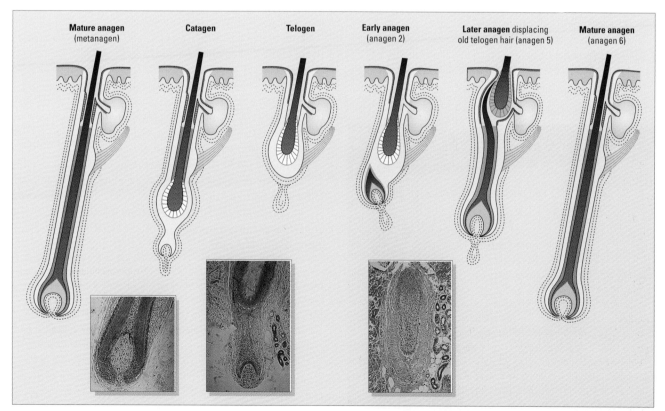

| Mature anagen (metanagen) | Catagen | Telogen | Early anagen (anagen 2) | Later anagen displacing old telogen hair (anagen 5) | Mature anagen (anagen 6) |

Fig. 1.12 The hair cycle.

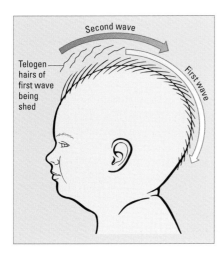

Fig. 1.13 Child aged 7 months demonstrating wave of hair fall which is progressing over frontoparietal regions.

which is running from the forehead to the occiput. Over the occiput the primary hairs do not enter telogen until 8–12 weeks after birth and then fall producing a well-defined area of alopecia. This has been described as occipital alopecia of the newborn and the only contribution of rubbing the head on the pillow (which is often blamed) is to facilitate release of telogen hairs (Fig. 1.14).

Following the first two synchronized moults of the child and towards the end of the first year of life there is a change in the relationship of adjacent hairs such that a random mosaic pattern emerges in which each hair follows its own intrinsic rhythm. This asynchrony continues throughout life, unless modified by pregnancy or illness. At any one time there will be a uniform distribution of hairs in each stage of the cycle reflecting the relative duration of the hair cycle phases.

On the scalp approximately 86% of hairs will be in anagen, 1% in catagen and 13% in telogen. As there are about 100 000 hairs on the scalp of which 13 000 are in telogen, and telogen lasts around 3 months, approximately 100–200 hairs are shed each day in times of health.

1.5 Systemic and local influences on the hair cycle

Circulating androgens increase both the rate of hair growth and the calibre of the hair (transforming vellus to terminal hairs) in androgen dependant sites such as the beard. Paradoxically in the scalp of a person genetically predisposed to androgenetic alopecia, androgens reduce both the rate of scalp hair growth and the calibre (transforming terminal to vellus hairs) of the hair, while antiandrogens partially restore it. It is not known why or how the same chemical can induce exactly opposite effects on different hair follicles. Despite these relatively site specific changes, most hairs on the body are relatively uninfluenced by androgens. This insensitivity is most likely due to the differences in follicular metabolism of androgens, possible related to regional variation in the distribution of 5α reductase isoenzymes.

Oestrogens reduce the rate of hair growth, but prolong the duration of anagen. This is best seen during pregnancy when there is decreased hair shedding. Post-partum, large numbers of hairs enter catagen and subsequently telogen, which is followed by sometimes massive shedding, approximately 3 months after the birth, known as telogen effluvium gravidarum.

Thyroxine hastens the onset of anagen in resting follicles and corticosteroids delay it. There is also a seasonal variation on the rate of hair growth in man such that it grows faster in summer and falls in winter. It is mediated through the pineal gland but the exact mechanism is obscure.

In regions of the body other than the scalp anagen is relatively short and telogen relatively long (Table 1.1). At any given time up to half the follicles in a particular region will be dormant. Events that cause epithelial hyperplasia such as wounds will also initiate a new anagen in a resting follicle. Interestingly the inflammation of a ringworm infection synchronizes hairs into telogen in the area surrounding the lesions, thus limiting extension of the infection.

Cutting or shaving has no influence on the rate of hair growth or on the calibre of the hair produced by the follicle. Maximum hair length is genetically determined. It depends on the duration of anagen and the rate of growth. Hair will not achieve its maximum length if it is intrinsically weak or extrinsically damaged.

Table 1.1 Approximate duration of anagen and telogen at various body sites.

	Anagen (weeks)	Telogen (weeks)
Scalp	150	12
Moustache	16	6
Finger	12	9
Arms	13	13
Leg	23	19

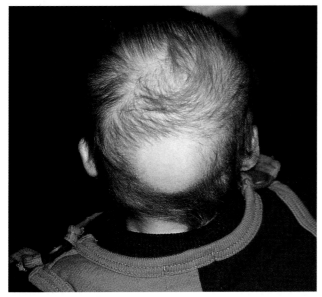

Fig. 1.14 Occipital alopecia in a child aged 9 months.

Changes in hair growth have been observed in skin affected by a variety of neurological abnormalities. Terminal hairs overlying a neural tube defect (faun tail) or around ectopic neural tissue on the scalp (the hair collar sign) are well recognized. Shorter hair was noted on the right side of the scalp in a patient with syringomyelia with impaired pain and temperature sensation in the region. Causalgia has been associated with decreased hair growth in affected areas, reflex sympathetic dystrophy may produce hypertrichosis, while denervation of skin can produce either decreased hair growth or hypertrichosis. The mechanism of these changes is not understood.

1.6 Physical properties of hair

Much information of the physical properties of hair has been derived from research on the keratin fibres in wool. The strength of human hair resides in the cortex where longitudinally orientated keratin fibres embedded in a sulphur rich matrix are packaged in cell envelopes. This composite structure allows hair to be deformed by mechanical stress and the energy dissipated evenly into the fibre at the fibre matrix interface. The cuticle also plays a vital role in hair resistance to external stress, as is evidenced by the relative fragility of weathered hair that has lost its cuticle.

Hair shaft dimensions show variation between races. Mongoloid hair is circular in cross-section and large with a mean diameter of 120 μm. Caucasoid hair is elliptical in cross-section and smaller. It has a mean diameter of between 50 and 90 μm with the variation being due to the larger calibre of dark hair compared to fair hair. Negroid hair is flattened, curled and oval in cross-section. Longitudinal grooving is common. The different cross-sectional shapes of hair correspond to the flat straight appearance of Mongoloid hair, the wavy fuller bodied Caucasoid hair and the tightly curled Negroid hair.

When dry hair is rubbed or combed static electricity is produced. This is associated with 'fly away' hair. Certain shampoos and conditioners decrease fly away hair and lessen the static charge by reducing the frictional force during combing and increasing hair moisture.

1.7 Hair colour, canites and poliosis

Hair without pigment is white due to reflection and refraction of incident light. This is accentuated by a broad medulla as found in the hairs of many arctic animals. The variety of colours seen in animal hair is due to the combinations of pigments produced which include porphyrins, carotenoids and melanin. In contrast the range of human hair colour is limited as it is produced entirely by melanin within the keratinocytes of the cortex with a small contribution from the medulla.

Melanocytes present in the hair bulb at the apex of the dermal papilla are able to produce two types of melanin pigment; eumelanin which is responsible for black and brown hair and pheomelanin which produces auburn and blond hair. Pheomelanin is unique to hair and is not found in the epidermis. It is produced by a modification of the eumelanin synthesis pathway that involves an interaction of dopaquinone with cysteine (Fig. 1.15). Usually an individual will only produce either pheomelanin or eumelanin throughout life, however, some people's hair colour changes spontaneously, and a number of blond children grow up to become brunettes.

Nonfunctional melanocytes are also present in the outer root sheath of the lower part of the follicle. They do not contribute to hair colour, but become involved in the repigmentation that occurs with resolution of vitiligo or with wound healing. Epidermal and hair melanocytes are independently involved in certain disorders. For example vitiligo can have pigmented hairs arising from depigmented skin. The reverse occurs in poliosis or canites, when hair turns grey.

Subtle variations in hair colour are due to variations in the number of melanocytes present in a follicle, the density of melanin formation within melanosomes and melanosome shape (oval melanosomes being more readily degraded), the transfer of melanosomes to hair matrix cells and the distribution and metabolism of the melanosomes within the hair cortex keratinocytes.

Melanocytes are only functionally active during anagen and lie dormant in telogen hairs. When anagen restarts, melanocytes reawaken and new melanocytes are produced by replication. Despite this proliferation of melanocytes, melanoma arising in the hair follicle does not seem to occur. Anagen hairs are usually uniformly pigmented. An exception to this is nose hair arising from the nasal mucosa,

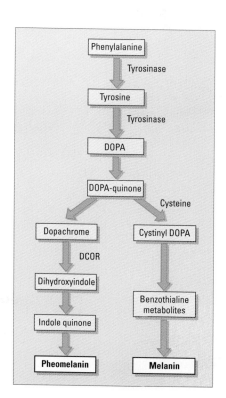

Fig. 1.15 Pathway of melanin production. (DCOR, dopachrome oxidoreductase).

which have a nonpigmented 2–3 mm tip, that gradually darkens.

Hair colour varies according to the body site with eyelashes being darkest. Scalp hair is usually lighter than pubic hair which often has a red tinge. A red tinge is also common in axillary and beard hair even in people with essentially brown hair on their scalp. Sunlight bleaches hair, and after death hair is slowly oxidized which lightens the colour.

Hormones such as melanin stimulating hormone (MSH) can darken light hair as can oestrogens and progestogens during pregnancy. Drugs that can change hair colour include: antimalarials such as chloroquine, mephenesin, triparanol, butyrophenone and phenylthiourea that all produce lightening, while carbidopa, bromocryptine, minoxidil and diazoxide tend to produce darkening.

Inheritance of hair colour is complex and appears to be controlled by multiple loci in the genome. A putative gene locus for red hair has been identified, but awaits further confirmation.

Greying of hair, or canites

This occurs in both man and primates (Fig. 1.16) and is a manifestation of ageing. It is due to a progressive reduction in

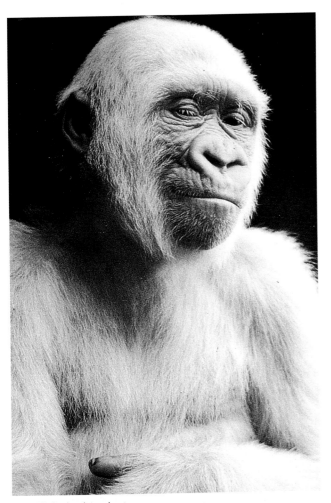

Fig. 1.16 Canites in a primate.

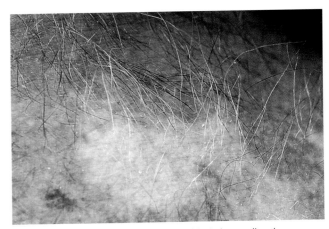

Fig. 1.17 Vitiligo showing depigmentation of the hair as well as the epidermis.

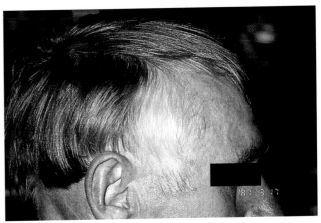

Fig. 1.18 Regrowth of white hair following alopecia areata.

melanocyte function rather than number. Canites can occur prematurely in autoimmune disorders such as pernicious anaemia, vitiligo, the premature ageing syndromes progeria, pangeria and Down's syndrome; and rare metabolic disorders such as prolidase deficiency. In addition when vitiligo directly involves the scalp or hair bearing skin (Fig. 1.17), depigmentation can occur within affected patches. Conversely darkening of the hair has been described in Addison's disease.

Greying commences in the third decade on the temples and spreads later to the crown and occiput. By the age of 50 years, 50% of the population have at least 50% grey hairs. Except in the earliest phases of canites and the early regrowth of alopecia areata (AA) (Fig. 1.18), greying is usually irreversible, however, there are anecdotal reports of repigmentation occurring following electron beam therapy and in porphyria cutanea tarda. Temporary repigmentation may also occur following large doses of para-amino benzoic acid.

Sudden overnight greying, as is reputed to have affected Marie-Antoinette on the eve of her decapitation, is due to a diffuse AA preferentially affecting the pigmented hairs (see Fig. 6.4).

Poliosis or piebaldism

This is a congenital, localized variant of albinism inherited as an autosomal dominant trait. The genetics have not yet been determined; however, affected individuals may be mosaic for the relevant gene. In the scalp there is a localized patch of white hair. The abnormality is due to either the absence of or a deficiency of melanin production in a group of neighbouring follicles. In addition pigment production is impaired in the surrounding interfollicular epithelium and melanocyte numbers appear to be reduced in affected skin and hair. While any part of the scalp can be involved, the most commonly affected site is the central frontal hairline of the forelock (Fig. 1.19), and this may be the only manifestation. The white area often extends forwards to the base of the nose.

On the trunk and limbs there may be additional patches of depigmented skin (Fig. 1.20) that remain fixed. Islands of normally pigmented skin often occur within the hypomelanotic areas.

Poliosis has been associated with congenital perceptual deafness and this may be a forme fruste of Waardenburg's syndrome. Poliosis also occurs in up to 60% of cases of tuberous sclerosis and may be the earliest manifestation. A patch of poliosis overlying a scalp neurofibroma in Von Recklinghausen's disease has been described.

The opposite of poliosis, a black hair naevus (Fig. 1.21), occurs as an isolated developmental anomaly.

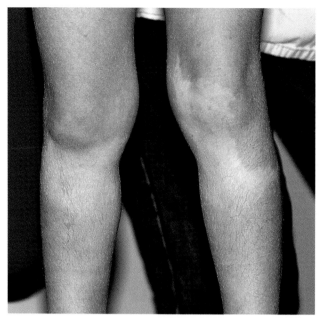

Fig. 1.20 Piebaldism—daughter of patient in Fig. 1.19 showing vitiligo-like areas of depigmentation.

Waardenburg's syndrome

This is the combination of a white forelock (present in 20%), lateral displacement of the medial canthi with dystopia canthorum, hypertrophy of the nasal root, confluent eyebrows, partial or total dyschromia of the iris, and perceptive deafness in about 20%. Abnormal patterns of hair growth, with a beard covering the entire cheeks and terminal hairs on the nose have been described as has premature canites.

Teitz's syndrome is a similar condition with generalized patches of white skin and hair associated with deafness and eyebrow hypoplasia. The Vogt–Koyanagi–Harada syndrome consists of bilateral uveitis, labyrinthine deafness, tinnitus, vitiligo, poliosis and AA. Alezzandrini's syndrome combines

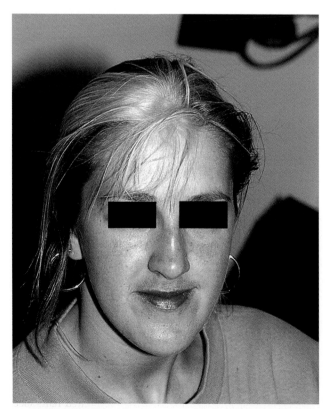

Fig. 1.19 Piebaldism.

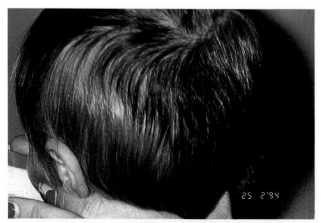

Fig. 1.21 Black hair naevus. (Courtesy of Dr M. Haskett, Melbourne.)

facial vitiligo, retinitis, and poliosis of the eyebrows and eyelashes.

Albinism

In both tyrosinase positive and tyrosinase negative autosomal recessive oculocutaneous albinism, the hair is yellowish-white in colour (Fig. 1.22), although it can be cream, yellow, yellowish-red or vibrant red on occasion.

Chediak–Higashi syndrome

This is an autosomal recessive defect of membrane-bound organelles in white cells, platelets and a variety of neuroectoderm derived cells including melanocytes. A lethal immune deficiency, oculocutaneous hypopigmentation, hepatosplenomegaly and lymphadenopathy occur as does an increased risk of lymphoma.

Phenylketonuria

Phenylketonuria, an inherited deficiency of phenylalanine hydroxylase, results in accumulation of the tyrosine precursor phenylalanine (Fig. 1.23) and a reduction in melanin formation. The skin is pale and the hair is fair.

1.8 Hair weathering

Hair weathering is defined as the microscopic changes in the hair shaft structure not seen at the root end and which become progressively more obvious or frequent towards the tip. It manifests as a progressive degeneration from root to tip of, initially, the cuticle, and later the cortex. Weathering occurs to some extent in all hairs (Fig. 1.24) allowed to grow long enough, in response to routine wear and tear.

Hairs with intrinsic structural defects are less able to withstand routine wear and tear and weather prematurely with the recognizable changes occurring close to the root. It is the proximity of these changes to the root that distinguishes these defective hairs from weathered hairs.

At the root end of normal hair, the cells of the cuticle are

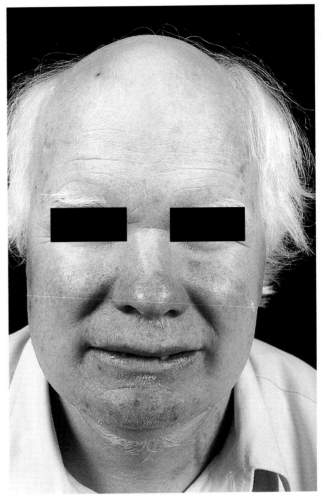

Fig. 1.22 Albino with white hair.

closely opposed to each other and to the underlying hair cortex. They are arranged with each cell partially overlapping the adjacent cell, akin to roof tiles (Fig. 1.24).

In normal hair the earliest manifestations of weathering can be seen within a few centimetres of the scalp. Exposed to the vigours of a variety of cosmetic and environmental stresses, the free margin of the cuticle cells lifts up and

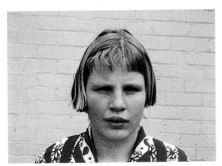

[a]

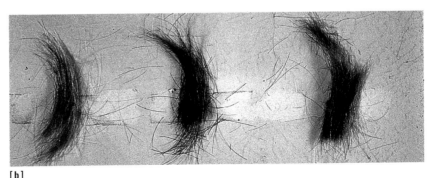

[b]

Fig. 1.23 (a) A child with phenylketonuria before dietary treatment. (Courtesy of Dr J. Brenan, Melbourne.) (b) Colour changes in phenylketonuria. Left to right: hair before dietary treatment; at completion of 6 months treatment; 15 months later.

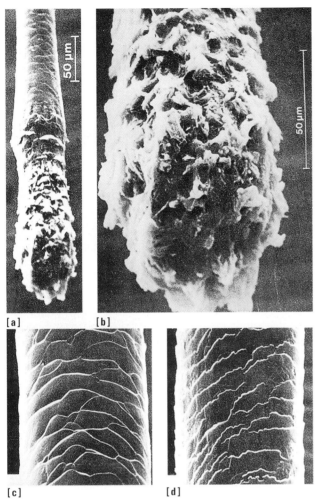

Fig. 1.24 Surface view of the proximal part of a club hair from the human scalp, the cuticular scales in the region adjacent to the club and the distal portion of the hair.

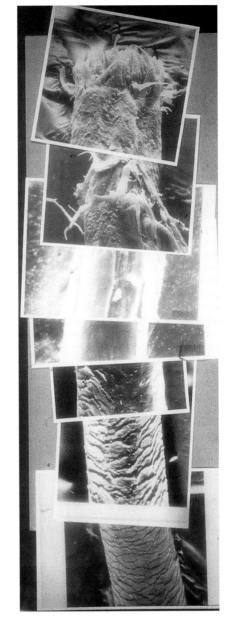

Fig. 1.25 Montage of electron microscope photographs showing the root to tip degeneration of the hair follicle. Initially the cortex is eroded and subsequently the exposed cortex is damaged and fractures.

breaks irregularly (Fig. 1.24). Progressive scale loss leads to areas of the hair shaft that are totally denuded of cuticle (Fig. 1.25). The exposed cortex is weak and fractures and produces nodes or frayed tips. Proximal to the terminal fraying, longitudinal fissures, otherwise known as split ends, may develop.

The tips of long hairs will have been subjected to considerable wear and tear and may show transverse fissures and nodes of the type seen in trichorrhexis nodosa. If the wear and tear has been excessive these changes will occur closer to the root, but rarely will they occur as close to the root as seen in the structural hair shaft disorders. The spectrum of changes that are seen is shown in Fig. 1.26 and Table 1.2.

As weathering occurs to some extent in all hair, longer hair exhibits a greater degree of terminal weathering. Weathering is also modified by a number of factors that are listed in Table 1.3.

1.9 Hair patterns

Regional variations in hair pattern are related to age (Table 1.4), genetic constitution and endocrine status. While eunuchs do not develop secondary body hair, and castration or hypogonadism of males results in a loss of body hair, there is not a direct relationship between the volume of body hair and the level of circulating free testosterone. In addition dark-haired people have both an increased amount and more noticeable body hair than their fair-haired counterparts.

Pubic hair

Three patterns of distribution of pubic hair based on the upper border of the pubic triangle have been described:

Table 1.2 The spectrum of changes seen in weathering.

Cuticular loss
Trichorrhexis nodosa
Trichoschisis
Trichoclasis
Trichoptilosis
Trichonodosis
Twisting dystrophy
Pseudomonilethrix
Frayed tips
Tapered hairs

Table 1.3 Factors that influence hair weathering.

Promoting factors	Protective factors
Brushing	Conditioner
Combing	Sebum
Bleaching	
Curling	
Perming	
Straightening	
Ultraviolet light	

Table 1.4 Presence of body hair in American boys.

Area	14 years (%)	16 years (%)	18 years (%)
Pubic	97	100	100
Axillary	40	97	100
Anterior leg	46	90	100
Anterior thigh	30	67	95
Forearm	14	37	80
Abdomen	14	37	75
Buttocks	14	33	50
Chest	3	7	40
Lower back	3	7	20
Upper arms	0	0	10
Shoulders	0	0	0

vidual and racial variation in the amount of hair developed. In about 20% of individuals with extensive chest hair, circular bare areas known as pectoral alopecia are present around the nipples. Such individuals frequently have accompanying hair on their shoulders and back.

Axillary hair

Terminal hair in the axilla usually appears 2 years after the first pubic hair, but there is much individual variation in this figure and axillary hair occasionally appears first. Mongoloids tend to have sparser hair than Caucasoids and it is not infrequently absent among older subjects of both sexes.

Most Caucasoids have a fairly extensive cover of hair over the extensor aspect of the arms. In about a quarter the hair is limited to the forearms and a small minority has no terminal hair.

The fingers tend to show hairs over the proximal phalanx, while in most people the middle phalanx is hairless. Hair over the proximal phalanx of the thumb and the middle phalanges shows individual and racial variation.

horizontal, acuminate and disperse. The horizontal pattern is found in 90% of women and 20% of males. The acuminate pattern is seen in 10% of women and 50% of men, while the diffuse pattern is generally only seen in middle-aged men with much terminal hair on their thighs and chest.

An acuminate pattern often reverts to a horizontal pattern in women following the menopause. A change to a horizontal from an acuminate pattern also occurs in men following oestrogen treatment for carcinoma of the prostate.

Chest hair

This appears in the normal male soon after puberty and continues to increase until the sixth decade. There is a wide indi-

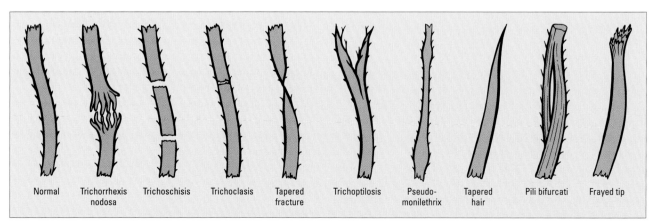

Normal   Trichorrhexis nodosa   Trichoschisis   Trichoclasis   Tapered fracture   Trichoptilosis   Pseudo-monilethrix   Tapered hair   Pili bifurcati   Frayed tip

Fig. 1.26 Terminology used in hair shaft disorders. (Courtesy of Dr D. Whiting, Dallas.)

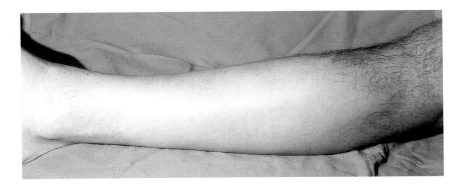

Fig. 1.27 Peroneal alopecia.

Peroneal alopecia

This refers to the bare areas over the anterolateral aspect of the lower leg (Fig. 1.27) It occurs in up to 35% of people and is probably unrelated to wearing socks, except that friction from socks may cause premature release of telogen hairs.

1.10 Trichoglyphics

Hair does not grow vertically but leaves the scalp at an angle that is precisely determined so that streams and patterns are formed. At certain sites the individual follicles are curved away from the axis of the emergent shaft to form whorls. Whorls and streams probably appear as early as 12 weeks gestation. They can be usually seen on the parietal region of the scalp, the inner canthus of the eye and other sites of skin depressions such as the axilla and back.

A single parietal whorl is seen in 95% of people and it is usually clockwise (Fig. 1.28). The remainder have two or rarely three whorls. A frontal cowlick due to a counter stream of hair from the forehead is present in 7%. Abnormal scalp hair patterns with absent or aberrant whorls may be seen on the heads of children with abnormal brain development, such as microcephaly. Multiple scalp whorls are more common among mentally retarded children.

The ridgeback anomaly (Fig. 1.29) is due to the hair waves growing towards the vertex rather than the normal spiral away from the crown. It too may be associated with intellectual impairment.

Displacement of the scalp line occurs in a number of syndromes. A congenitally low anterior line occurs in Cornelia de Lange syndrome (Fig. 1.30), lipoatrophic diabetes, fetal hydantoin syndrome and Rubinstein–Taybi syndrome (Fig. 1.31), while a low posterior line occurs in Noonan's and Turner's syndromes. A congenitally high anterior line is seen in myotonic dystrophy (Figs 1.32 & 1.33).

1.11 Investigation of hair and hair follicle diseases

Accurate diagnosis of hair disorders is important for management. Even if therapy is limited for a specific condition, advice regarding the natural history of the condition, associ-

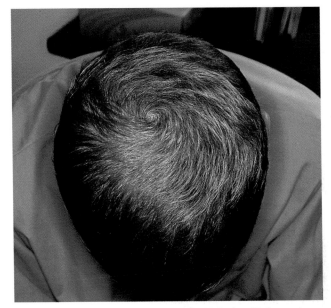

Fig. 1.28 Single parietal whorl. (Courtesy of Dr M. Haskett, Melbourne.)

ated manifestations of the disorder and genetic counselling for hereditary disorders can be of enormous value to the patient.

Following clinical assessment of a disorder the clinician should have established whether the condition is congenital or acquired, diffuse or focal; and in the case of alopecia, scarring or nonscarring. Any associated abnormalities of skin, nails and teeth should be noted and if virilism is suspected a directed history, examination and biochemical investigations are appropriate (p. 41).

The hair pull test (Fig. 1.34) is an easy method of confirming that abnormal hair loss is occurring and also its distribution. To do this test a clump of hairs are grasped at their base between the thumb and forefinger. Firm traction is then applied, being careful not to produce pain, as the examiner's hand slides along the hairs from the base to the tip. This can be repeated at various sites in the scalp. Normally 2–5 telogen hairs will be obtained after five or six passes done in this way, depending on when the scalp was last shampooed.

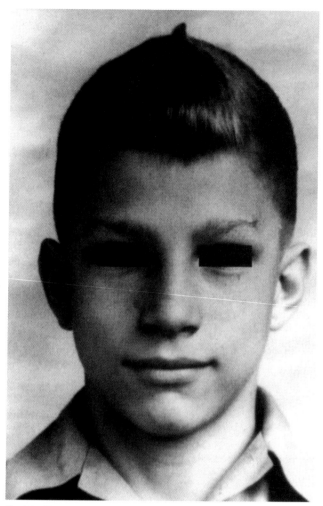

Fig. 1.29 Ridgeback anomaly.

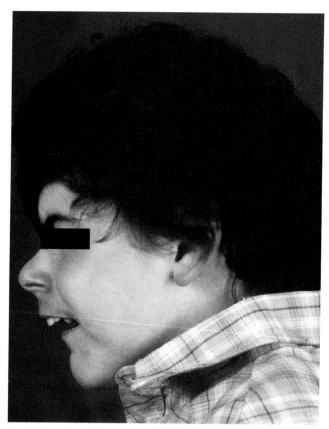

Fig. 1.30 Low frontal hair line in Cornelia de Lange syndrome. (Courtesy of POSSUM.)

Telogen hairs can be recognized with the naked eye by their nonpigmented tip.

Except in loose anagen syndrome (p. 178), protein calorie malnutrition, anagen effluvium, occult poisoning, and occasionally early diffuse AA, normally only telogen hairs should be obtained as normal anagen hairs are firmly anchored in the scalp. Occasionally patients swear their hair is falling out but a hair pull test is normal. In such cases it is valuable to ask the patient to collect all the hairs shed during the course of a day in the shower, sink, pillow, brush, etc. and to count them. The normal loss is less than 100 per day. In active telogen effluvium it can be several hundred per day.

In cases where one wishes to establish anagen/telogen ratios (a trichogram), for example, in attempting to differentiate androgenetic alopecia from telogen effluvium, a hair pluck should be performed. For accuracy the scalp should not be washed for 3–6 days before the procedure (as this removes telogen hairs) and at least 50 hairs should be plucked. The best instrument for this is a haemostat with the tips covered with rubber tubing. The hairs are grasped at the base and extracted with a sharp quick pluck, as slow traction deforms the morphology of the root and prolongs the discomfort (Fig.

1.35). The hairs can be mounted between two glass slides for microscopic examination either using double sided sticky-tape or cyanoacrylic glue that will allow the hair slide to be kept permanently for future reference. In the absence of glue, immersion oil can be used and gives a clear image as it has the same refractive index as glass. The normal scalp anagen to telogen ratio in children is over 90% while in adults it is approximately 85%. Dysplastic anagen hairs are a nonspecific finding in many alopecias and can be produced by slow extraction of the hair.

For fungal microscopy only half a dozen or so hairs need be plucked. If the suspected pathology is increased hair shaft fragility, it is important to examine both plucked and cut hairs to avoid over diagnosing artefacts from the act of plucking. Plucked hairs allow assessment of an abnormality in relation to its distance from the hair root. Any abnormality occurring within the first 2 cm is likely to be of intrinsic origin, while distal abnormalities will simply reflect extrinsic weathering.

The epiluminescence hand-held microscope (dermatoscope), more commonly used for examination of pigmented naevi, can also be of use (without the oil) in examining the scalp for hair shaft defects. In patchy disorders such as monilethrix the optimal site to obtain hair for microscopy can be determined. In addition the dermatoscope can

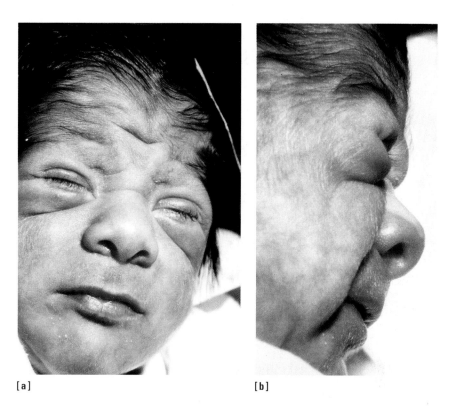

Fig. 1.31 (a), (b) Low frontal hair line in Rubinstein–Taybi syndrome. (Courtesy of POSSUM.)   **[a]**   **[b]**

be used with oil in the assessment of scarring alopecias (Fig. 1.36).

Light microscopy of hair allows visualization of structures larger than 0.2 µm and has a narrow depth of focus. Transmission electron microscopy gives very high resolution down to 2 nm and has a depth of focus of 100 nm. A diamond knife is required for cutting ultra-thin sections of hair without distortion, and the hair is then stained with a heavy metal such as gold to give anatomical detail. Scanning electron microscopy gives a wealth of information about surface architecture. However, for many conditions, sufficient diagnostic information is gained from light microscopy.

Polarized light microscopy gives additional information regarding the structural composition of the hair and makes fine structural abnormalities more obvious, but is not essential. Striking alternating dark and light bands (reminiscent of a tiger's tail) are seen on polarized microscopy in the sulphur deficient hairs of trichothiodystrophy (p. 168).

Scalp biopsy (Fig. 1.37) relies on good technique to provide useful histological information. The site of biopsy is important, and the active edge of a scarring alopecia is likely to yield more information than the 'burnt-out' centre. Often multiple 3 or 4 mm punch biopsies are more useful than a single incisional biopsy. The biopsy should be angled in the direction of hair growth to avoid transecting hairs, and must include subcutaneous fat in order to include anagen hair bulbs. Because follicles in a biopsy specimen tend to bend before hardening, cross cutting is common. This can be avoided by placing the biopsy face down on a piece of cardboard, before putting it in the formalin. The scalp is very vascular and biopsies will usually need to be sutured. Horizontal

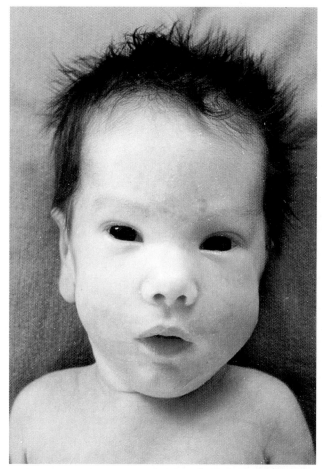

Fig. 1.32 High anterior frontal hair line in an infant with myotonic dystrophy. (Courtesy of POSSUM.)

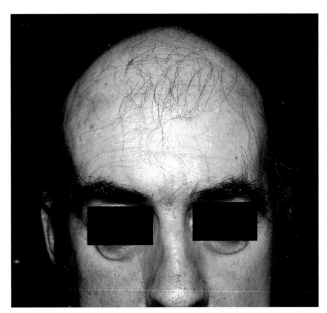

Fig. 1.33 High anterior frontal hair line in an adult with myotonic dystrophy.

1.12 The psychological importance of hair

An appreciation of the special psychological significance of the hair is important for those involved in the assessment and management of diseases of the hair and scalp. Hair is central to our perceptions of beauty and attractiveness. Either too little hair on the scalp or too much hair on the face of a woman can make her feel unattractive, self-conscious and miserable. It is not uncommon for such people to be and feel stared at in public and as a consequence shy away from personal contact. Perhaps the greatest testimony to the importance of hair is the time and money spent in hairdressing salons around the world and the multibillion dollar annual turnover of the hair cosmetic and trichology industries. Disorders of hair frequently produce profound anxieties out of keeping with their objective severity or physiological importance.

The association of hair with attractiveness can be confirmed by even the most superficial surveys of the visual arts, literature and advertising in magazines. Unfortunately fashion magazines portray an inaccurate stereotype for women, and this contributes to the common misconception that women do not go bald.

Many societies associate shaving of the head with celibacy or chastity, as seen in monks and nuns of Buddist and Christian faith as well as Hindu priests and women. Covering the hair among Catholic nuns and in Muslim and orthodox Jewish society has a similar connotation. Today shaving the head may be simply a fashion statement (Fig. 1.38).

Some societies cut women's hair as punishment for adultery. Similar punishment was handed out in Europe after the Second World War for women who had consorted with soldiers of occupying armies.

processing often gives complementary information to the traditional longitudinal biopsy particularly regarding follicle type and density and anagen to telogen ratios, but requires an experienced pathologist for interpretation.

Scalp histology is necessary to establish the diagnosis in scarring alopecia and is also useful in trichotillomania and unexplained diffuse hair loss. It has also been used to determine the potential for regrowth in long-standing apparent nonscarring alopecias. Elastin stains are useful to assess scarring. Immunofluorescence of fresh or frozen tissue should be performed if lupus erythematosus or a bullous disorder is suspected.

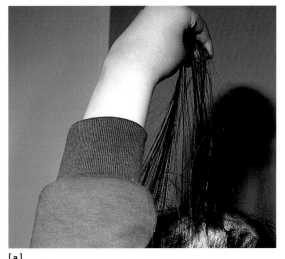

[a]

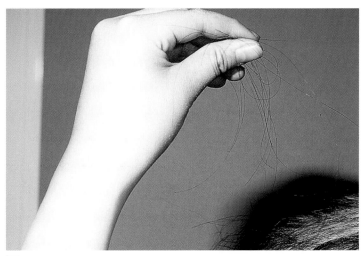

[b]

Fig. 1.34 (a), (b) The hair pull test. Around 10 hairs are grasped firmly at the scalp and traction is applied as the hairs are pulled along their length.

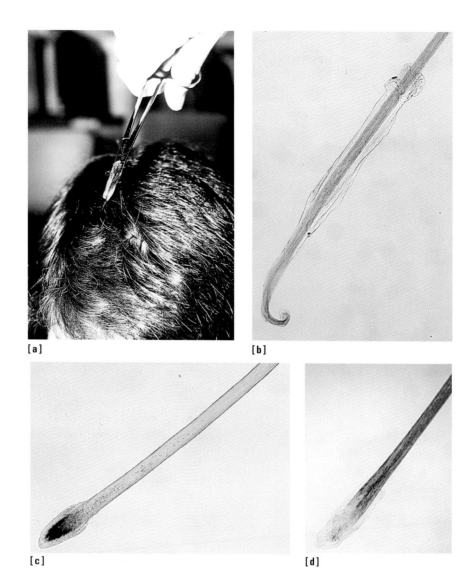

Fig. 1.35 The hair pluck. (a) The hairs are extracted with a sudden firm pull using a haemostat with rubber tubing to minimize artefactual changes. Plucked hairs (b) anagen, (c) catagen, (d) telogen.

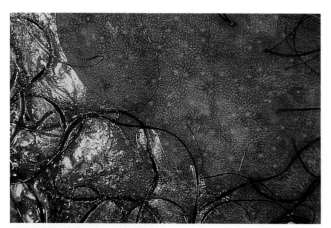

Fig. 1.36 Dermatoscopic image of the scalp in a case of scarring alopecia due to lichen planopilaris. The pale dots correspond to a focal decrease in melanin overlying the fibrous tract remnants of destroyed follicles. (Courtesy of Professor S. Kossard, Sydney.)

The importance placed on short hair by the military reinforces the popular association between short hair and authority and discipline. Beards and moustaches come in and out of fashion. At various times they are associated with masculinity, maturity, good looks, and self-confidence, while at other times they are considered unattractive, indicating the wearer has something to conceal.

Matted uncut hair is seen as a withdrawal from worldly concerns and vanities, in the Hindu Sadhu. Long hair can be seen as a religious requirement and source of identification among Rastafarians and in the Sikh religion. Dreadlocks, made popular by the Rastafarians are now fashionable among white as well as black people.

Classical paintings from the 15th to the 19th century do not show any body hair on female nudes. Axillary hair, considered normal and attractive on women in parts of continental Europe, may be regarded as ugly or a sign of blatant feminism in the UK and USA.

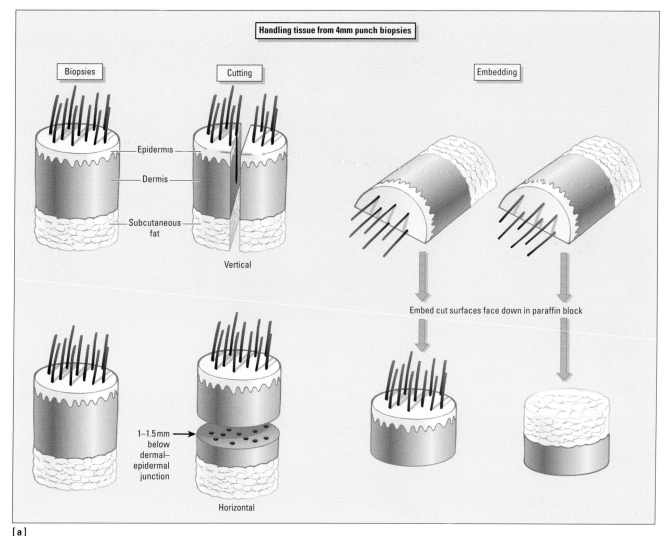

Fig. 1.37 Vertical and horizontal sections of scalp biopsies. (Courtesy of Professor D. Whiting, Dallas.) (a) Diagrammatic representation, (b) vertical, (c) horizontal.

Disorders of the hair can be triggered by major stress such as divorce or a death in the family. This is the case with some examples of telogen effluvium and AA, although diffuse alopecia should not be glibly attributed to the minor stresses that with perseverance can be elicited in most people.

Disorders of hair may result from somatization of psychological disorders. Artefacts, or self-inflicted lesions are uncommon on the scalp but usually reflect a severe underlying personality disorder. Trichotillomania (p. 85), consists of plucking the hair to produce bald patches. It frequently develops as a habit tic in children and is seldom of serious psychiatric significance. In contrast the systematic plucking of all the hair by an adult indicates a very severe disturbance, usually of personality in a female and of mood in a male.

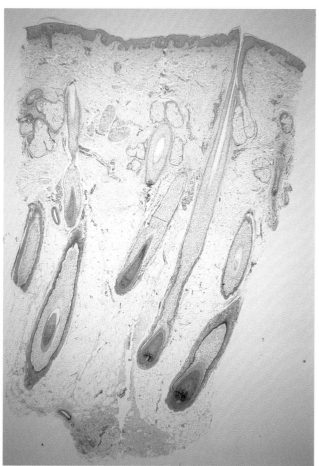

[b]

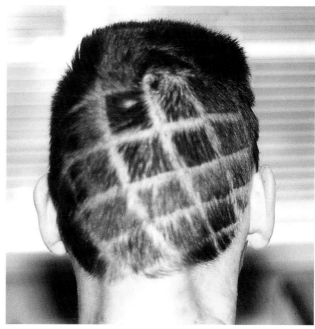

Fig. 1.38 Hair sculpture.

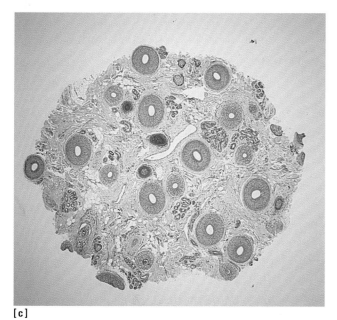

[c]

Fig. 1.37 Continued.

Section B
Excess Hair

Chapter 2

Hypertrichosis

2.1 Circumscribed hypertrichosis

Hypertrichosis occurs in both sexes. It is defined as excessive growth of hair on sites not normally hairy. The hairs may be of the lanugo or vellus type and some of these hairs evolve into terminal hairs. Hair may be excessive in density or length and the condition may be localized or generalized. The process is not androgen dependant.

The normal hair patterns have previously been discussed (p. 15). Localized hypertrichosis occurs as an isolated finding or in association with a number of neurological, endocrinological and naevoid disorders.

Hairy ears

Hereditary development of coarse hairs on the pinna of the ear (Fig. 2.1) occurs most frequently and with the longest, most dense hairs in Indians. It first appears at around 20 years of age and thereafter increases in incidence and severity such that by the age of 70 years, 70% of men in Madras are affected. Normally only males are affected, and hypertrichosis of the pinna is believed to be a sex-linked recessive trait. The combination of hairy ears and azoospermia has been proposed as the only known Y chromosome-linked disorder.

Congenital hairy ears occur in babies born to diabetic mothers (unrelated to maternal diabetic control), babies with XYY syndrome and in some normal infants. Acquired hairy ears have been observed in AIDS, and often accompany trichomegaly of the eyelashes and eyebrows.

Hairy eyebrows

Extremely long eyebrows or eyelash hair, or eyebrows that join in the centre (synophrys) (Fig. 2.2) are usually familial. In infants it may occur as a localized problem or rarely as part of a syndrome such as Cornelia de Lange (Fig. 2.3), Rubinstein–Taybi (Fig. 1.31), congenital hypertrichosis lanuginosa or congenital trichomegaly with dwarfism, mental retardation or pigmentary degeneration of the retina.

Long eyebrows are commonly the most pronounced aspect of the drug-induced acquired hypertrichosis occurring with cyclosporin (Fig. 2.4), minoxidil and diazoxide. AIDS can also induce eyebrow growth.

Hairy palms

Localized patches of hair on the palms and soles have been reported in two families as an autosomal dominant trait. The hypertrichosis was associated with increased pigmentation and textural changes in the skin. This could represent hypertrichosis in association with a connective tissue hamartoma as histology shows an increased amount of disorganized elastic tissue.

Hairy elbows

In familial hypertrichosis cubiti, excessive hair growth develops in infancy over the lower third of the upper arm and the upper third of the forearms. The hypertrichosis is progressive for a few years before partially regressing around puberty. The mode of inheritance is uncertain, and both autosomal recessive and autosomal dominant patterns have been suggested. An association with short stature is seen in 10%. An increased proportion of anagen hairs (>90%) are seen histologically, suggesting that this condition is caused by prolongation of anagen.

Becker's naevus

This condition is an androgen-mediated hyperplasia that first appears at puberty as a unilateral localized area of hyperpig-

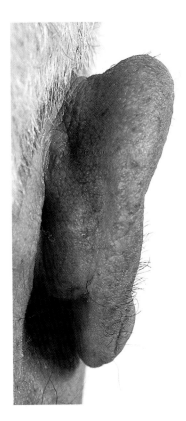

Fig. 2.1 Hairy ears.

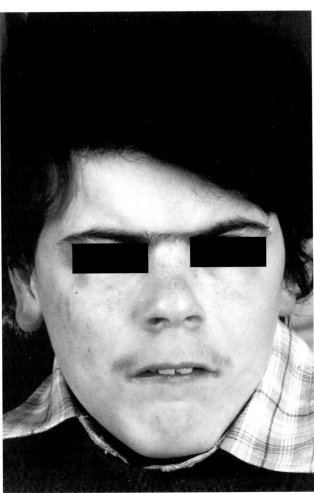

Fig. 2.3 Cornelia de Lange syndrome in a 12-year-old boy.

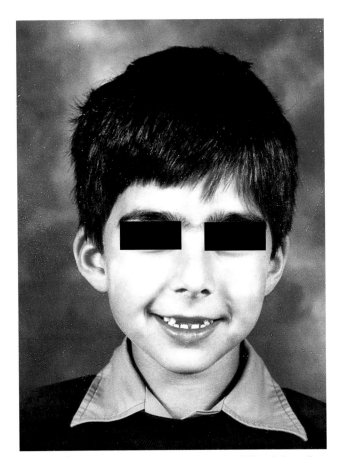

Fig. 2.2 Eyebrows that join in the centre in a normal child born in Australia to Indian parents.

mentation. In 50% of cases it is followed by hypertrichosis. The hairs are predominantly terminal hairs (Fig. 2.5). Acne occasionally develops within a Becker's naevus. The incidence is about 0.5% and the male to female ratio is 10 : 1. About half occur on the shoulder and the rest on the trunk and a few on the limbs or face. Multiple lesions are rare as are familial cases. The term naevus requires qualification, as there is no increase in the number of melanocytes and histology simply shows acanthosis with basal hyperpigmentation. An increase in smooth muscle bundles in the dermis is sometimes noticed.

Uncommon associated abnormalities include ipsilateral breast hypoplasia, spina bifida, pectus carinatum, accessory nipples, morphoea and ipsilateral leg hyperplasia. Electrolysis has been used with mixed success to treat the hypertrichosis, but the pigmentation is very difficult to treat.

Congenital melanocytic naevus

Both congenital and acquired naevi can develop hypertrichosis, usually consisting of terminal hairs. The presence of hairs does not help to determine if a pigmented lesion is benign or malignant as a melanoma may arise at the edge of a

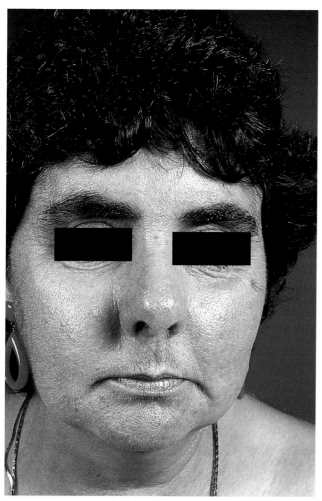

Fig. 2.4 Cyclosporin A induced hypertrichosis of the eyebrows.

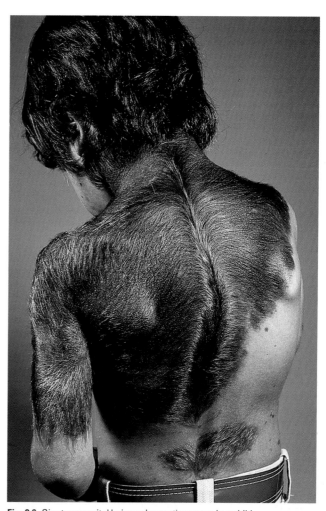

Fig. 2.6 Giant congenital hairy melanocytic naevus in a child.

hairy naevus and in addition loss of hairs tends to be a late feature in the development of melanoma. Congenital pigmented hairy naevi are probably the commonest cause of localized hypertrichosis in infancy. The German term *Tierfellnevus* (animal skin naevus) has been used to describe a particularly hairy variant and is an apt morphological description (Figs 2.6 & 2.7).

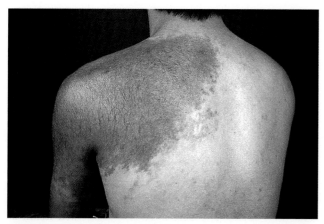

Fig. 2.5 Becker's naevus with hypertrichosis.

Faun tail

A congenital midline dorsal patch of hypertrichosis or faun tail is an important clue to a possible occult spinal abnormality that may in time produce neurological deficits. It consists of a tuft of long silky hair in the sacral area usually overlying normal skin (Fig. 2.8).

Occasionally there will be a sinus or a dimple within the faun tail and rarely a lipoma or a capillary naevus will be found beneath it. Sinuses are usually 1–2 mm wide and can connect directly with the spinal cord. They are a potential portal of entry for infection and they can be associated with a cystic dilatation within the spinal cord that produces neurological deficits.

Spinal dysraphism (failure of spinal fusion) occurs beneath the faun tail four times more frequently in girls than boys. In association with this the cord can be transfixed by a bony spicule (diastematomyelia), or the cauda equina may be tethered by fibrous cords. With time this produces traction damage to the cord as a result of differential growth of the vertebra and the cord. Neurological deficits are not present at birth, but gradually develop over the first 5 years. If

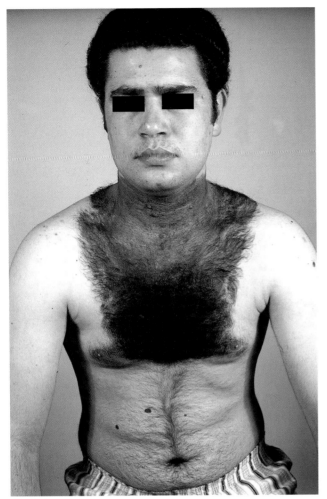

Fig. 2.7 Giant congenital hairy melanocytic naevus in an adult.

identified early permanent damage can be prevented by prophylactic surgery.

Midline hypertrichosis can occur anywhere along the back associated with cervical, thoracic or lumbar dysraphism. The stimulant for hair growth is presumably a growth factor secreted by neural tissue, however, none has been identified.

Hair collar sign

In 1989 Commen described a distinctive collar of hypertrophic hairs that palisaded around a bald nodule containing heterotopic brain tissue (Fig. 2.9, see also Fig. 13.3). The nodule usually overlies an embryonic fusion line. The collar of long terminal hairs grows faster, earlier and longer than the rest of the infant's scalp hair. It has also been described in a number of other neuroectodermal defects including dermoid cysts, dermal sinus tumours, encephalocele, sequestrated meningocele, and leptomeningocele. If the cyst fills when the baby cries this suggests an intracerebral communication.

The hair collar sign is an important clue alerting the clinician to the possibility that the lesions extend intracranially and a computed tomography (CT) or magnetic resonance imaging (MRI) scan is required, particularly if a biopsy is being considered. Ultimately the central nodule will flatten to form a circular smooth patch of rubbery hairless skin and the collar of hypertrophic hair will blend in with the adjacent scalp hair as it grows. The palisading hairs are then discernible only on close inspection.

Naevoid hypertrichosis

Hypertrichosis of a limited extent occurs as an isolated developmental defect (Figs 2.10 & 2.11). It can also occur over a patch of thickened parchment-like skin or complicate a benign tumour such as a neurofibroma or a smooth muscle hamartoma. Smooth muscle hamartomas show transient piloerection when stroked.

Congenital hemihypertrophy with hypertrichosis

This rare syndrome present at birth becomes more pronounced at puberty. Other possible associations include mental retardation, multiple naevi, telangiectases and internal malignancies.

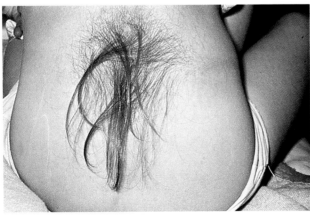

Fig. 2.8 Faun tail.

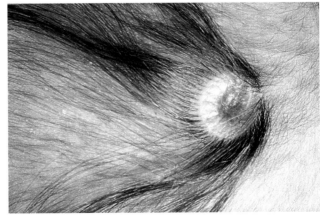

Fig. 2.9 Collar of hypertrophic hair surrounding a bald scalp nodule; a dermoid cyst in this case. (Courtesy of Dr C. Darley, Brighton.)

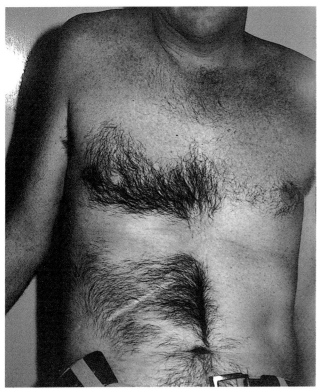

Fig. 2.10 Multifocal naevoid hypertrichosis with sharp cut-off in the midline in a distribution reminiscent of Blashko's lines. (Courtesy of Dr A. Callen, Melbourne.)

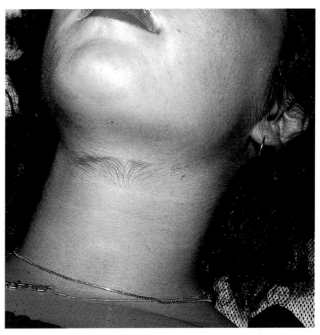

Fig. 2.11 Naevoid hypertrichosis. (Courtesy of Dr A. Callen, Melbourne.)

2.2 Congenital hypertrichosis lanuginosa

Introduction

This rare autosomal dominant disorder is characterized by the retention and continued synchronized growth of fetal lanugo hair. Names such as apeman, dogman, manlion and wildman were used in older literature to describe this condition. The incidence is estimated at 1 in 10^9 live births.

Clinical features and investigation

The infants are either born with or develop within the first few months, a fur consisting of a thick coat of fine silky hair that can be up to 5 cm long and which covers the entire nonglabrous surface (Fig. 2.12). The terminal scalp hairs are easily distinguished from the extensive silvery-grey body hair that only spares the palms, soles, lips, glans penis and the terminal phalanges.

During childhood the condition usually progresses, but occasionally it may regress or even stay the same. At puberty there is growth of sexual hair but without the usual conversion to terminal hair. Thus longer lanugo hairs grow in the pubic, axillary and beard areas.

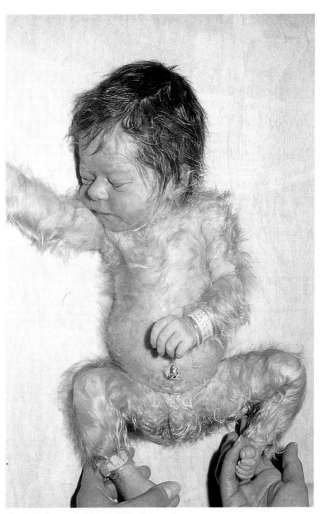

Fig. 2.12 Congenital hypertrichosis lanuginosa.

There are generally no associated features, although neonatal teeth and pyloric stenosis have been described. This condition should be distinguished from hypertrichosis with gingival hyperplasia (see below).

Management

The striking appearance of affected individuals has lead to their exploitation over the centuries as side-show freaks. Psychological support of the patient and family is an important part of the management. Shaving is often the only feasible means of controlling the hair growth at present, although the new, non-q-switched ruby lasers may prove to be effective.

Key points

A complete pelage of fine silvery hair makes this hereditary condition unmistakable.

2.3 Other congenital syndromes with prominent hypertrichosis

Hypertrichosis with gingival fibromatosis

Hypertrichosis in association with gingival hyperplasia and epilepsy was recognized as a rare autosomal dominant condition before the introduction of phenytoin. Eighty per cent of cases are familial and the condition has been associated with Cowden's disease, suggesting genetic linkage.

The hypertrichosis usually appears at birth and mainly affects the face, arms and back. During infancy it mimics congenital hypertrichosis lanuginosa, but the hair darkens with puberty. The gingival fibromatosis may not be noticed until the age of 10 years, but usually is detected earlier if the epilepsy is severe. The hypertrophy of the gums buries emerging teeth in a mass of redundant tissue. It has been suggested that phenytoin induced gingival hyperplasia relates to poor dental hygiene, however, it is not known if the same holds true for familial cases.

Hypertrichosis with osteochondrodysplasia

This is an autosomal recessive condition combining generalized congenital hypertrichosis with a constellation of skeletal abnormalities that include a narrow thorax, generalized osteopaenia, hypoplastic pubic rami and premature growth arrest of the femur (Fig. 2.13).

X-linked hypertrichosis

This X-linked dominant condition is characterized by hypertrichosis predominantly over the face, back, upper chest and pubic regions. The facial growth obscures the eyebrows and sometimes only the eyes and lips are visible beneath a dense growth of dark black hair (Figs 2.14 & 2.15).

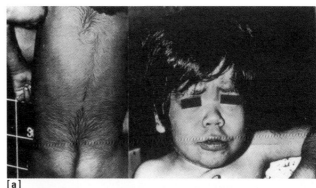
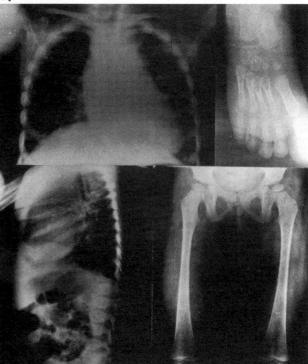

Fig. 2.13 Osteochondrodysplasia with hypertrichosis. (a) Clinical appearance of a girl aged 4½ years. (b) X-rays of the same girl demonstrating a narrow thorax and cardiomegaly platyspondyly and ovid vertebral bodies, hypoplastic ischiopubic rami, small abdurator foramina and enlarged medulla of Erlenmeyer flask-shaped femora which show bands of growth arrest. (Courtesy of Professor J.M. Cantu, Guadelajara.)

Prepubertal hypertrichosis

This is a nonfamilial hypertrichosis, present at birth, that increases in severity during early childhood. As it occurs equally in people of Asian or European descent, the term racial hypertrichosis is inappropriate. There is growth of terminal hairs on the temples spreading across the forehead, bushy eyebrows, and marked growth on the upper back and proximal limbs (Fig. 2.16). In contrast to the synchronized growth of lanugo hairs in congenital hypertrichosis lanuginosa, the hair growth in this condition is unsynchronized. In adolescence this form of hypertrichosis is often confused with hirsutes. Misdiagnosis of this condition is the

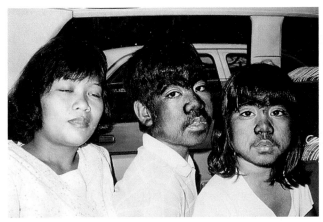

Fig. 2.14 X-linked hypertrichosis affecting two brothers but sparing the sister.

reason why some so-called 'hirsute' women fail to respond to antiandrogen therapy.

Coffin–Siris syndrome

This syndrome combines generalized congenital hypertrichosis, prominent eyebrows and eyelashes and sparse scalp hair with profound mental and growth retardation and congenital absence of the distal phalanges and nails of the fifth fingers and toes. Characteristic facies and abnormal dentition, have also been described. The inheritance of this syndrome has not yet been established.

Cornelia de Lange syndrome

Hypertrichosis is a constant and distinctive feature of this rare syndrome. In addition to the mild generalized hypertrichosis there is abundant scalp hair with low frontal and nuchal hair lines (Fig. 1.30). The eyebrows are bushy and meet in the centre and the eyelashes are long and curled. Other features are variable and include physical and mental retardation, characteristic facies, cutis marmorata, short digits, syndactyly of the second and third toes, a high arched palate, an unusual cry, increased susceptibility to infection and a constellation of ocular, dental and skeletal abnormalities.

Leprechaunism

This entity is characterized by grotesque elfin facies with thick large lips, large low set ears, breast enlargement and prominent genitalia. Absence of subcutaneous tissue gives rise to excessive folding of the skin. Generalized hypertrichosis is seen in three-quarters of cases and is most prominent on the forehead and cheeks.

Other syndromes that produce hypertrichosis

• Gorlin syndrome, with patent ductus arteriosus, hy-

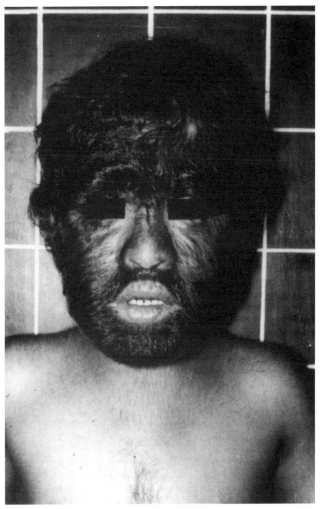

Fig. 2.15 X-linked hypertrichosis in a boy aged 8 years. (Courtesy Professor J.M. Cantu, Guadalajara.)

poplasia of the teeth, eyes and labia majora and craniofacial dysostosis;
• Lissencephaly, with growth and mental retardation and a smooth brain without sulci and gyri;
• Rubinstein–Taybi syndrome with broad thumbs, physical and mental retardation cryptorchidism and characteristic facies;
• Schinzel–Gideon syndrome with club feet, skeletal abnormalities and characteristic facies with redundant folds of skin overlying a short neck;
• Lawrence–Seip syndrome with congenital lipoatrophy and juvenile onset insulin-resistant diabetes, hyperlipidaemia and hepatosplenomegaly;
• Hunter's, Hurler's and Winchester's mucopolysaccharidoses syndromes;
• Fetal alcohol syndrome with mental and physical retardation, microcephaly, cardiac anomalies, joint defects, unusual facies and capillary haemangiomas.
• POEMS syndrome is an acronym for *p*eripheral neuropathy, *o*rganomegaly, *e*ndocrine dysfunction, *m*onoclonal gam-

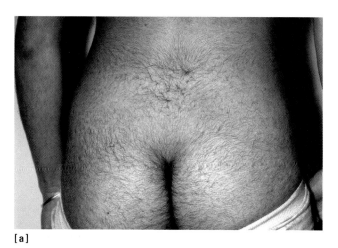
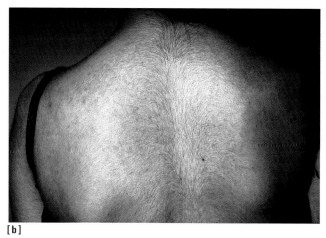

[a] [b]

Fig. 2.16 Hypertrichosis with an onset in early childhood in an otherwise healthy 18 year old female.

mopathy and skin changes. The main skin changes include hypertrichosis on the extensor surfaces, malar region and forehead, hyperpigmentation and oedema. Scarring alopecia on the abdomen has been described.

• Wardenburg's syndrome (p. 13) is associated with terminal hair on the tip of the nose and a beard that extends over the entire surface of the cheeks.

2.4 Acquired hypertrichosis lanuginosa

Introduction

This rare condition is characterized by the rapid growth of long, fine, downy lanugo hairs particularly over the face, but also on the body. It is a paraneoplastic phenomenon often seen late in the course of an internal malignancy; a so-called malignant down. The importance of this condition is that it may be the presenting sign of the malignancy and can appear up to 2 years prior to other manifestations. A hair growth factor produced by the tumour has been postulated but not identified.

Clinical features and investigation

Acquired hypertrichosis lanuginosa has an age range of 19–69, with a female predominance of 3:1. The extent and degree of lanuginose transformation varies considerably. In early cases the growth of down on the forehead and temples is the only abnormality. In others the striking feature is the rapidity with which obvious hypertrichosis develops. Hair appears on the forehead, eyelids, nose (Fig. 2.17a), ears (Fig. 2.17b) and torso (Fig. 2.17c) giving the patient a simian appearance. The palms, soles, pubic regions and scalp tend to be spared. Balding scalps are rejuvenated by a dense growth of hair, albeit lighter and finer than the neighbouring hair. Hairs may grow as fast as 2.5 cm per week and achieve a length of 15 cm, but more commonly are about 1 cm long.

Other cutaneous abnormalities that may coexist include

keratotic lesions on the palms, soles and limbs, glossitis (Fig. 2.18), acquired ichthyosis and acanthosis nigricans with tripe palms.

The malignancies most often associated with this condition are carcinoma of the lung, colon, uterus and lymphoma.

Management

In order to detect an occult cancer a detailed history and examination, including rectal and pelvic examination with a cervical smear are required. This should be complemented by a full blood examination, a mammogram, colonoscopy and chest X-ray. If available an abdominal and pelvic CT scan can be performed, however, an abdominal ultrasound may suffice. If these investigations are negative, continued vigilance is required and a thorough examination should be repeated regularly.

Successful removal of the underlying cancer has resulted in regression of the hypertrichosis.

Key points

Malignant down occurring on the face late in the course of a malignancy is common. Rarely, the hypertrichosis predates the diagnosis of the cancer. In these cases the rapid appearance of fine downy hairs on the body and face of an apparently healthy person should alert the physician to the probable presence of an occult malignancy.

2.5 Other acquired syndromes with prominent hypertrichosis

Porphyria

Hypertrichosis occurs in all forms of porphyria except acute intermittent porphyria. It is most prominent in congenital porphyria, certain forms of acquired porphyria cutanea tarda (PCT) (Fig. 2.19) and erythropoietic porphyria. Photosensitivity plays a role, particularly as the hypertrichosis

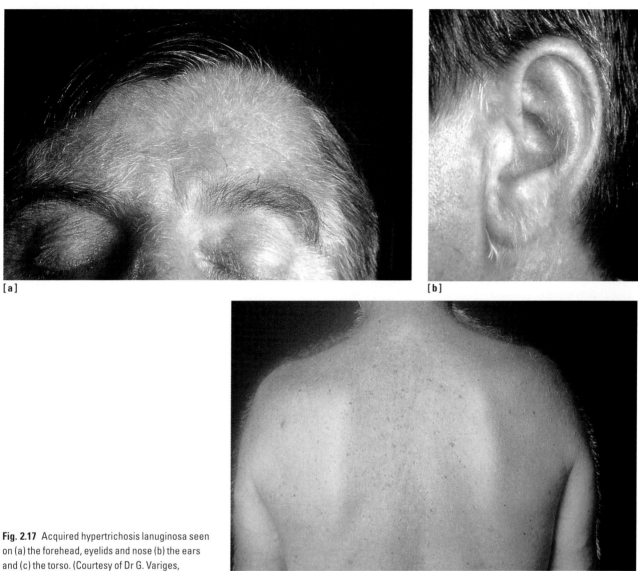

Fig. 2.17 Acquired hypertrichosis lanuginosa seen on (a) the forehead, eyelids and nose (b) the ears and (c) the torso. (Courtesy of Dr G. Variges, Melbourne.)

[a]

[b]

[c]

Fig. 2.18 Glossitis in a patient with acquired hypertrichosis lanuginosa.

usually appears on the exposed sites such as the face and hands.

The facial hair is most prominent along the temples, cheeks, eyebrows and hairline and the hair is generally soft and pigmented. In black people hypertrichosis is an important sign of PCT as blistering is uncommon.

The combination of photosensitivity, milia and scarring on the hands or face and hypertrichosis presents little diagnostic difficulty and requires a blood, urine and faecal porphyrin screen to confirm the diagnosis and elucidate the subtype. The absence of hypertrichosis in pseudoporphyria, epidermolysis bullosa acquisita, Hutchinson's summer prurigo, drug-induced photosensitivity, chronic renal failure and frusemide therapy allow these clinical look-alikes of PCT to be distinguished.

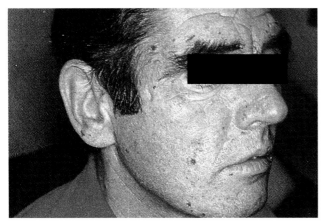

Fig. 2.19 Porphyria cutanea tarda with hypertrichosis and clustered lesions on the face. (Courtesy of Dr M.M. Black, London.)

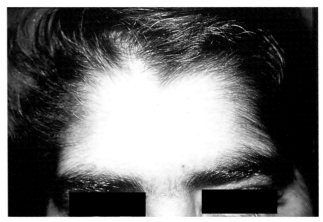

Fig. 2.20 Minoxidil hypertrichosis of the forehead and eyebrows.

Thyroid disease

Diffuse hypertrichosis affecting the temples, back, shoulders and limbs occurs as a manifestation of congenital hypothyroidism and is often associated with converging eyebrows. It usually remits with thyroxine therapy. At puberty the pubic and axillary hair fail to develop. More usually hypothyroidism is associated with a diffuse alopecia of the scalp (p. 69). In Grave's disease localized hypertrichosis can also occur over plaques of pretibial myxoedema.

Anorexia nervosa

Malnutrition from malabsorption, starvation and anorexia nervosa can cause hypertrichosis of the limbs and trunk that in some cases is striking.

Drug-induced hypertrichosis

It is important to distinguish between iatrogenic hirsutism, where new hair occurs in a male sexual distribution and drug-induced hypertrichosis, which is generalized. Minoxidil, diazoxide, phenytoin, cyclosporin A, psoralens and ultraviolet A therapy (PUVA), prednisolone, streptomycin, acetozolamide, benoxaprofen, penicillamine and fenoterol have all been reported to induce hypertrichosis in a proportion of users. The mechanism of hair induction is not known and the same mechanism is not involved in all cases.

Minoxidil and diazoxide are vasodilators that produce hypertrichosis in 80% of recipients predominantly over the face (Fig. 2.20), shoulders, arms and legs. The hair falls out several months after cessation of therapy. Minoxidil is also active topically and has been used to treat androgenetic alopecia. The resultant hairs that appear on the scalp after oral minoxidil are often fine, poorly pigmented indeterminate type hairs of marginal cosmetic significance (Fig. 4.18).

Cyclosporin A, an immune modulator, may induce a switch from telogen to anagen in hair. In humans it produces a diffuse growth of hair across the shoulders, back, upper extremities, face, scalp, eyebrows (Fig. 2.4) and earlobes. It begins within a few weeks of taking cyclosporin in upwards of 60% of recipients. Hypertrichosis is more common in childhood and adolescence and reverses about 1 month after stopping treatment.

In about 10% of people receiving phenytoin an excessive growth of hair develops after 1–2 months across the extensor aspects of the limbs and subsequently on the face and trunk. It remits within a year of cessation of therapy. This hypertrichosis does not appear to be related to dose or duration of therapy.

Prolonged administration of cortisone can induce hypertrichosis that is most marked on the forehead, the temples and the sides of the cheeks. It also occurs on the back and the extensor surface of the arms. Steroid-induced acne may be associated (Fig. 2.21).

PUVA induces hair in exposed sites as does benoxaprofen following the induction of drug-induced photosensitivity. Penicillamine tends to produce lengthening and coarsening of hair on the trunk and limbs.

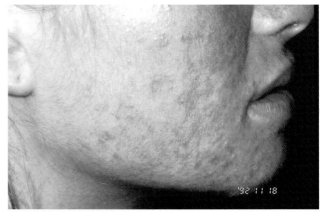

Fig. 2.21 Prednisolone induced hypertrichosis. (Courtesy of Dr M. Haskett, Melbourne.)

Head injuries

Approximately 4 months after a severe head injury or encephalitis, children may experience a temporary generalized hypertrichosis. Neither the mechanism nor the cerebral structures affected by the injury have been determined.

Miscellaneous conditions

Other conditions in which hypertrichosis has been reported include reflex sympathetic dystrophy in the affected limb, lichen simplex chronicus, overlying a bony fracture treated in plaster of Paris and juvenile dermatomyositis.

Chapter 3

Hirsutes

Definition

In general hairy men are called hairy, while hairy women are called hirsute. There is a considerable individual and racial variation in the degree of body hair people grow. To distinguish hirsutes from normal hair growth along a spectrum of biological variation is often difficult, particularly as many women will have already taken effective steps to disguise or remove the unwanted hairs.

Epidemiology

Facial and body hair is less pronounced on Mongoloids, Negroids and American Indians than on Caucasians; and amongst Caucasians, those of Mediterranean ancestry have a heavier growth than those of Nordic origins.

Aetiology

Investigation of the hirsute patient should distinguish idiopathic hirsutes from the less common ovarian and adrenal causes of increased circulating androgens (Table 3.1). Idiopathic hirsutes is presumed due to end-organ hypersensitivity to normal amounts of circulating androgens.

Pathogenesis

Hirsutes results from the transformation of fine vellus hairs into coarse, thick, heavily pigmented terminal hairs with a longer anagen growth phase. This transformation is driven by androgens. Follicular androgen excess may be the result either of overproduction of circulating androgens by the ovaries or adrenal gland, underproduction of sex hormone binding globulin by the liver, enhanced conversion of circulating testosterone into the more potent dihydrotestosterone (DHT) or increased androgen receptor sensitivity within the follicles. Conversion of testosterone to DHT is catalysed by the enzyme 5α reductase. Hirsute skin may demonstrate increased 5α reductase activity *in vitro*.

Normal levels of circulating androgens in men are sufficient to maximally stimulate the hairs and individual variations in the hairiness of men are presumed due to differences in follicular sensitivity.

Not all follicles are sensitive to androgens and androgen excess typically induces excess hairs to develop in the same pattern and sequence as hair appears in the postpubertal male (Fig. 3.1). Paradoxically follicles on the vertex of the scalp respond to androgen excess by miniaturization, with transformation of terminal hairs into vellus hairs. The reason for this is not known.

Clinical features

Excessive hair growth occurs in women, this is usually coarse and deeply pigmented. The transformation of vellus follicles into terminal follicles occurs in women in the same pattern and sequence as that which develops in the postpubertal male (Fig. 3.1). However, as most females develop hair at puberty in an identical pattern to males that is quantitatively inferior, what differs is not that females grow hair in these sites but rather the degree and quality of the growth.

The clinical presentation is influenced by the cause of the hirsutes.

Conditions associated with hirsutes

Polycystic ovary syndrome (PCO)

Stein and Leventhal described a syndrome consisting of obesity, amenorrhoea, hirsutes and infertility combined with bilaterally enlarged polycystic ovaries (Fig. 3.2). As this syndrome is defined by the appearance of organs that are difficult to visualize, and because the pathogenesis of the cysts and their relationship to the state remains controversial the definition of this syndrome varies from text to text. Most patients seen by a dermatologist will be overweight and have acne and hirsutes and menstrual abnormalities (Fig. 3.3). A moderate elevation in luteinizing hormone (LH), serum testosterone and androstenedione are common. Weight loss in these women often results in regulation of menses, a reduction in hirsutes and normalization of the hormone profile.

Congenital adrenal hyperplasia

A deficiency of the enzyme 21β hydroxylase in the pathway of adrenal and ovarian synthesis of cortisol and aldosterone results in a redistribution of precursors to adjacent pathways

Table 3.1 Causes of hirsutes in adults.

Ovarian causes

Polycystic ovary syndrome
Ovarian androgen secreting tumours
 Gonadal stromal tumour
 Thecoma
 Lipoid tumour
Postmenopausal hirsutes

Adrenal causes

Congenital adrenal hyperplasia
 Early onset 21β-hydroxylase deficiency
 Late onset 21β-hydroxylase deficiency
 11β-hydroxylase deficiency
 3β-dehydrogenase deficiency
Cushings disease
Adrenal adenoma
Adrenal carcinoma

Pituitary causes

Cushings syndrome
Prolactinoma

Obesity related

HAIR-AN syndrome

Drugs
Glucocorticosteroids
Anabolic steroids
Minoxidil*
Diazoxide*
Cyclosporin A*
Phenytoin
Psoralens*
Penicillamine
Streptomycin

Idiopathic

*More commonly produces *hyper*trichosis.

and a consequent overproduction of androstenedione and testosterone (Fig. 3.4). Complete deficiency is incompatible with life. Severe reduction presents in childhood with dehydration and a salt losing state (cortisol deficiency) combined with virilization (androgen excess). Partial deficiency leads to a late onset congenital adrenal hyperplasia that presents with postpubertal hirsutes and such patients account for 3–6% of women presenting with hirsutes. Menstrual cycles may be normal and differentiation then relies on endocrine investigations. Treatment is with a nocturnal dose of 5 mg of prednisolone that both replaces the under produced cortisol and suppress the pituitary secretion of adrenocorticotrophic hormone (ACTH) that is driving the excessive androgen production. A similar process can be due to other rarer deficiencies in this pathway, such as an 11β hydroxylase or a 3β hydroxylase deficiency.

Androgen secreting tumours

Approximately 10% of adrenal adenomata and carcinoma present with virilization and hirsutes, while only 1% of ovarian tumours do. While tumour is a rare cause of hirsutes it should be suspected when there is a rapid development of hair combined with other features of virilization. In particular oligomenorrhoea or amenorrhoea, alopecia and cliteromegaly are often present and most will have an elevated serum testosterone and/or dehydroepiandrosterone sulphate (DHEAS) level.

Cushing's syndrome

Excessive ACTH produced either by a pituitary adenoma or ectopically as a paraneoplastic phenomenon stimulates the adrenals not only to produce excess cortisol, but also excess androgens and this causes hirsutes (Fig. 3.5). Iatrogenic Cushing's syndrome due to oral steroids produces a combination of hypertrichosis and hirsutes. Acromegaly also causes hirsutes.

Hyperprolactinaemia

The amenorrhoea–galactorrhoea syndrome is frequently associated with hirsutes. This can be due either to prolactin directly stimulating adrenal androgen production, attenuating hair follicle 5α reductase activity or to a frequent association of hyperprolactinaemia with PCO.

HAIR-AN syndrome

HAIR-AN is an acronym for hyperandrogenization, insulin resistance and acanthosis nigricans and is found in around 7% of women presenting with hirsutes, particularly obese women. Such women may have a marked degree of virilization with a muscular physique, acne, and alopecia.

Premature adrenarche

Hirsutism in a prepubertal child must always be taken seriously, and presumed to be due to either an androgen-secreting tumour or congenital adrenal hyperplasia until proved otherwise. Nevertheless most commonly the appearance of axillary and pubic terminal hair heralds the onset of an early puberty with adrenarche preceding the other signs.

Physiological postmenopausal hirsutes

Postmenopausal women paradoxically develop thinning of axillary and pubic hair but hirsutes at other sites. This is related to a change in the androgen to oestrogen ratios (Fig. 3.6).

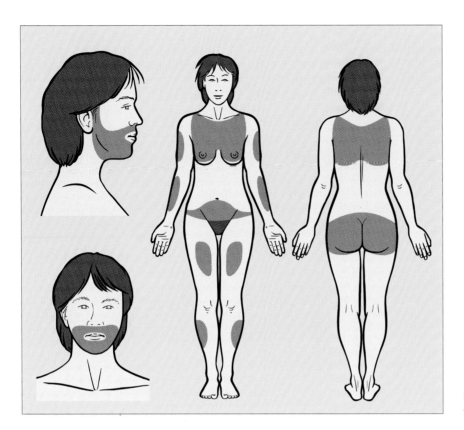

Fig. 3.1 Sites of development of hirsutes in women.

Idiopathic hirsutism

This term is applied when no underlying endocrinological cause for hirsutes is found. The incidence varies with the curiosity of the clinician and the criteria used to diagnose PCO. Subtle variations in androgen synthesis and metabolism exist which are not always detectable by routine laboratory techniques, due to the large overlap with normal values. Detailed investigations suggest that many hirsute women synthesize increased daily amounts of androgens (3.5–5-fold), and that their androgens are secreted as testosterone rather than DHEAS. Also there are lower levels of sex hormone binding globulin (SHBG) resulting in more available free testosterone. In women for whom no biochemical abnormality is found the abnormality resides in the hair follicle itself. Such follicles show increased 5α reductase activity that converts circulating testosterone into the more potent locally active dihydrotestosterone (DHT).

Investigation

While hirsutes is most commonly produced by end-organ hypersensitivity to circulating androgens, in some women it is due to an endocrine disorder associated with androgen hypersecretion. The yield of routinely screening all hirsute patients for an endocrinological abnormality is low, and while a full history and examination is suggested for all patients only a minority will require further biochemical investigations.

Screening investigations are recommended for patients who have early (prepubertal) onset or severe and rapidly progressive hirsutes, and for those who have associated features of hyperandrogenism. Such features include menstrual irregularity, acne, androgenetic alopecia, male habitus, deepening of the voice and cliteromegaly.

For most cases the screening tests in Table 3.2 will be sufficient and cost effective. The main aim of investigation is to exclude a tumour. A second aim is to diagnose congenital adrenal hyperplasia as this may be treated differently from other causes of hirsutes. A third aim is to distinguish between polycystic ovary syndrome and idiopathic hirsutes, but this is of lesser importance as the management of these two conditions is similar. For this reason a SHBG level looking for a subtle alteration in free testosterone is not routinely required.

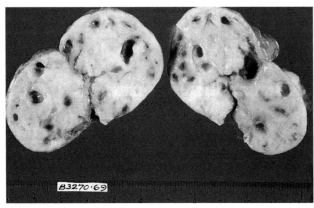

Fig. 3.2 Polycystic ovaries.

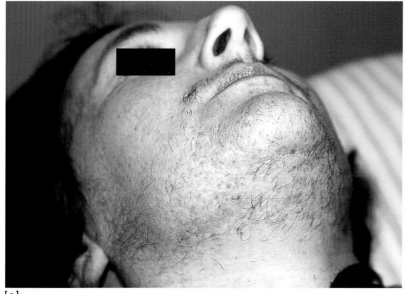

[a]

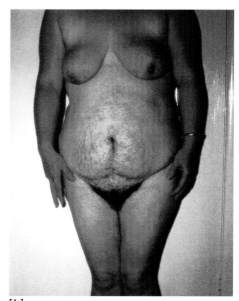

[b]

Fig. 3.3 A patient with polycystic ovarian syndrome demonstrates hirsutes (a) of the face and neck, and (b) of the body.

Table 3.2 Initial investigation of hirsutes.

Serum testosterone (+/–SHBG)	Uniform marked elevation in ovarian tumours Occasional marked elevation in adrenal tumours Small to moderate elevation with PCO Normal in idiopathic hirsutes, CAH (and some PCO)
Serum DHEAS	Uniform marked elevation in adrenal tumours Occasional marked elevation in ovarian tumours Usually elevated in congenital adrenal hyperplasia Normal or small to moderate elevation in PCO
Serum 17α hydroxyprogesterone	Will detect a proportion of patients with mild CAH otherwise missed by serum DHEAS and serum testosterone estimation alone. The low yield and relatively high expense make routine testing unnecessary.

	Reference range		
Screening test	Age	Normal values	Cost ($US)*
Serum testosterone		0.25–0.95 ng/ml	88.50
SHBG		20–106 nmol/l	59.25
Serum DHEAS	20–29 years 30–39 years 40–49 years 50–59 years 60–69 years 70–79 years	70–450 μg/dl 50–410 μg/dl 40–350 μg/dl 30–270 μg/dl 20–180 μg/dl 10–90 μg/dl	89.75
17α hydroxyprogesterone	prepubertal follicular luteal postmenopausal	<200 ng/dl <80 ng/dl 30–290 ng/dl <50 ng/dl	92.25

PCO, Polycystic ovary syndrome; CAH, congenital adrenal hyperplasia; DHEAS, dihydroepiandrostendion sulfate; SHBG, sex hormone binding globulin.
*The information regarding the cost in $US is from Sperling and Heimer, June 1993. In Australia the recommended fee for the first test is $AU 31.55 and each subsequent test $11.00. All four tests would cost $AU 64.55.

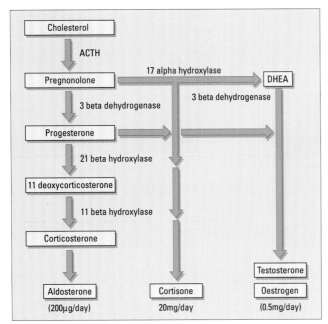

Fig. 3.4 Major pathway of adrenocortical hormone biosynthesis. Deficiency of either 21β hydroxylase or 11β hydroxylase will disrupt both aldosterone and cortisone synthesis. Deficiency of 3β dehydrogenase will disrupt aldosterone, cortisone and testosterone and oestrogen synthesis. Because the daily cortisone production is more than an order of magnitude greater than androgen synthesis, even a minor diversion of cortisone precursors to androgen synthesis would substantially increase the testosterone output. In addition decreased cortisol production stimulates ACTH production, which in turn enhances pregnenolone production. ACTH, adrenocorticotrophic hormone; DHEA, dehydroepiandrosterone.

If there is a very high index of suspicion of virilization or the screening tests are grossly abnormal, with value twice the upper limit of normal, then a referral to an endocrinologist may be appropriate. This is especially important for women of child bearing age for advice regarding their future fertility.

Diagnosis

Hirsutes must be distinguished from hypertrichosis which refers to excess hair that is usually fine and uniform over the body. Hypertrichosis is not the result of androgen excess.

Associated conditions

Hirsutes may be associated with low self-esteem and occasionally frank depression. Low fertility is an important association, and whether nulliparous women should be alerted to this possibility is contentious. Other associated features will vary with the cause of the hirsutes and have already been discussed.

Pathology

Hirsutes is rarely biopsied. The features are an increased number of terminal hair follicles without inflammation.

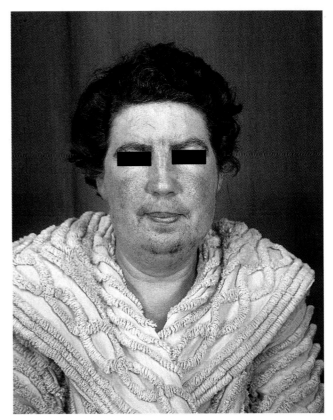

Fig. 3.5 Cushing's disease.

Prognosis

Untreated idiopathic hirsutes tends to be slowly progressive. Tumours tend to produce a more rapid progression.

Treatment

Not all patients who have unwanted hair seek treatment. The desire for treatment is influenced by the subjective perception of the woman and by racial, cultural and social factors as well as the distribution of the hair. Terminal hairs on the face, chest and upper back are more likely to induce a woman to seek medical advice than hairs on covered sites such as the limbs and buttocks.

Hirsutism of sufficient severity to seek medical attention has social and psychological influences on women. Women need reassurance that they are not turning into men or becoming excessively masculine. They also need advice on cosmetic measures to remove hair. A minority will require pharmacological treatment of hirsutism either directed at an underlying cause or, in cases of idiopathic hirsutes, towards lowering the impact of normal levels of circulating androgens on the hair follicle

Cosmetic measures for the removal of hair

Bleaching with hydrogen peroxide is the easiest measure, but may produce an unacceptable yellow hue. Plucking and

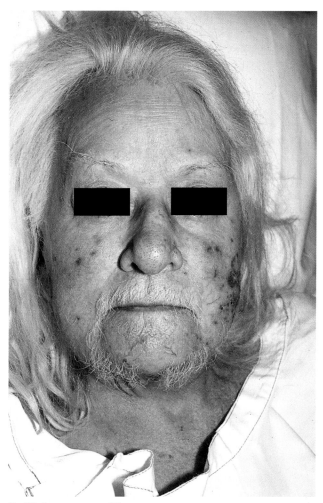

Fig. 3.6 Postmenopausal hirsutes.

hairs, but only those that were previously in anagen regrow. Many women object to shaving but as facial hair has a long telogen phase this is a good preliminary to plucking. Depilatory creams act by dissolving keratin and often irritate the interfollicular epidermis. Home epilators are in reality no more effective than plucking.

Electrical epilation by high frequency short wave diathermy or galvanic electrolysis offers permanent methods of hair removal. Galvanic electrolysis is time consuming and has been largely superseded by electrical epilation, which is loosely referred to as 'electrolysis'. Electrical epilation requires insertion of a fine needle through the ostium of the hair follicle to the root where a brief pulse of electricity is delivered with the intention of cauterizing the dermal papilla. In skilled hands it is safe, but time consuming, mildly painful and expensive. Individual hairs often need multiple treatments to disappear, and up to 80% regrowth can be expected after a single treatment. In unskilled hands it can be complicated by folliculitis and scarring (Fig. 3.8).

A number of lasers have been adapted to treat unwanted hair. The non-q-switched ruby laser and Alexandrite laser show the most promise and are designed to thermally destroy the pigmented anagen hair bulbs. The risk of scarring with these new techniques appears to be low. However, hypopigmentation is a potential problem so these treatments are most appropriate for women with dark hair and fair skin. Hair regrowth is inevitable but delayed by six or more months with the currently available lasers.

Pharmacological methods

Since hirsutes is a condition mediated by androgens, attempts have been made to ameliorate the growth of hair with drugs that reduce androgen bioactivity. These drugs interact at a number of sites (Table 3.3). It is important that hirsute women are carefully selected prior to initiating treatment and are given realistic expectations of the potential improvement. This is important because it can take 6–9

waxing stimulate the root into anagen resulting in only a short delay before the new hair emerges. Waxing is painful and sometimes produces a folliculitis. In addition the use of hot wax can burn the patient (Fig. 3.7). Shaving removes all

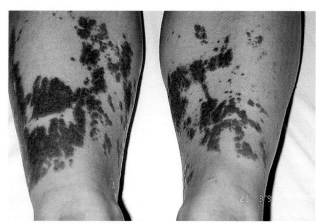

Fig. 3.7 Waxing burns can develop if the epilating wax is too hot. (Courtesy of Dr M. Haskett, Melbourne.)

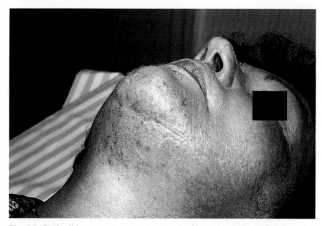

Fig. 3.8 Folliculitis secondary to electrolysis. (Courtesy of Dr A. Callen, Melbourne.)

Table 3.3 Pharmacological treatment of hirsutism.

Androgen receptor antagonists	Spironolactone Cyproterone acetate Flutemide
Follicular 5α reductase inhibitor	Finasteride
Free testosterone reducer (by increasing SHBG and inducing hepatic metabolism of androgens)	Oral contraceptives
Suppression of adrenal androgen production (by reducing pituitary ACTH secretion)	Prednisolone
Adrenal and gonadal steroid synthesis inhibitor	Spironolactone

SHBG, sex hormone binding globulin; ACTH, adrenocorticotrophic hormone.

months before any effect on hair growth is detectable and only partial improvement is to be expected. Additionally, because these drugs are suppressive and not curative, their effects wear off a few months after ceasing therapy. They therefore need to be taken indefinitely to sustain any improvement.

First line therapy consists of either spironolactone or cyproterone acetate. Spironolactone is a synthetic steroid structurally related to aldosterone that acts as an antiandrogen by altering steroidogenesis in the adrenals and the gonads through inhibition of cytochrome p450, a coenzyme for 17α-, 11β- and 21β-hydroxylases. Additionally it affects the target organ response by competitively blocking cytoplasmic receptors for dihydrotestosterone. The 7α-thio substituted metabolite of spironolactone is thought to be the active molecule.

Premenopausal women should take it together with an oral

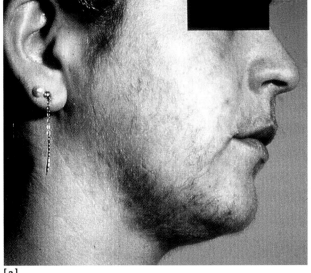

[a]

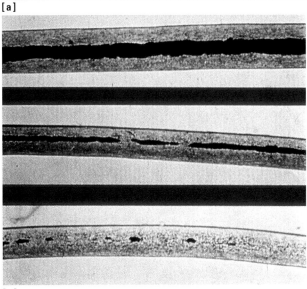

[c]

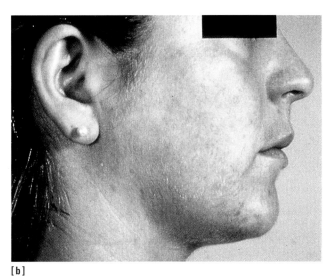

[b]

Fig. 3.9 (a) Before and (b) after treatment of hirsutes with cyproterone acetate (CPA). (c) Hair diameter decreases, and hair colour lightens, with cyproterone acetate treatment. The medulla is intact (top), fragmented (middle) and almost lost (bottom). (Courtesy of Oxford Clinical Communications.)

contraceptive to prevent a pregnancy (complicated by masculinization of a female fetus) and menstrual irregularities, that otherwise occur in 80%. Suitable contraceptives are those with minimal androgenic effects such as those containing either desogestrel (Marvelon®), norethisterone (Brevinor®), or cyproterone acetate (Dianette®). The main side effects are breast soreness and enlargement, decreased libido and menstrual irregularities on stopping therapy. Hypotension does not seem to be a problem, and hyperkalaemia is rarely significant in the absence of coexisting renal impairment. An initial dose of 100 mg spironolactone daily is recommended. If the response at 3 months is unsatisfactory the dose can be increased to 150 mg daily and after a further 3 months to 200 mg daily. Measurement of the baseline renal function should be considered in postmenopausal women, and it is prudent to advise patients to avoid potassium supplements. Serum potassium levels are recommended to be checked every 6–12 months.

Cyproterone acetate is a hydroxyprogesterone derivative that can be used in combination with ethinyl oestradiol 35 µg daily for 21 days in every 28 days (Fig. 3.9). If the response is inadequate after 3 months then an additional 50 mg of cyproterone acetate can be taken daily for days 5–15 of the menstrual cycle. After a further 3 months, should the response still be unsatisfactory, the dose of cyproterone acetate can be further increased to 100 mg daily for days 5–15. This particular regimen is used, otherwise the long half-life of cyproterone disrupts the menses. Side-effects are similar to aldosterone. The role of the additional cyproterone acetate is to hasten the response rather than to increase the magnitude of the ultimate reduction in hair density and diameter.

While spironolactone and cyproterone acetate can be used to treat hirsutes associated with congenital adrenal hyperplasia, corticosteroids are an alternative and were previously used for all types of hirsutes. Flutamide, a potent antiandrogen and finasteride, a specific 5α reductase inhibitor show promise in clinical trials, but at this stage they are only recommended for recalcitrant cases.

Section C
Nonscarring alopecia

Chapter 4

Androgenetic alopecia

Definition

Androgenetic alopecia (AGA) is also known as common baldness. It is a patterned, progressive and until recently largely irreversible loss of an excessive amount of hair from the scalp.

Epidemiology

Significant androgenetic alopecia occurs in 50% of men by the age of 50 and 50% of women by the age of 60 years, while limited androgenetic alopecia affects all men and women progressively as they age. This may manifest only as an alteration in the frontal hair line. Excessive or premature hair loss thus represents an exaggeration of a normal physiological process rather than a disease *per se*.

Aetiology

Prerequisites for androgenetic alopecia are a genetic predisposition and the presence of sufficient circulating androgens. Between 95% and 100% of the population possess the inherited predisposition, but far fewer develop significant alopecia due to variable gene expression.

The evidence in support of androgenetic alopecia being due to the local effects of androgen excess are listed below.
1 Androgenetic alopecia does not occur in eunuchs castrated prior to puberty, but can be induced by the administration of testosterone to those genetically predisposed. If the testosterone is discontinued the alopecia does not progress, although it does not reverse either.
2 Virilization produces androgenetic alopecia in women with a genetic predisposition combined with acne, hirsutes and menstrual irregularity.
3 Antiandrogen therapy slows the progression of androgenetic alopecia. It may also partly reverse hair miniaturization.
4 The 5α reductase enzyme that converts testosterone into the more active dihydrotestosterone (DHT) is found in the dermal papilla cells, as are the androgen receptors that bind DHT. Two subtypes of 5α-reductase have been identified, both of which appear to be present on the scalp.
The response of hair to androgens is site specific. While vellus hair follicles on the prepubertal pubis, axilla, beard and chest react by enlarging into terminal hairs, the terminal hairs on the frontoparietal region of the scalp react to these same androgens by miniaturizing into vellus hairs. These two events are independent of each other and there is no correlation between the degree of baldness and the density of hair patterns on the trunks and limbs of males. There is no satisfactory explanation for this differential effect, nor for the reason many other hair follicles, including the occipital scalp hairs, are relatively unaffected by androgens.

Regional variation exists in distribution of subtypes of 5α-reductase, the activity of 5α-reductase and the density of androgen receptors in the dermal papillae, with greatest levels being found in the frontoparietal areas of the scalp corresponding to the areas of development of androgenetic alopecia. Very high levels are also found in the pubic region and other areas of secondary sexual hair development. The possibilities that different regional receptor subtypes or different second messenger processing of the signal account for the different effects require further investigation.
5 Orentreich demonstrated that punch grafts taken from the occiput of men with androgenetic alopecia and transferred to the frontoparietal area behave like the adjacent hairs from the donor site and maintain their resistance to androgenetic alopecia after transplantation. This implies that the interpretation of the androgen signal locally by the individual follicle is relatively more important than the amount of circulating androgen. This principle of donor dominance forms the basis for successful hair transplantation.
Men have sufficient circulating testosterone to maximally stimulate hair follicles so that all genetically predisposed men will develop androgenetic alopecia. In contrast, androgen levels in the normal female range will only induce balding in premenopausal women with a strong genetic predisposition. In women with a lesser genetic predisposition, baldness develops when androgen production is increased or drugs with androgen-like activity are taken.

Seborrhoea may be associated with common baldness, but is not a factor in the aetiology.

Pathogenesis

Three events combine to produce androgenetic alopecia:
1 progressive prolongation of the telogen phase of the hair cycle, associated with shortening of duration of anagen;
2 development of a latent phase in the hair cycle following shedding of the telogen hair;
3 follicular miniaturization that reduces the calibre of the anagen hairs produced.
The latent phase may last a number of months before anagen recommences and produces empty follicles. Scarring is not a feature of androgenetic alopecia and on biopsy there is no

actual reduction in the number of follicles on the scalp. Loss of pigmentation of the hairs further diminishes their cosmetic significance. This process does not occur evenly over the scalp but follows a pattern of progression that has been described and graded by Hamilton (and later modified by Norwich) and Ludwig.

The follicular miniaturization is global affecting the papilla, the matrix and ultimately the hair shaft. Terminal hairs initially transform into indeterminate hairs and later into vellus hairs that ultimately become so short they do not reach the follicular ostium (Fig. 4.1). These 'secondary' vellus follicles differ from *de novo* vellus follicles in that they still have the remnants of their arrector pili muscle attached to them.

Clinical features

Male pattern baldness

Hamilton described the distinctive pattern of progression of hair loss in men and graded the severity on a scale from I to VIII (Fig. 4.2). Alteration of the frontal hair line with bitemporal recession occurs first and is followed by balding of the vertex. Eventually a more uniform frontal recession joins the bald areas and the entire frontoparietal region bears only inconspicuous secondary vellus hair. The posterior and lateral scalp margins are spared even in advanced cases.

Hamilton's type I describes the normal prepubertal pattern (Fig. 4.3), and postpuberty this may still be seen in some women, but is rare in adult men. Progression to type II occurs in at least 96% of men. It is usually detectable clinically by the age of 17, however, many men do not notice it until their thirties. Types V to VIII occur in 60% of men over the age of 50 years and the balding progresses continuously until death (Figs 4.4–4.6).

Even before alopecia is evident, an increase in the number of terminal hairs less than 4 cm long is detectable due to the progressive curtailment of anagen, producing shorter and shorter hairs with each subsequent hair cycle. Ultimately the hairs fail to emerge from the follicular ostium and all that is seen on the surface of the skin is the pore. The hair pull test becomes positive in the affected areas as the proportion of vellus hairs increases.

Female pattern baldness

Hamilton pattern balding also occurs in women (Fig. 4.7). Hamilton suggested 79% of women develop Hamilton II alopecia after puberty and 25% of women develop Hamilton V by the age of 50, after which time there is minimal progression, but the true incidence is somewhat less than this. Bitemporal recession tends to be less prominent in females than males and is likely to go unnoticed until the late twenties.

Although male pattern alopecia occurs in women, more commonly females develop a hair loss over the crown with preservation of the frontal hair line. This pattern of alopecia was first described by Ludwig and the most useful grading scale for women bears his name (Fig. 4.8).

The earliest change (Ludwig grade I) is thinning of the hair on the crown (Fig. 4.9). This produces an oval area of alopecia encircled by a band of variable breadth with normal hair density. Frontally the fringe is narrow (1–3 cm) while at the sides the margin is 4–5 cm wide. Progression to Ludwig grade II results in further rarefaction of the crown with preservation of the fringe (Fig. 4.10). Grade III is near complete baldness of the crown (Fig. 4.11).

The relative incidence of Ludwig vs. Hamilton pattern alopecia among balding women has been determined. Ludwig pattern I–III occurred in 87% of premenopausal women while Hamilton stage II–IV occurred in 13%. Among postmenopausal women, Ludwig I–III occurred in 63% while Hamilton II–V occurred in 37%.

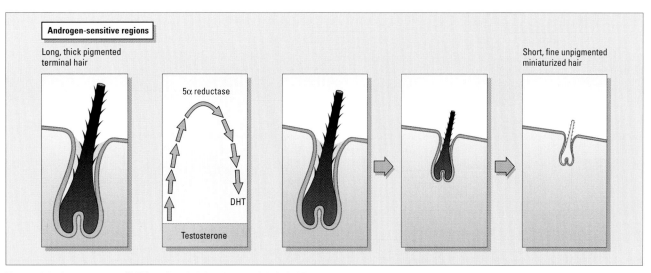

Fig. 4.1 Dihydrotestosterone (DHT) mediated miniaturization of the hair follicles with each successive hair cycle.

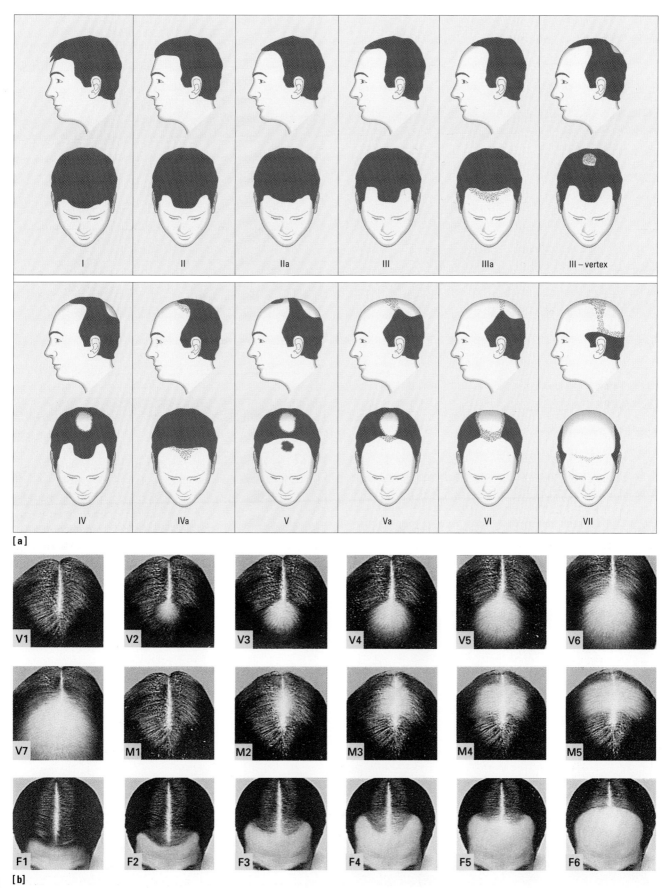

[a]

[b]

Fig. 4.2 (a) The pattern of alopecia in a male (after Hamilton and Norwood). (b) The Savin scale for assessment of male pattern androgenetic alopecia.

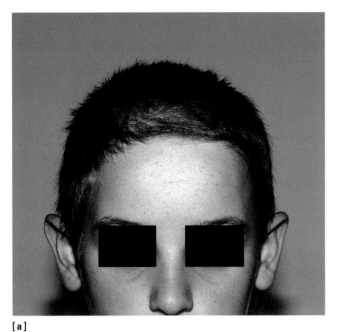

[a]

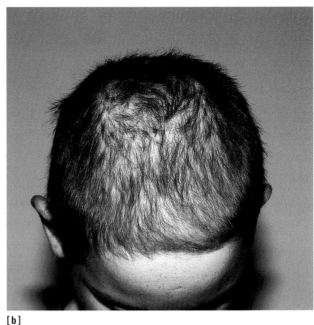

[b]

Fig. 4.3 (a), (b) An intact frontal hairline consistent with Hamilton type I in a prepubertal boy. This 13 year old had androgenetic alopecia in a Ludwig pattern. This is the least common pattern of androgenetic alopecia seen in men.

Investigation

The presence or absence of assciated virilization of females with androgenetic alopecia cannot be inferred from the pattern of alopecia, be it Hamilton or Ludwig. More useful is the rate of development of the alopecia, its severity and any associated evidence of androgen excess such as hirsutes, acne, menstrual irregularities and cliteromegaly. The vast majority of women do not require any investigation for virilization other than a directed history and examination. The causes and investigation of virilization have already been

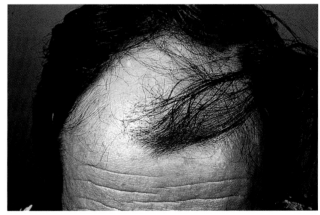

Fig. 4.5 Androgenetic alopecia Hamilton type V.

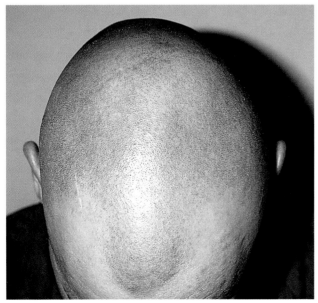

Fig. 4.4 Androgenetic alopecia Hamilton type III.

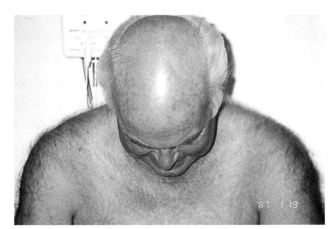

Fig. 4.6 Androgenetic alopecia Hamilton type VII in a man with numerous terminal hairs on the shoulders. (Courtesy of Dr M. Haskett, Melbourne.)

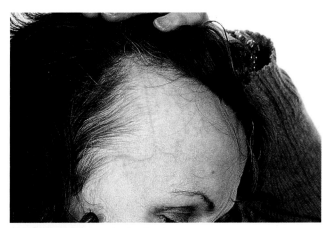

Fig. 4.7 Temporal recession in a female.

discussed (pp. 38–45). It is usually more relevant to direct investigations towards excluding other causes of a diffuse alopecia, especially in patients with early androgenetic alopecia when the pattern of loss is difficult to discern.

Diagnosis

The diagnosis of androgenetic alopecia is a clinical one and is based on recognizing the pattern of hair loss. A hair pull test may demonstrate loss of an increased number of telogen hairs from the frontoparietal region, but not the occiput, in keeping with the pattern of the altered trichogram. In doubtful cases analysis of the trichogram of clumps of plucked hairs from different regions of the scalp will further support the diagnosis.

In the early stages of androgenetic alopecia in a woman, the hair loss may be diffuse. In such cases a drug history, thyroid function tests and a serum ferritin estimation will be required to exclude other causes of a diffuse alopecia. While a scalp biopsy is only rarely required in a male, it may be the only way to distinguish early androgenetic alopecia in a female from chronic telogen effluvium (pp. 64–7).

Associated conditions

Premature balding also occurs in progeria and Werner's syndrome and early frontoparietal recession with greying is seen in myotonic dystrophy. Other signs of these disorders will allow a specific diagnosis. Occasionally a diffuse alopecia can coexist with androgenetic alopecia and will be suggested by a history of rapid deterioration and a positive hair pull test from all over the scalp. In such circumstances a drug history (see Table 5.2, p. 72), thyroid function tests and a serum ferritin measurement are indicated.

Pathology

A scalp biopsy is helpful in difficult cases, but is not required routinely. At scanning magnification the histology shows a decreased number of terminal hair follicles, and an increased number of vellus follicles. The sebaceous glands appear large and solar elastosis may be apparent. Streamers (remnants of

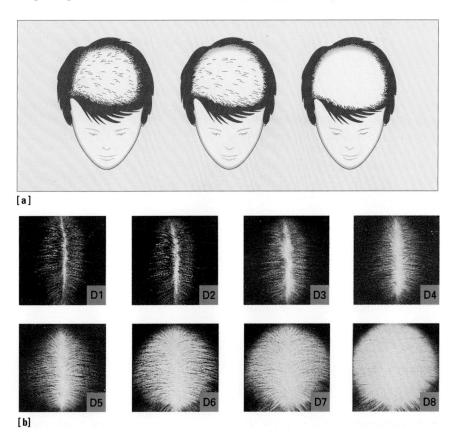

Fig. 4.8 (a) Ludwig classification of scalp hair distribution in females. (b) Savin scale.

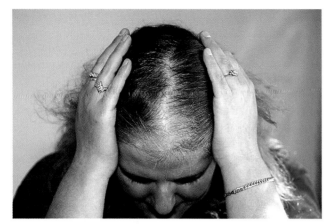

Fig. 4.9 Androgenetic alopecia, Ludwig grade I.

involuted anagen hairs) and a lymphohistiocytic inflammatory infiltrate around the hair follicle at the level of the sebaceous duct (Figs 4.12 & 4.13) and also around the superficial dermal capillaries may be seen.

Prognosis

Androgenetic alopecia is a progressive disorder. The age of onset is variable, but always follows the onset of puberty. The rate of progression is also variable with some men taking 10 years and others 30 or more years to advance to Hamilton VI and VII. The rate of hair loss also fluctuates with periods of excessive shedding punctuated by periods of minimal loss.

The prepubertal hair density of the scalp is approximately 200 terminal hairs per cm² and a reduction of 30% to 140 terminal hairs per cm² is required before balding is apparent.

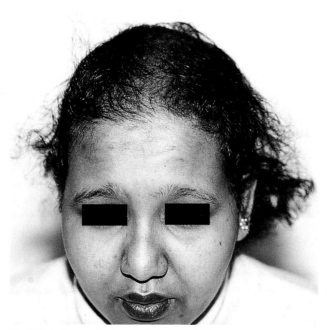

Fig. 4.10 Androgenetic alopecia, Ludwig grade II.

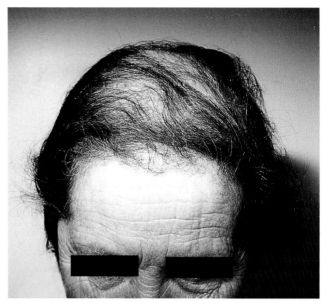

Fig. 4.11 Androgenetic alopecia, Ludwig grade III.

Once balding is obvious loss of terminal hairs (also referred to as nonvellus hairs in some studies) tends to progress at a rate of 10% per year, and total hair loss at a rate of 5%.

Until recently it was accepted dogma that the miniaturization of hairs was an irreversible process. The dramatic, but exceptional regrowth that has been documented with minoxidil has led to a reappraisal of this and motivated a large research effort into finding the key to unravel the complex series of events that will reverse androgenetic alopecia.

Treatment

The treatment of androgenetic alopecia is considered in terms of conservative therapy and wigs, medical management and surgical management.

Conservative management

Camouflage is the simplest, easiest, cheapest and most effective way of dealing with mild androgenetic alopecia. Balding becomes most noticeable when the scalp can be seen through the hair. Camouflage treatments dye the scalp the same colour as the hair, and give the illusion of thicker hair. Numerous brands are available, in pressurized spray cans in a number of different colours (Fig. 4.14) and they are often combined with a holding hair spray (and sunscreen). The hair is dried and styled before the dye that matches the patient's hair colour is sprayed onto the base of the hair. Although many of the newer agents are water resistant, problems may still arise in the rain if the hair gets wet and the dye runs. In addition patients should avoid touching their hair as the dye will colour their hands. Towels and pillow cases may stain, but these come out in the wash. Patients are advised to

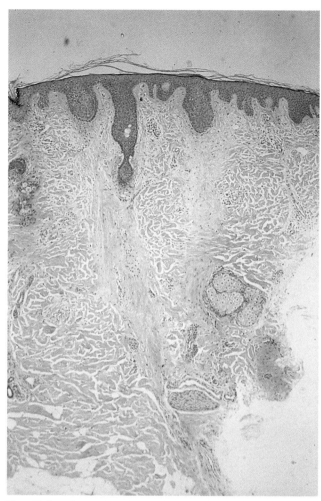

Fig. 4.12 Scanning power photomicrograph of androgenetic alopecia shows a reduction in the number of follicles. In addition anagen hair follicles are decreased in size, relative to the sebaceous glands and lie superficial in the dermis suggesting they are vellus-like hair follicles. (Courtesy of Dorevitch Pathology, Melbourne.)

remove the dye each night by shampooing and to reapply the dye each morning.

Wigs

Many men and women with diffuse alopecia prefer wigs to medical treatments or scalp surgery (Fig. 4.15). Wigs can either be interwoven with existing hair or worn over the top of existing hair. Interwoven wigs tend to lift as the hair beneath grows and require adjustment every few weeks. This may add considerably to the expense.

Wigs are made from either a synthetic acrylic fibre or natural fibre. The most commonly used natural fibres are human hair, which may be Asian hair or European hair. Each has different advantages. Natural fibre wigs look better and last longer, but are more expensive. Wigs can be styled and washed and the manufacturer usually gives the recipient detailed instructions on wig care.

Attachment to the scalp may be by either adhesive tape, glue or by suction. Suction attachments are made by taking a mould of the completely bald (or shaved) skull upon which a hairpiece is constructed by hand (Fig. 4.16). Such wigs tend to remain well fixed to the skull and can be worn during all activities including water sports. One drawback of wigs is that they may get excessively hot in the summer.

In general the only wigs people tend to notice are the bad ones and many people require encouragement to visit a wigmaker. Excellent advice on wigs and wigmakers is usually available from patient support groups such as Hairline International in the UK, the National Alopecia Areata Foundation in the USA and the Alopecia Society in Australia. Clinicians are wise to familiarize themselves with the services local organizations offer.

Medical management

Currently available pharmacological therapy for women consists of antiandrogens and topical minoxidil. Antiandrogens may feminize males and are therefore not an appropriate

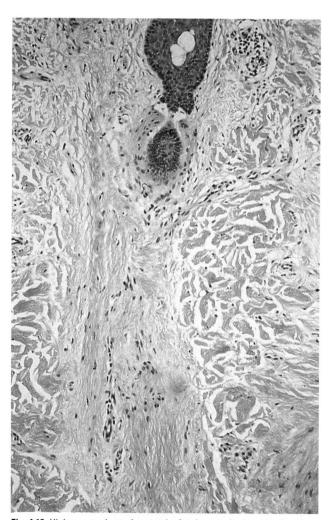

Fig. 4.13 High-power photomicrograph of androgenetic alopecia, showing the perifollicular mononuclear cell infiltrate.

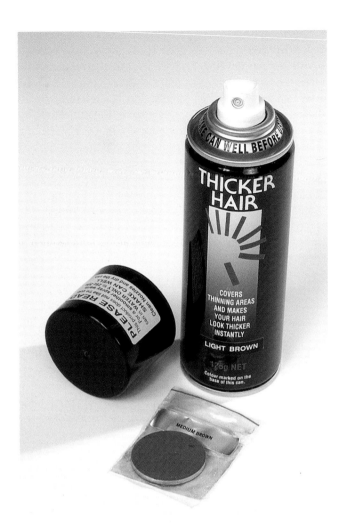

Fig. 4.14 Coloured hair spray and lacquer.

therapy for balding men. Until recently the only effective pharmacological treatment for men was topical minoxidil. The recent introduction of oral finasteride has revolutionized the treatment of male AGA.

Minoxidil

This is a vasodilator that was developed for the treatment of hypertension. Hypertrichosis mainly of the body and to a lesser extent of the scalp was noticed as a side-effect, and subsequently a topical preparation for use in androgenetic alopecia was developed.

Numerous dosing studies have been done. The minimum concentration that will increase nonvellus hair counts is 0.1%. The minimum concentration that will produce cosmetically acceptable regrowth is 1% and the optimal result is obtained with 2%. It remains controversial whether there is added long-term benefit from using 5%; however, a more rapid initial response may be noted. One millilitre should be applied directly to the bald area twice daily and gently massaged into the scalp. The scalp must be dry when minoxidil is

applied and the hair should not be wetted for 1 hour after the application. Once daily use is not sufficient for maintenance therapy, and there is no extra benefit with applications more frequently than twice daily.

If successful, after 2 months of continuous minoxidil use, hair shedding decreases; hair regrowth may be detected at 4–8 months. The hair counts usually stabilize after 12–18 months whereas control groups continue to progressively lose hair at 5% per year. Occasionally regrowth does not begin for up to 12 months and the treatment should not be abandoned due to lack of efficacy before then. Most people will get a regrowth of indeterminate hairs, but for many this is not cosmetically significant and insufficient to warrant the expense of treatment (Fig. 4.17). Very occasionally there is a dramatic response with near reversion to normal, but this is unpredictable.

Patients need to be warned that in the initial stages there may be an increased amount of hair shedding due to stimulation of telogen follicles to re-enter anagen. If this occurs it is usually an indication that the patient is likely to respond well to the treatment.

Other useful prognostic factors for regrowth are the severity and the duration of the alopecia. Good prognostic factors are:
1 a brief history of balding (fewer than 5 years);
2 limited alopecia on the vertex (less than 10 cm diameter);
3 more than 100 indeterminate hairs in the treated area.

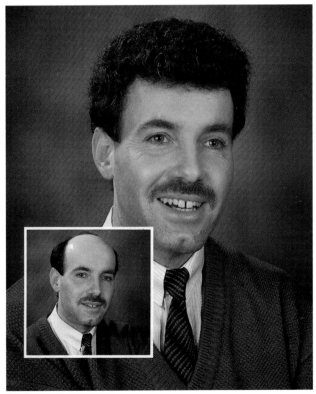

Fig. 4.15 Natural looking wig for male pattern baldness.

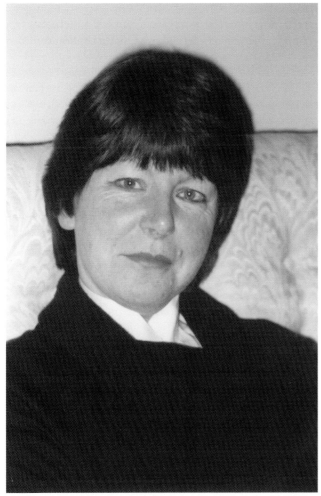

Fig. 4.16 For total alopecia, wigs may be held in place by suction. (Courtesy of Positively Hair, 23 Green Lane, Woodstock, Oxford OX20 1JZ.)

Approximately 50% of users find their hair loss stabilizes, while an additional 10% notice significant regrowth. If successful, treatment needs to be continued indefinitely because once stopped the new hairs fall out and regression to the pretreatment state occurs within 3 months (Fig. 4.18).

Minoxidil has also been used together with tretinoic acid to enhance penetration, however, this combination produces greater scalp irritation and the benefits are minimal.

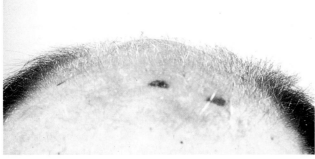

Fig. 4.17 Indeterminate hairs, regrowing following minoxidil therapy.

The side-effects of topical minoxidil include pruritus, a contact irritant dermatitis and occasionally contact allergic dermatitis can develop. Hypotension does not occur with topical treatment because there is minimal systemic absorption. Oral minoxidil has also been used, however, it appears to be no more effective than topical minoxidil. In addition the systemic side-effects make its routine use for androgenetic alopecia inappropriate.

Spironolactone

Used primarily as a potassium sparing diuretic, spironolactone is an aldosterone antagonist. It is also an antiandrogen that can be used to treat androgenetic alopecia in women. It appears to inhibit the interaction between dihydrotestosterone and the intracellular receptor, as well as inhibiting ovarian androgen production. The dose range is 50–200 mg per day; however, the optimal dose of spironolactone is 100 mg daily. This tends to slow the progression of balding without reversing the process. Much of the data on spironolactone relates to its use in hirsutes and few trials have been conducted on its use in androgenetic alopecia. A contraceptive pill is not mandatory with this agent, but women of child-bearing age should be warned against becoming pregnant while on this medication due to the risks of feminizing a male child.

Cyproterone acetate

Systemic antiandrogen therapy with cyproterone acetate (as described for hirsutes on p. 45) decreases hair shedding but there is generally no cosmetically significant regrowth. In premenopausal women a contraceptive pill should be used with this agent. The effects are generally not noticed for 3–6 months after commencing treatment and they tend to continue only for as long as the tablets are taken. About one-third to one-half of women taking 100 mg of cyproterone acetate notice a major reduction in hair fall (Fig. 4.19). Lower doses do not appear to work as effectively. The trial data presently available is limited and should be interpreted cautiously. Comparative trials, with pretreatment biopsy to exclude women with chronic telogen effluvium are required to judge the relative benefits of aldosterone and cyproterone acetate in androgenetic alopecia.

Finasteride

Finasteride, a selective inhibitor of the type 2 isoenzyme 5α reductase has been shown in clinical studies in a dose of 1 mg per day to effectively treat androgenetic alopecia in men, with minimal side-effects. Dose ranging studies have demonstrated no additional benefit from higher doses, however, side-effects are more common. Circulating levels of testosterone are minimally affected and there is no obvious feminization. Alteration of libido is seen in 1.8% of males receiving finasteride, compared to 1.3% in the placebo group

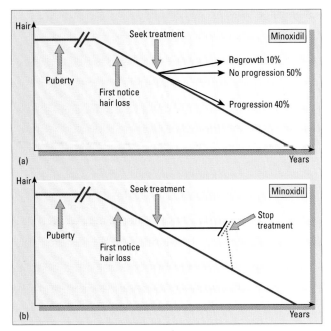

Fig. 4.18 (a) Response rates to minoxidil superimposed on the natural history of AGA and (b) effect of cessation of treatment.

and erectile dysfunction was seen in 1.3%, compared to 0.7% in the placebo group.

Preliminary trials in postmenopausal women failed to demonstrate efficacy and premenopausal women are cautioned against taking it as finasteride is a potential teratogen that may induce hypospadius or feminization of a male fetus. The amount of finasteride potentially absorbed from sperm through the vagina of a pregnant woman is too low to pose a risk to the fetus.

In the trials a number of measures of efficacy were used, however, the most persuasive was standardized macrophotography (Fig. 4.20). The macrophotography results of the phase III studies showed that after 2 years hair loss on the vertex of the scalp is arrested in one-third of patients, another one-third achieve minimal regrowth (sufficient to be detected by clinical photography) while another one-third achieve marked or moderate regrowth. Only 1% of the men who received finasteride had progression of their hair loss (Fig. 4.21a–c).

Frontal hair loss also responds to finasteride, albeit less well. Half the patients showed no further hair loss, about 40% had minimal regrowth and only 4% had moderate regrowth. No patients had marked regrowth and 5% had further progression of their frontal hair loss (Fig. 4.21d).

It is not possible to predict in advance which patients are more likely to respond to finasteride. Unlike minoxidil where a short duration of hair loss and limited extent are favourable prognostic features, some men with advanced hair loss were among the best responders to finasteride (Fig. 4.22).

In the placebo group 33% of men had obvious progression of their hair loss, 60% remained unchanged and 7% had

increased hair. This demonstrated the marked variation in the rate of progression in androgenetic alopecia and the fact that for many men hair loss progresses slowly. It also confirms that the amount of hair lost fluctuates on a week to week or month to month basis, with periods of accelerated loss punctuated by periods where the loss plateaus. During the plateau phases it is not uncommon for there to be some reversal of the hair loss which is detected as improvement using the macrophotographs.

Upon commencing finasteride, patients who have previously been aware of excessive hair shedding can expect to notice a reduction in hair shedding within 4 months. While regrowth may be noticed within 4 months this is exceptional, and only about 20% will be aware of regrowth at 12 months and about 40% at 24 months. Upon stopping the finasteride, the process continues, however, the rapid correction seen with minoxidil does not occur (Fig. 4.21a).

A major difficulty is effective monitoring of patient progress in the clinical setting. Without access to global photography patients with arrested progression of androgenetic alopecia and patients with minimal regrowth may be unable to determine whether the treatment is working or not, and one suspects that without the appropriate pretreatment counselling to ensure they have realistic expectations, and ongoing reassurance by their physician, a significant proportion of these men will abandon an effective treatment. Patient photography may prove to be a useful tool to enhance long-term patient compliance.

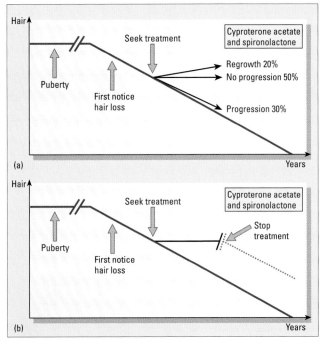

Fig. 4.19 (a) Response rates to spironolactone and cyproterone acetate superimposed on the natural history of AGA and (b) the effect of cessation of treatment.

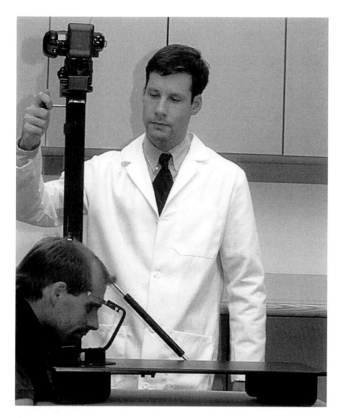

Fig. 4.20 Global photography of vertex.

The combination of topical minoxidil with systemic antiandrogens or finasteride may be more efficacious than either used alone. Properly conducted trials to verify this clinical suspicion are awaited.

Surgical management

Androgenetic alopecia in women presents with a thinning of hair over the vertex. It rarely produces bald patches suitable for corrective surgery, and the techniques discussed here apply predominantly to men.

All surgical procedures aim to use androgen insensitive parietal and occipital hairs to cover the bald areas. Relocated hairs behave as they did prior to moving, showing little tendency to miniaturize in their new home. Numerous different techniques have been used and include those described below.

Scalp reduction surgery

This involves the excision of an ellipse of central bald skin. Tissue expanders can be used to increase the harvest, but require insertion up to 3 months prior to the procedure to give the tissue time to expand. Postoperatively some of the initial gain is ultimately lost as scalp laxity returns and the area of alopecia may enlarge due to 'stretch-back'. This

technique is ideal for patches of nonprogressive scarring alopecia.

Rotation flaps

Rotation flaps, such as the Juri flap are used to swing in vascularized tissue to recreate the frontal hair line (Fig. 4.23). Flaps have the advantage of achieving a high density of hair growth, although sometimes it is too dense and looks unnatural (Fig. 4.24). In addition there is less postoperative telogen effluvium than occurs post-transplantation. One disadvantage of flaps is that they represent an uneconomical use of a restricted supply of donor tissue. Furthermore, if the patient has a large bald spot there may not be enough parietal and occipital skin available to cover the defect. The same applies if the patient returns 5 or 10 years later with progression of his androgenetic alopecia looking for a second graft. Another problem with flaps is with their orientation. Hairs grow in their original direction, and simple rotation directs hair growth posteriorly, exposing the scar and appearing unnatural. Newer techniques, such as tunnel flaps are designed to address this. Potential complications of the procedure include unsightly donor scars and flap devitalization with consequent loss of valuable donor tissue.

Hair transplantation

This takes advantage of donor dominance (the Orentreich principle), which is the tendency of transplanted hairs to maintain the growth characteristics of their original (donor) site, independent of the character of the recipient site. Thus occipital and parietal hairs from the scalp margin do not fall victim to androgenetic alopecia when placed on the crown. *Punch grafting* used to be the most commonly used technique. Multiple 4 mm punch biopsies are taken from the scalp margins and inserted into the bald areas. The donor sites can be individually glued, sutured or left to heal by secondary intention. The recipient site is prepared to receive the grafts by creating 3.5 mm circular holes in the bald skin with another punch biopsy. Slightly better results are achieved with smaller recipient holes, as the grafts tend to shrink after they are removed, while the recipient holes tend to enlarge slightly. Because the blood supply to the grafts is compromised if they are placed too close together, the final result may look artificial with discrete tufts of hair separated by bald areas.

This technique can be used to provide hair cover for large areas of bald scalp, the limiting factor being the availability of donor tissue. It is axiomatic that donor plugs should be taken from the hairy areas with the best prospect of retaining their hair during the patient's lifetime. The zone of androgen responsive hair is variable between individuals and may be too narrow to provide complete coverage of the defect. Often doubtful hair has to be used and for this reason balding recurs in the transplanted hair in the ensuing 5–10 years necessitating a further procedure. This possibility

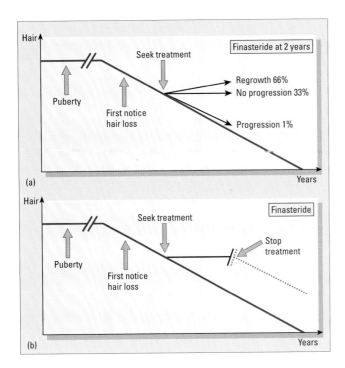

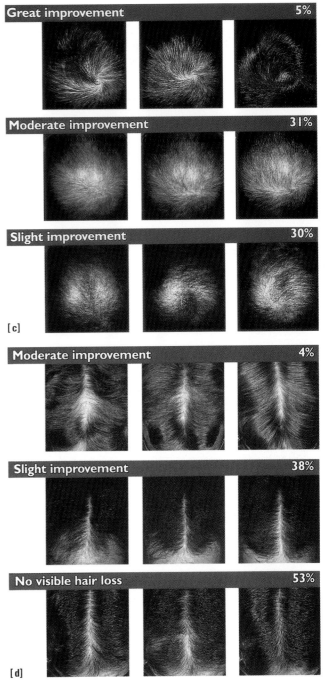

Fig. 4.21 (a) Response rates to finasteride and (b) the effect of cessation of treatment. (c) Vertex studies; (d) anterior mid-scalp study.

should be carefully explained to the patient in advance. Nevertheless many patients feel 5–10 years of hair in some areas is worth the moderate discomfort and significant expense.

The state of the art surgery for baldness is *single follicle transplantation*. This has gradually replaced punch grafting. The technique involves harvesting strips of hair bearing skin from areas likely to be less sensitive to androgenic alopecia. When harvesting the donor tissue, the surgeon must be careful to angle the incision to conform to the direction of hair

growth so as to not transect follicles. The donor site is sutured and the grafts are then dissected by a technician into individual hairs using a scalpel and jeweller's forceps. These hairs are then placed obliquely into holes made with an 18-gauge hypodermic needle or slits made with a fine scalpel blade that are orientated according to the desired direction of hair growth. Three or four sessions (of 300–600 grafts) are usually required to achieve the desired hair density, producing a more gradual return of hair growth (Fig. 4.25). The cost to the patient is approximately $US 5–10 per hair.

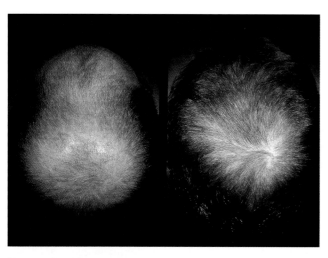

Fig. 4.22 Men with advanced hair loss were among the best responders to finasteride.

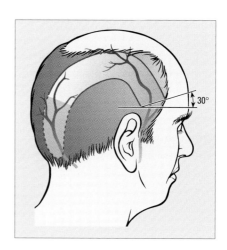

Fig. 4.23 Diagram of the Juri flap.

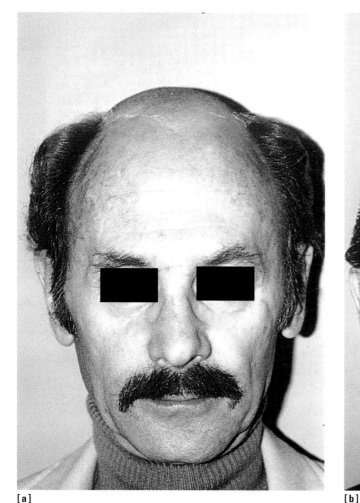

[a]   [b]

Fig. 4.24 Photographs taken (a) before and (b) after of a patient who had a Juri flap. (Courtesy of Dr R. Sheil.)

Single follicle grafts are particularly useful when treating 'early' androgenetic alopecia in men and can also be used for females with androgenetic alopecia as the grafts can be fed in between existing follicles to increase hair density. There is minimal damage to the recipient site using this technique, while punch grafting would require removal of some hair bearing scalp tissue.

However, used as the sole method of covering a large patch

of alopecia, single follicle grafts are very time consuming and expensive. Some prefer to use a combination of small punch grafts and single follicle grafts, with the single hairs placed in between the punch grafts to soften the effect. Alternatively single grafts can be used to recreate the fringe, and punch grafts used for the main defect.

The best candidates for grafting are those with light, fine hair, good residual hair density over frontal regions, and minimal contrast between the colour of the hair and the skin. Orientation of the grafted hairs is important as the hairs will grow in the direction they have been inserted. Shortly after inserting the grafted hairs they undergo a telogen effluvium and it takes between 6 and 12 months before a good cosmetic result is achieved.

A detailed postoperative instruction leaflet (Box 4.1) is required so that the patient can know what to expect. Apart from early mild pruritus and scalp oedema, postoperative problems are uncommon. The major complications of grafting include hypertrophic scarring, hyperaesthesia, haematoma formation, arteriovenous fistula formation and postoperative infection.

Attempts to increase the pool of donor hairs have not yet

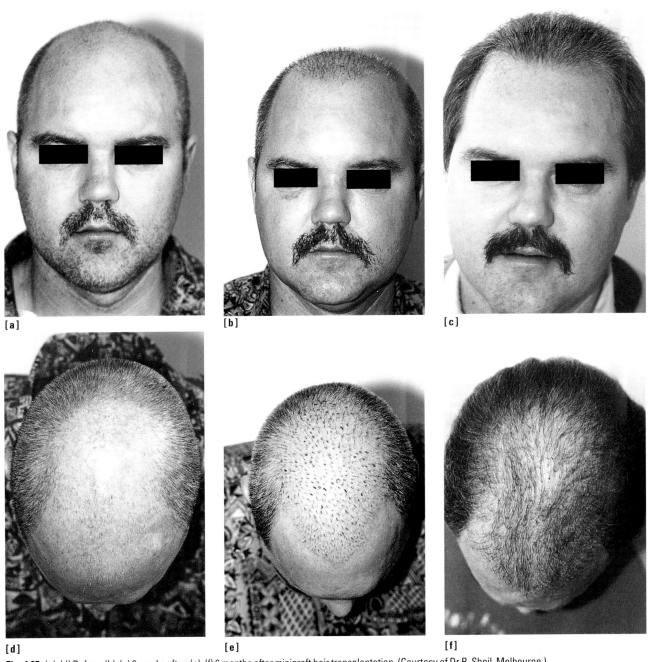

Fig. 4.25 (a), (d) Before; (b), (e) 6 weeks after; (c), (f) 6 months after minigraft hair transplantation. (Courtesy of Dr R. Sheil, Melbourne.)

Box 4.1 Instructions for patients following hair transplantation

The first 24 hours

1 You will feel drowsy after the operation so you should make arrangements for someone else to drive you home.

2 Take care getting in and out of the car while your scalp is numb. If you bump your head you may dislodge some grafts.

3 On reaching home, rather than lying down it is suggested you rest in an upright position until your normal bedtime.

4 Postoperative pain is not usually a problem, but if necessary you can take any of the commonly available 'pain killers'. The donor site at the back and side of your scalp is often the most uncomfortable and may remain tender for some days.

5 The bandage and dressing can be removed on the day following the operation. This is best done in the shower and you can lightly shampoo the scalp. An electric drier should be used to dry the hair.

6 If you have a hair piece this can be replaced after drying the scalp, but try to leave this off as much as possible during the first 2–3 weeks.

7 Some of the grafts may appear a little raised at first. This is quite normal and generally subsides after a few weeks. The grafts will usually become flat within 6 months, but occasionally this may take longer.

8 Rarely there is some spotting of blood through the bandages overnight. It is usually only necessary to add a further layer of padding and bandages. If the bleeding persists please call me.

The first 3 weeks

9 No special treatment is required for the grafts, but it is suggested that you wash your scalp daily with shampoo until the crusts have separated. Normal scalp washing can then be resumed.

10 There may be slight oozing from the donor region at night so it is suggested that you cover your pillow with a towel until this settles. The stitches in the donor site will dissolve in time. If they become annoying these can be removed after 7 days.

11 After grafting to your frontal region you might expect some swelling around the eyebrows, forehead and occasionally the eyelids. On rare occasions one or two black eyes develop. The swelling usually develops on the third day after the operation and subsides over the next 2 or 3 days. The swelling is a natural response to the operation and no treatment is necessary although the regular application of ice packs will give relief.

12 Light jogging can be resumed 2 days after surgery. Swimming in the sea is permissible after 5 days, but be careful not to sunburn the areas. More vigorous sports should not be resumed before 10 days.

13 Infection of the grafts is rare but if you should develop swelling or tenderness beneath any of the grafts after a few days, sponge the area with an antiseptic solution and squeeze gently as for a pimple or boil. Antibiotics are rarely necessary but if the condition is not improving please call me.

14 Occasionally some tender swellings are detected behind the ears. These are enlarged lymph glands and will subside in a few days.

15 Crusts will form over each graft within 2–3 days. These generally come away after 2–3 weeks taking many of the graft hairs with them. You can assist the process by gently rubbing but do not use force. Temporary loss of the graft hairs is expected and these hairs will regrow.

16 If vigorous bleeding should occur at any time use a clean handkerchief or towel and apply firm pressure to the bleeding point for 10 minutes. Please call me if the bleeding persists.

The first 12 months

17 After the graft hairs have been lost there will be a period of several weeks when the transplants are bare and dormant. The new hair will begin to appear after approximately 12 weeks. At first only a few hairs will be seen and these will then grow at the normal rate of 1 cm per month. The number of new hairs will continue to increase for 12 months. Occasionally the graft hairs do not fall out but continue to grow.

18 With second and subsequent operations the onset of the new hairs can be delayed and on rare occasions may not commence until 18 weeks.

19 Often the new hair is a little darker and coarser than the pre-existing hair. The new hair may also have a slight crinkle but the texture returns to normal with continued growth.

20 You may have some persistent numbness over the donor and newly grafted regions. This will gradually improve over several months as the cut nerve fibres regenerate.

If you require any further advice or information please call me on . . .

Courtesy of Dr R. Shiel

---

proved successful. Hairs grown in culture are only viable for a few weeks and hair cloning is still hazardous. Hair cloning involves transversely bisecting a single donor hair into two pieces through the bulge and implanting the two bisected donors into the scalp in the hope that two new hairs will regenerate from a single donor. The problem with hair cloning is the low survival rate of the transected donors, and this technique needs further refinement.

Chapter 5

Diffuse hair loss

5.1 Classification of diffuse hair loss

The normal hair cycle results in the replacement of every hair on the scalp every 3–5 years, with the consequence that between 50 and 150 telogen hairs are shed each day (see Chapter 1). While there is some seasonal variation in the amount of hair lost each day, this amount remains fairly uniform throughout life. Most of this hair loss passes unnoticed, particularly when the hair is short.

Disease states that cause large numbers of hairs to fall out may be classified according to whether the the scalp is scarred or not and whether the hair loss is patchy, patterned or diffuse (Table 5.1). Diffuse hair loss may be further classified according to the type of hairs that are shed, be they anagen or telogen hairs. As telogen hairs have a depigmented bulb, examination of the shed hairs with the naked eye will determine which type of hairs are being lost (Fig. 5.1).

Diagnostic difficulty may occur when the pattern of the loss is not yet clear. This occurs in early androgenetic alopecia in women, making it hard to distinguish this condition from chronic telogen effluvium. However, the diagnosis can usually be established by biopsy.

5.2 Acute telogen effluvium, telogen gravidarum and chronic telogen effluvium

Definition

Telogen effluvium is a self limiting, nonscarring, diffuse hair loss from the scalp that usually occurs 3–6 months following a severe illness or other similar trigger. It usually, but not always, resolves over 3–6 months with restoration of the hair to its normal state. Telogen gravidarum is the name given to a telogen effluvium that follows childbirth.

Chronic telogen effluvium is much less common. This chronic diffuse alopecia is said to occur when the increased hair shedding persists beyond 6 months.

Epidemiology

Telogen effluvium is one of the most comon causes of diffuse hair loss; however, many patients do not seek medical attention, which makes the precise incidence difficult to establish. It is estimated that telogen gravidarum affects one-third to one-half of all women following childbirth. Again many more cases are subclinical.

For reasons that are not entirely clear, chronic telogen effluvium virtually only occurs in women.

Aetiology

A wide variety of triggers have been implicated for acute telogen effluvium. Severe febrile illness, pregnancy (as per telogen gravidarum), chronic systemic illness, a change in medication, a large haemorrhage, a crash diet or sudden starvation, accidental trauma, surgical operations or severe emotional stress are the most common.

While chronic telogen effluvium may follow an acute telogen effluvium, more commonly no trigger is evident.

Pathogenesis

The physiological daily shedding of a few telogen club hairs from the scalp is a natural consequence of the hair cycle. Follicles normally retain telogen hairs until they have re-entered anagen. Eventually the new anagen hair pushes the old telogen hair out. This shedding does not produce alopecia and does not alter the trichogram.

Telogen effluvium occurs if a significant number of anagen hairs are triggered to prematurely stop growing and enter catagen and then telogen. Excessive hair shedding occurs

Table 5.1 The nonscarring alopecias.

Anagen hair loss		Telogen hair loss	
Diffuse	Circumscribed	Diffuse	Patterned
Anagen effluvium	Alopecia areata	Telogen effluvium	Androgenetic alopecia
Drug induced	Loose anagen syndrome	Telogen gravidarum	Occipital alopecia of the newborn
Radiotherapy	Postoperative occipital alopecia	Chronic telogen effluvium	
Poisoning	Syphilis	Early androgenetic alopecia	
Diffuse alopecia areata	Traction alopecia	Drug induced	
	Trichotillomania	Iron deficiency	
	Tinea capitis	Malnuitrition/malabsorption	
		Hypothyroidism	
		Hyperthyroidism	
		Diffuse alopecia areata	
		Syphilis	
		Systemic lupus erythematosus	
		Chronic renal failure	
		Hepatic failure	
		Advanced malignancy	

some 2–3 months after the initial event. A temporary alopecia develops as the long club hairs are replaced by short, cosmetically insignificant, new anagen hairs. Provided the insult is not repeated, the alopecia resolves as the new anagen hairs grow.

Telogen gravidarum occurs because the high circulating placental oestrogens prolong anagen and lead to a very full head of hair during pregnancy. The withdrawal of these trophic hormones at delivery causes all the overdue anagen hairs to simultaneously enter catagen. Telogen hairs are then shed a few months later.

The cause of this chronic telogen effluvium is uncertain, but may be due to shortening of the anagen phase of the cycle. It has been suggested that shedding is not noticeable until anagen is reduced by 50%, however, formal studies are not available.

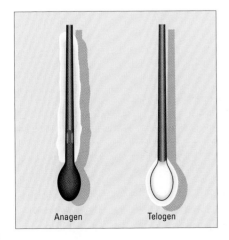

Fig. 5.1 Inspection with the naked eye can distinguish anagen from telogen hairs. This diagram illustrates the important features which are pigmentation of the bulb and the presence or absence of an inner root sheath.

Anagen   Telogen

Clinical features

Approximately 2–3 months after the triggering event there is a period of dramatic hair loss. It is lost diffusely from the scalp and continues for a few weeks to months

The diffuse hair fall may produce marked thinning of the scalp hair (Fig. 5.2). Patients often do not relate these events to their recent illness and become concerned that they are going to go bald. The hair pull test is strongly positive with clumps of telogen hairs being extracted with ease from both the vertex and the margins of the scalp.

The presentation of chronic telogen effluvium tends to be distinctive. Affected women are between the ages of 30 and 50 and have a very full, thick head of hair (Fig. 5.3). Frequently there is a history of being able to grow their hair very long in childhood, suggesting a particularly long anagen phase. They complain of an abrupt onset of hair shedding often sufficient to block the drain after a shower with thinning of their hair.

On examination there is prominent bitemporal recession (Fig. 5.4) and a positive hair pull test equally over the vertex and occiput, but it is difficult to be convinced of any hair thinning. There is no widening of the central part (Fig. 5.5) as is common in androgenetic alopecia. Nevertheless, patients are adamant that they previously had more hair and are distressed by the prospect of going bald. Usually there is no family history of early onset androgenetic alopecia and scalp biopsy shows only a few miniaturized vellus-like hair follicles.

Investigation

A full blood count, serum ferritin and thyroid function tests should be performed in all cases to exclude other causes of diffuse hair loss. Syphilis serology, antinuclear antibodies

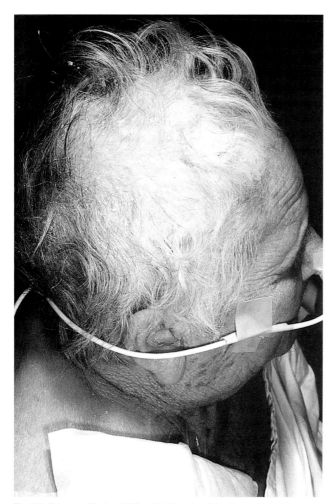

Fig. 5.2 Telogen effluvium. Diffuse hair loss involving the scalp margins as well as the vertex.

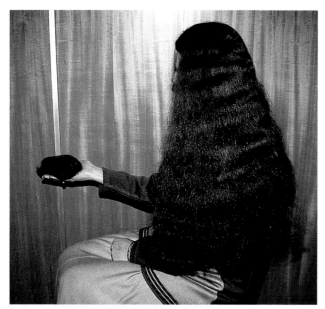

Fig. 5.3 Chronic diffuse global alopecia of women. This woman attended complaining of hair loss!

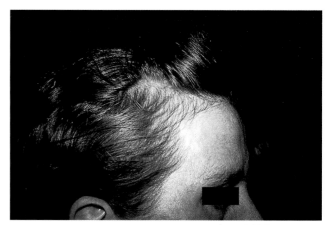

Fig. 5.4 Bitemporal recession associated with chronic telogen effluvium.

and a serum zinc level should be performed if there are other features on history or examination to suggest these conditions. A drug history should be taken and in particular a change in the oral contraceptive pill 3 months earlier should be enquired about as this is a relatively common cause of a short-lived telogen effluvium and is easily overlooked.

A scalp biopsy is usually required in cases of chronic telogen effluvium, mainly to exclude early androgenetic alopecia.

Diagnosis

Diagnostic difficulty occurs when the insult is prolonged or regularly repeated. Chronic telogen effluvium can be difficult to distinguish from early androgenetic alopecia, especially as periods of progression in androgenetic alopecia are preceded by increased shedding of telogen hairs.

Chronic diffuse alopecia areata (AA) is very rare (p. 75). Acute forms are generally seen in rapidly evolving alopecia totalis and exclamation mark hairs are usually present. In the absence of exclamation mark hairs the diagnosis of diffuse AA cannot be made clinically and a biopsy is required.

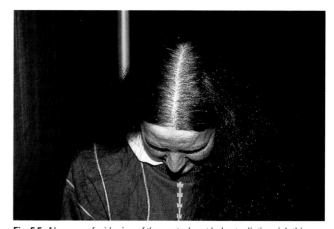

Fig. 5.5 Absence of widening of the central part helps to distinguish this condition from androgenetic alopeica.

Associated conditions

Beau's lines of the nails may coexist on occasion. More usually there are no associated conditions, unless manifestations of the triggering event persist.

Pathology

In acute telogen effluvium, the trichogram is abnormal with greater than 25% telogen hairs and this can be useful in difficult cases to distinguish telogen effluvium from early androgenetic alopecia (Table 5.1). A biopsy is rarely required in acute cases, although it will provide reassuring prognostic information in a patient who is particularly anxious.

The histology of acute telogen effluvium shows an increased number of telogen hairs without inflammation.

The histology of chronic telogen effluvium closely resembles that of the normal scalp. In particular there is no follicular miniaturization, no loss of terminal hairs and no increase in the vellus hair count. There may be a mild increase of telogen hairs, but less marked than in acute telogen effluvium or androgenetic alopecia. Trichograms from the occiput and the crown show similar slight increases in the telogen count. In contrast the trichogram in early androgenetic alopecia should show an increase in telogen hairs on the vertex, but not on the occiput.

Prognosis

Acute telogen effluvium and telogen gravidarum are self limiting over 3–6 months. Most women get full restoration of their hair, while the hair in a small proportion of cases remains thin, possibly due to unmasking of underlying androgenetic alopecia. Such cases may benefit from a biopsy to further delineate the prognosis.

It has been suggested that, following telogen gravidarum, some hairs may not revert to the asynchrony in hair growth normally seen over the human scalp and cause generalized or regional episodic hair loss in the future.

The prognosis for women with chronic telogen effluvium is less certain, but it appears the hair shedding follows a fluctuating course, that they do not go bald and the condition usually resolves spontaneously after 3–4 years.

Treatment

Mere reassurance that they are not going bald, that the telogen effluvium is temporary and that the hair will regrow is sufficient. Some patients require a wig whilst awaiting regrowth. Empirically, topical minoxidil may hasten resolution by prolonging anagen and stimulating telogen hairs to re-enter anagen, however, evidence for this is lacking.

Key points

Telogen effluvium is an acquired, self-limiting, reversible, nonscarring, diffuse alopecia due to excess shedding of telogen hairs. A precipitating event can usually, but not always be identified.

5.3 Iron deficiency and other nutritional causes of diffuse alopecia

Definition

Iron deficiency with or without anaemia is an occasional finding in the investigation of diffuse alopecia. In some of these cases iron replacement therapy causes cessation of hair loss and regrowth. In many other cases replenishment of the body's iron stores does not produce an improvement. In these cases the iron deficiency is probably an incidental finding and these people have an alternative cause of their hair loss such as early androgenetic alopecia or chronic telogen effluvium.

Epidemiology

Iron deficiency anaemia has been reported in as many as 72% of women presenting with diffuse telogen hair loss, but this figure is an overestimate. There are numerous cases in the literature where patients treated with oral iron had regrowth of their hair associated with normalization of their iron stores. On cessation of iron replacement therapy the anaemia and hair loss returned, confirming that at least in some cases the iron deficiency is a causative factor in their alopecia (Fig. 5.6).

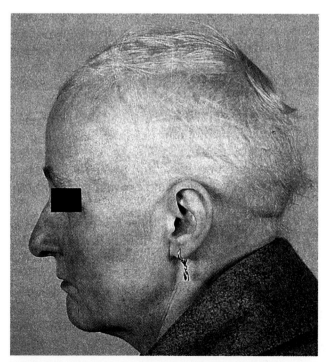

Fig. 5.6 Telogen effluvium secondary to iron deficiency anaemia.

Pathogenesis

As iron is an essential cofactor for ribonuclease reductase which is involved in DNA synthesis, it has been proposed that iron deficiency reduces proliferation of matrix cells. However, this would not readily explain a chronic telogen effluvium.

Clinical features

Patients present with diffuse telogen hair loss. Iron deficiency may also be an aggrevating factor in other forms of alopecia, particulary androgenetic alopecia and may be missed unless specifically looked for. In about 20% of cases the iron deficiency occurs in the absence of anaemia and manifests solely with a serum ferritin below 20 μg/l.

Investigation

Iron deficient patients should be investigated as to the cause of the deficiency, and referral to a general practitioner or internal physician may be appropriate.

Diagnosis

There are a number of other dietary causes of diffuse telogen hair loss. Sudden weight loss can precipitate a telogen effluvium. Chronic starvation, and in particular marasmus, may result in dry, lifeless, fine, straight hair that is sparse and easily plucked. The colour of the hair can also change producing light coloured or reddish hair. Dystrophic changes in the anagen bulb can be seen with light microscopy. Kwashiorkor results in periods of interrupted hair growth that either sends the hair into telogen or if less severe affects the calibre of the hair more so than its linear growth hence producing multiple Pohl Pinkus lines (p. 180). Changes in hair colour are another prominent feature. Dark hair changes to brown or red, whilst brown hair becomes blond. This colour change together with the periodic constrictions produces the so-called flag sign of kwashiorkor. Essential fatty acid deficiency can also produce marked telogen hair loss combined with a lightening of hair colour. Zinc deficiency, both hereditary (Fig. 5.7) and acquired (Fig. 5.8) leads to sparse, dry, brittle hair and the hair loss is an important clue to the diagnosis.

Associated features

The patient may be pale, easily fatigued and lethargic due to anaemia. Disease states producing blood loss may be apparent or occult. Multiple vitamin deficiencies may be present in patients on poor diets or with malabsorption.

Pathology

The pathology is indistinguishable from telogen effluvium.

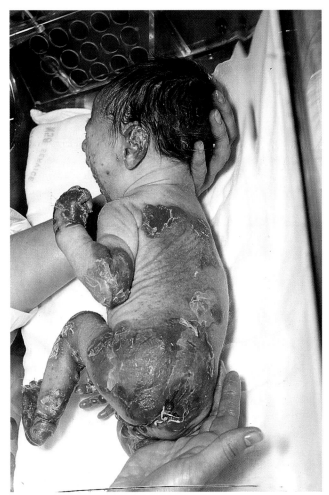

Fig. 5.7 Acrodermatitis enteropathica.

Prognosis

Alopecia will improve in some, but in many others it will not and an alternative cause for the hair loss, such as androgenetic alopecia should be sought.

Treatment

Patients should be treated with oral iron supplements until their ferritin rises above 40 μg/l.

Key points

All patients with diffuse telogen hair loss should have their serum ferritin estimated and, if this is low, the patient should be investigated for the cause of the iron deficiency and treated with oral iron supplements.

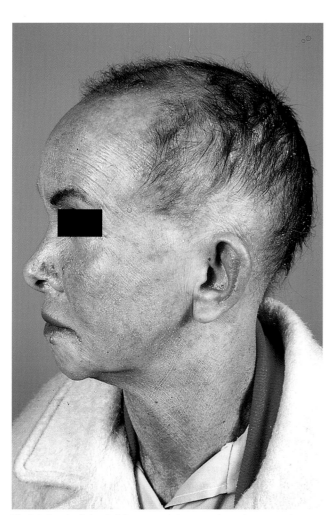

Fig. 5.8 Acquired zinc deficiency secondary to prolonged parenteral feeding produced this diffuse alopecia.

5.4 Thyroid disease and other metabolic causes of a diffuse alopecia

Definition

Diffuse telogen hair loss may occur in association with both hypo- and hyperthyroidism.

Epidemiology

Loss of the outer third of the eyebrows is seen in approximately 25% of patients with hypothyroidism, while diffuse scalp alopecia occurs in about one-third of hypothyroid patients.

Hyperthyroidism, when severe, is said to cause a diffuse alopecia in up to 50% of affected individuals, although this figure is contested.

Pathogenesis

Hypothyroidism inhibits cell division both in the epidermis and the skin appendages. In a proportion of patients this inhi-

bition of mitosis induces catagen and delays re-entry of telogen hairs into anagen. The mechanism of hair loss in hyperthyroidism is unknown.

Clinical features

Hair loss may precede other clinical manifestations and is an important clue to the diagnosis (Fig. 5.9). Drug-induced hypothyroidism also produces alopecia in a similar proportion of patients. The alopecia has a very gradual onset and continues indefinitely until the thyroid disease is treated. Marked hair loss can occur.

Investigation

Thyroid function tests are part of the routine work-up in the assessment of diffuse alopecia.

Pathology

Both the trichogram and hair microscopy reveal an increased proportion of telogen hairs. The histopathology is identical to that of telogen effluvium.

Diagnosis

Other causes of a telogen effluvium need to be considered and iron deficiency anaemia excluded. Other metabolic, inflammatory and infectious causes of telogen effluvium that should be considered are included in Table 5.1

Chronic renal failure and dialysis is associated with dry, brittle, sparse scalp hair and loss of body hair, including pubic and axillary hair. Chronic liver failure can produce a diffuse alopecia as can advanced malignancy. The mechanism for this is not known. Pancreatic disease and upper gastrointestinal disorders associated with malabsorption may also be associated with diffuse alopecia.

Diffuse hair loss occurs in secondary syphilis (Fig. 5.10, p. 71) producing the classical moth-eaten appearance, however, this is not always present. A telogen effluvium often occurs 2–3 months after a primary infection or after successful treatment as a feature of the Jarisch–Herxheimer reaction. Connective tissue disorders, in particular systemic lupus erythematosus (p. 102 and Fig. 5.11) and dermatomyositis (p. 121) may also produce a nonscarring diffuse alopecia.

Associated features

While, most commonly, the features of the metabolic disorder are apparent at the time of diagnosis, there is often a history of the hair loss preceding the other manifestations of the condition by many months. There appears to be no relationship between duration or severity of hypothyroidism and the degree of alopecia.

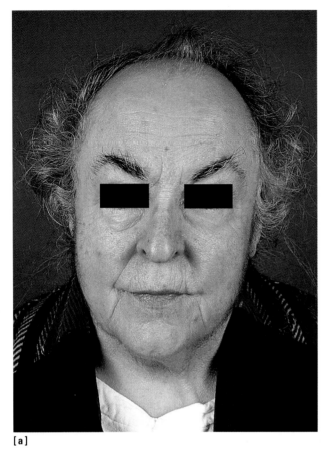

[a]

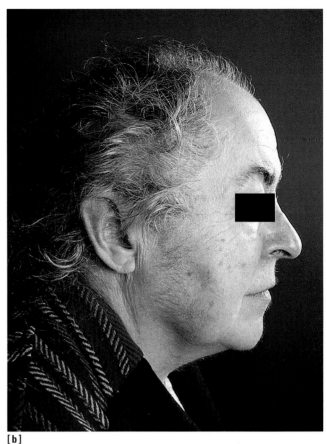

[b]

Fig. 5.9 Diffuse alopecia in association with hypothyroidism.

Hair loss in hyperthyroidism is usually a relatively late sign and the diagnosis has usually already been made by the time the hair loss is apparent.

Prognosis

With thyroxine replacement the hairs rapidly re-enter anagen and the telogen count falls. Replacement therapy generally leads to regrowth of hair within a few months. An exception to this occurs when the hypothyroidism has been present many years and the hair follicles have atrophied. Nevertheless, failure of a biochemically hypothyroid patient to respond to therapy usually suggests an alternate or coincident cause of alopecia, most commonly androgenetic alopecia.

Hair loss in the hyperthyroid patient usually stops within a few months of becoming euthyroid.

Treatment

Referral to an endocrinologist for treatment may be appropriate. Rapid replacement therapy in a patient with long-standing hypothyroidism may precipitate myocardial infarction, and the management of hyperthyroidism is complex.

Key points

Hypothyroidism-induced alopecia is relatively common, often unsuspected clinically and reversible. All patients with diffuse scalp alopecia require thyroid function tests, especially if there is associated loss of the outer one-third of the eyebrows, a family history of autoimmune disease or other signs of hypothyroidism.

5.5 Drug-induced telogen hair loss

Definition

Drugs can induce alopecia through loss of either anagen or telogen hairs. Anagen hair loss is usually dramatic, with the patient rapidly developing total alopecia, and is discussed in the next section (p. 74).

Epidemiology

Hair loss affects everyone who receives high-dose chemotherapy. It is very common with etretinate and acitretin and is dose related. It is much less common with isotretinoin. Hair loss is frequently seen following either the cessation or commencement of oral contraceptive pills, and is

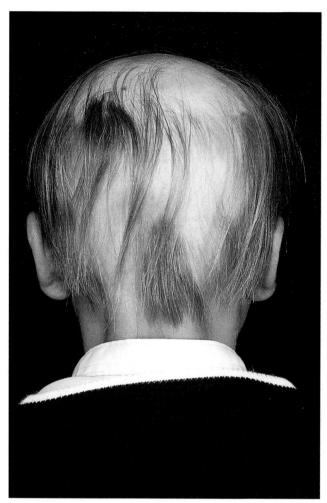

Fig. 5.10 Diffuse hair loss as a manifestation of secondary syphilis.

Aetiology

The long list of drugs reported to have caused hair loss is shown in Table 5.2. Many of these reports are not conclusive in that other causes have not been adequately ruled out.

Pathogenesis

Some medications act by exacerbating androgenetic alopecia, while others produce a telogen effluvium. Most drugs that produce an anagen effluvium in high doses can also produce a telogen effluvium in low dose (Fig. 5.12). Antithyroid drugs (including amiodarone) and antilipid medications may act by producing a deficiency state.

Minoxidil has been reported to produce increased telogen shedding, however, this is due to dormant follicles re-entering anagen and pushing out the old club hair and is not a true alopecia.

The mechanism of hair loss with retinoids (Fig. 5.13) is complex. There appears to be a reduction in the duration

more common with high-dose preparations and those that have a high progestogen to oestrogen ratio. The incidence of hair loss associated with a host of other implicated drugs is unknown.

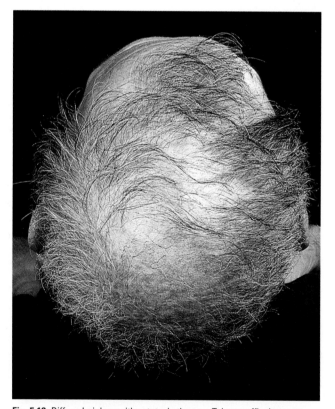

Fig. 5.12 Diffuse hair loss with cytotoxic therapy. Telogen effluvium may produce hair loss most noticeable over the vertex, which resembles a Ludwig grade III androgenetic alopecia. The rapid onset of the hair loss occurring a few months after chemotherapy and in association with Beau's lines in the nails and Pohl Pinkus lines in the hair helped to confirm the diagnosis. This pattern may represent an unmasking of subtle androgenetic alopecia in cases where regrowth may not be complete. In such cases the prognosis must be guarded.

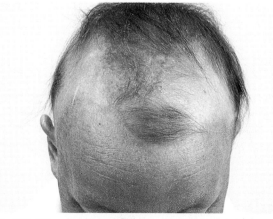

Fig. 5.11 Diffuse hair loss with systemic lupus erythematosus may occur with or without the short wiry lupus hairs along the frontal hair line.

Table 5.2 Drug induced alopecia.

Telogen effluvium

Heparin
Warfarin
Propranalol/metoprolol
Captopril/enalopril
Allopurinol
Boric acid
Phenytoin
Glibenclamide
Amphetamines
Levadopa
Bromocryptine
Methysergide
Interferon
Albendazole/mebendazole
Cimetidine
Colchicine (low dose)
Sulphasalazine
Penicillamine
Gold

Antithyroid action

Carbimazole
Propylthiouracil
Amiodarone
Lithium

Prothryoid action

Thyroxine

Hypolipidaemic agents

Clofibrate
Triparanol

Proandrogen action

Oral contraceptive pill
Danazol
Testosterone
Anabolic steroids

Lichenoid cicatricial alopecia

Chloroquine
Mepacrine
Proguanil

Anagen effluvium*

Radiation
Cyclophosphamide
Doxorubicin
Colchicine (high dose)
Thallium/mercury/arsenic
Cantharadin
Azathioprine
Methotrexate

*Almost all chemotherapeutic agents can provoke an anagen effluvium.

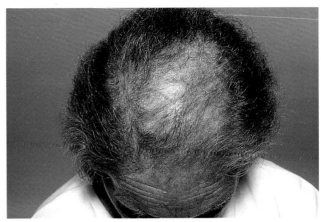

Fig. 5.13 Diffuse hair loss secondary to etretinate. The mechanism of loss is complex.

of anagen as well as a telogen anchorage defect. There is no evidence of an anagen effluvium.

Clinical features

Drug-induced telogen alopecia usually presents with diffuse hair loss leading to thinning which may be profound. The alopecia tends to begin about 6–12 weeks after starting treatment and is progressive while the drug is continued.

Diagnosis

The diagnosis is based on demonstrating the correct chronology of relevant drug use and hair loss and the exclusion of other causes.

Investigation

Patients should be investigated to exclude other causes of a diffuse telogen hair loss which could be exacerbating factors such as iron deficiency anaemia, hypothyroidism and androgenetic alopecia.

Pathology

The pathology reflects the nature of the trigger (see Table 5.2).

Associated features

Other features of the drug eruption may be present. Retinoids also have other unrelated effects on hair, namely inducing straight hair to curl (Fig. 5.14). The mechanism of this is unknown, but could relate to intrafollicular keratinization. It usually reverts to normal spontaneously around 6 months after the treatment is stopped.

Prognosis

With the exception of drug-induced androgenetic alopecia, and cicatricial alopecias caused by drugs, regrowth of hair

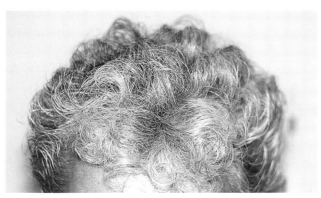

Fig. 5.14 Curly hair secondary to etretinate.

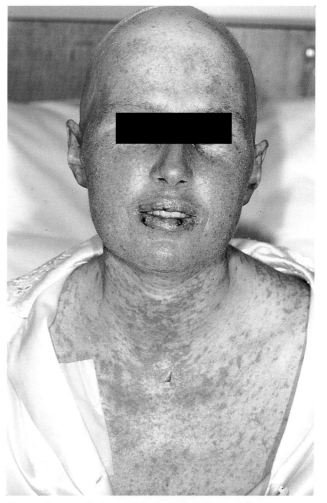

Fig. 5.16 Anagen effluvium secondary to X-ray therapy given immediately prior to bone marrow transplantation. The monomorphic acne is related to prednisolone and cyclosporin A.

occurs after the medication is stopped if the drug is truly the cause of the alopecia. Occasionally patients have persistent thinning of their hair and a few notice continued shedding. This is most common after retinoid-induced hair loss and the mechanism is not well understood.

Treatment

Cessation of the offending drug is advised.

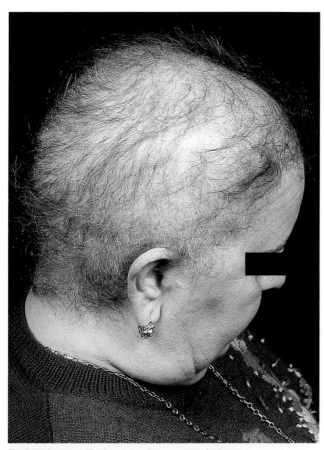

Fig. 5.15 Anagen effluvium secondary to cytotoxic therapy.

Fig. 5.17 Anagen effluvium occuring in acute graft vs. host disease (aGVHD). The hair had begun to regrow following the bone marrow transplant and was lost with the onset of the aGVHD.

Key points

Drug-induced alopecia is suggested by a diffuse hair loss developing in the absence of an alternative explanation while the patient is receiving a medication, and regrowth occurring on cessation of that medication. Reappearance of the alopecia on rechallenge helps to establish the drug, rather than the illness for which it was prescribed, as the cause of the hair loss. Certain drugs are well known to produce this side-effect. Many other drugs have been reported to cause hair loss, but the details provided in the case reports are insufficient to allow firm conclusions to be made.

5.6 Anagen effluvium

Introduction

A direct toxic insult to rapidly dividing keratinocytes in the hair matrix produces an arrest of mitosis. Consequent to this abrupt interruption of hair growth, anagen hairs narrow, fracture and are shed *en masse*. The classic causes are cytotoxic drugs and radiotherapy.

Clinical features

The hair loss usually occurs within a few days of the insult (Table 5.2). All the anagen hairs on the scalp (about 85% of the total) are rapidly shed (Fig. 5.15). The hairs do not come out with the bulb, but rather fracture at the base of the partially keratinized hair shaft. Light microscopy of plucked hairs shows either a tapered proximal end where the hair has fractured on extraction or a characteristic dystrophic root. Once the insult stops, the hairs are still in anagen and are able to recommence growth immediately. This is different to telogen effluvium where regrowth requires the hair to exit telogen and re-enter anagen.

Radiation-induced anagen effluvium (Fig. 5.16) can be prolonged, as in addition to the disruption to mitosis causing immediate shedding, hairs enter catagen precipitating a telogen effluvium some months later, from which recovery is prolonged. Single doses of around 4 Gy will produce a generalized shedding of anagen hairs in around 20% of subjects, and repeated doses will affect a greater proportion. If high doses (>10 Gy) are administered to the scalp, permanent alopecia may occur.

Heavy metal poisoning with thallium in particular, is an easily overlooked cause of a diffuse anagen effluvium. Thallium availability is now restricted after a vogue in the 1960s when this colourless, flavourless, odourless agent was a popular hemlock. Acute graft vs. host disease also sometimes produces an anagen effluvium (Fig. 5.17), which must be distinguished from the effects of the preceding chemo- and X-ray therapies. During the initial phases of a rapidly progressive alopecia areata anagen hairs are shed and this may produce a similar clinical picture.

Treatment

The commonest cause of anagen effluvium is drugs. Stopping the drugs produces a rapid recovery. Even cyclical chemotherapy regimens do not produce permanent alopecia. If hair loss is anticipated prior to a course of chemotherapy, ice packs producing local scalp cooling may lessen the amount of hair fall.

Key points

Anagen effluvium produces a rapid and dramatic hair fall. It is due to cessation of mitosis in the bulb and fracture of the proximal shaft. Total alopecia is common but recovers rapidly once the trigger is removed.

Chapter 6

Alopecia areata

Definition

Alopecia areata (AA) is an autoimmune, nonscarring, multi-focal disorder of hair growth characterized by circular bald areas, that contain pathognomonic exclamation mark hairs and which occur on any hair-bearing site of the body.

Epidemiology

Alopecia areata is said to occur in approximately 0.15% of the population. Based on these figures approximately 90 000 people are affected in the United Kingdom alone. This is almost certainly an underestimate as many patches, particularly when they occur away from the scalp go unnoticed.

Most will only have an occasional patch that spontaneously heals. Overall 30% will develop alopecia totalis or universalis during the course of their lives. The chance of progressing to alopecia totalis is higher if the onset is in childhood (50%, compared with an adult onset of 25%), if there is associated Down's syndrome (50%) or atopy (50–75%), and once alopecia totalis has developed only 1% of children and 10% of adults will achieve complete regrowth.

The age of onset for AA has a bimodal distribution with the first peak occurring at the age of 5 years and a second peak at the age of 30. Onset before 1 year of age is exceptional. Atrichia congenita should be considered in the differential diagnosis when alopecia totalis occurs in the first year, and a biopsy should be performed for prognostic purposes if diagnosis is unclear. Overall around 40–50% of patients develop AA before the age of 21 years and in only 20% does it begin after 40 years. The sex incidence is equal.

Aetiology

The exact cause of AA is unknown. A positive family history is present in 10–30% of patients and AA appears to be inherited as an autosomal dominant trait with variable penetrance, although a polygenic inheritance is not excluded. A familial component is more common in those patients with an early age of onset. Mild cases frequently go unnoticed, particularly when the hair loss occurs away from the scalp. In alopecia totalis patients definite HLA associations include HLA-DRB1*1104, HLA-DQB1*03 and HLA-DQB1*0301 (relative risk 30.2) This very strong HLA association has led some to

postulate that the gene for AA is on chromosome 6 near the HLA locus.

In persons with the prerequisite genetic predisposition, a second event or cofactor is required for disease expression. This cofactor is occasionally a major life crisis, but more commonly it is an unidentified trigger that precipitates the immunological attack on anagen hair follicles that produces alopecia. Alopecia areata differs from most other known autoimmune disorders in that no permanent tissue destruction occurs. This has lead some to suggest the immunological target may be a trophic factor or its receptor as occurs in Grave's disease.

The incidence of AA is increased, and the prognosis for regrowth is worse when atopy or Down's syndrome coexist. Atopy has been found in about 50% of patients with AA, compared to a general incidence of atopy of 20–30%. Atopics presenting with a patch of AA tend to go on to develop alopecia totalis more frequently.

The incidence of AA in Down's syndrome (Fig. 6.1) is around 6% compared with 0.1% in mentally retarded controls. About 50% of Down's patients go on to develop alopecia totalis. The incidence of AA in autoimmune polyglandular syndrome type 1, which is also known as mucocutaneous candidiasis is around 30%. The gene for this syndrome has been recently localized to the long arm of chromosome 21 at 21q22.3. This association has implicated chromosome 21 in the search for the gene for AA.

An immunological mechanism is considered likely based on the response of AA to immunosuppressive treatments and its association with other organ-specific autoimmune disorders such as thyroid disease, vitiligo, Addison's disease and pernicious anaemia. There is also an increased incidence of lupus erythematosus, rheumatoid arthritis, scleroderma, ulcerative colitis, myasthenia gravis, lichen planus, and diabetes mellitus.

In AA, early anagen hairs show aberrant expression of HLA class I antigens. Perhaps this enables immune recognition of hair antigens by T lymphocytes which subsequently attack these putative antigens located on the transient portion of the hair follicle. HLA class II and ICAM-1 expression on anagen hair bulbs then occurs in response to cytokines released by these lymphocytes. This further augments the immunological attack on the hair. The basal lamina that normally protects the hair bulb is damaged, but

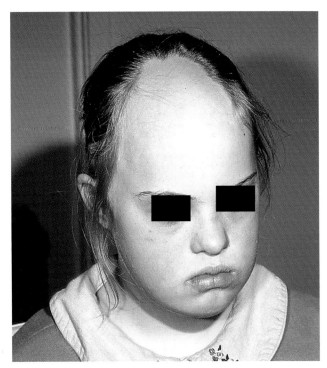

Fig. 6.1 Alopecia areata in a patient with Down's syndrome.

zone reaches the surface of the skin (Fig. 6.2), producing a rapid alopecia. Having entered telogen these fractured hairs are then eventually extruded as exclamation mark hairs, which are about 3 mm long. Light microscopy of exclamation mark hairs reveals a broken tip, below which the hair tapers towards a small but otherwise normal club hair (Fig. 6.3). As these hairs are telogen hairs, they are easily extracted from the scalp.

Hairs in anagen III (p. 9) are preferentially affected and are lost first, although all anagen hairs are eventually shed in a wave running across an affected patch. Follicles continue to cycle, but as soon as a new anagen hair reaches the anagen III stage, it is damaged by the inflammatory infiltrate and sent straight back into catagen. Histology of an established lesion shows that about 70% of hairs are either in catagen or telogen.

Anagen III is also the stage during which hair bulb melanin is transferred to cortical keratinocytes, and a number of pigmentary abnormalities occur in AA. Firstly the process seems to spare nonpigmented (grey) hairs in the initial phases (Fig. 6.4). Secondly the dystrophic anagen hairs that are also seen in this condition show variable pigmentation, and thirdly regrowth after resolution of a patch of AA occurs initially with grey hairs (Fig. 6.5).

Clinical features

Alopecia areata appears in a variety of patterns. The most common is one or more circumscribed totally bald, smooth patch (Fig. 6.6), often noticed first by the hairdresser. If grey hairs are present then they are usually spared at least initially. Multiple 3–4 mm long exclamation mark hairs may be present at the margin (Fig. 6.7). These exclamation mark hairs as well as normal looking hairs at the margin are easily extracted. Exclamation mark hairs are not always present, but if seen are diagnostic, and help distinguish it from secondary syphilis, a condition that can closely mimic AA. Trichotillomania may also simulate AA, and the short stubble of broken hairs can be mistaken for exclamation mark hairs. Plucking a suspected exclamation mark hair helps differentiate these two conditions. The broken hairs in trichotillomania are anagen hairs and firmly rooted to the scalp, whereas the true exclamation mark hairs are easily extracted telogen ones.

Some patients complain of irritation, tenderness or paraesthesia immediately preceding the development of a new patch, but more often they are asymptomatic. The first patch is on the scalp in over 60% of cases, although patches elsewhere are more likely to go unnoticed (Fig. 6.8). The occiput and the frontovertical areas of the scalp are common sites for the initial patch (Fig. 6.9). The eyebrows and eyelashes are commonly lost and may be the only site affected. Whether the first patch is on the scalp or elsewhere has no prognostic implications.

When regrowth occurs, it is at first fine and unpigmented (Fig. 6.5), but usually the hairs resume normal colour and

this appears to be a secondary event. The dermal papilla is another possible primary immune target in AA, and further work exploring this aspect of AA is required.

Humoral immunity does not seem to be important in the pathogenesis of AA and the asymmetrical distribution of patches of AA makes a neural aetiology unlikely.

Emotional stress in the form of a major life event such as divorce, death of a parent or spouse has long been recognized as a precipitant of AA, although the mechanism is not understood. Anecdotes of patients' hair turning grey overnight (due to the preferential loss of pigmented hairs) are an example of this. Most episodes of AA however, are not triggered by severe stress and neither the patients nor their families are more likely than normal to have a primary psychological disorder. Unfortunately secondary depression and anxiety consequent to hair loss, occur commonly.

Pathogenesis

In this condition there is invariably a dense peribulbar and intrafollicular lymphocytic infiltrate (predominantly CD4 positive phenotype) associated with aberrant HLA class I and class II antigen expression on the cells in the precortical matrix and presumptive cortex. This infiltrate disappears with resolution of the alopecia.

The perifollicular inflammation weakens anagen hairs at the keratogenous zone of the developing hair shaft and at the same time precipitates premature entry of the follicle into catagen. The weakened hairs break when the keratogenous

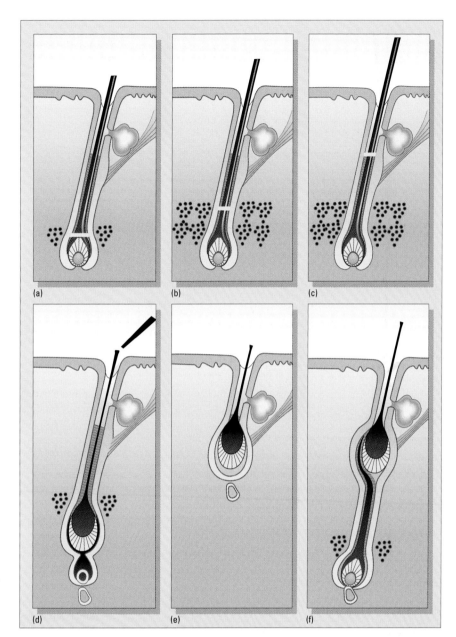

Fig. 6.2 The pathogenesis of exclamation mark hairs. (a) Lymphocytes accumulate around the hair bulb. The white line marks the time of the attack on the growing hair. (b) The hair continues to grow, although the hair shaft is thinned by the effects of the inflammation on the hair matrix. (c) The hair continues to grow, whilst progressively thinning. (d) The hair stops growing and enters catagen. Around this time, the weakened hair reaches the skin surface where it withstands external trauma poorly and snaps off. (e) The hair enters telogen. (f) After an appropriate delay, anagen resumes and the exclamation mark telogen hair is extruded.

calibre after a short period of time. Over the ensuing years almost 100% will relapse, however, this may not occur for many years.

Further patches often appear after a few weeks. New patches can develop even while the initial patch is resolving. Discrete patches may coalesce with loss of the intervening hairs to produce either a reticulate pattern (Fig. 6.10), alopecia totalis, with loss of all the hairs on the scalp (Fig. 6.11) or alopecia universalis, with loss of all the hairs on the body.

Other patterns of hair loss occur. Alopecia oophiasis describes a band-like loss of hair around the periphery of the scalp (Fig. 6.12). It has a particularly poor prognosis for regrowth. Acute diffuse AA may be the initial presentation of a rapid onset alopecia totalis (Fig. 6.13), which can develop within 48 hours. As pigmented hairs are affected first, their preferential loss can produce overnight greying (Fig. 6.4) Chronic diffuse loss is very rare and requires either the finding of exclamation mark hairs or supportive histology to distinguish it from the telogen effluvium, chronic diffuse global alopecia of women or trichotillomania. Peri-naevoid AA is another uncommon presentation. It is characterized by the development of alopecia around naevi. The opposite of this has also been described, with the hairs within hairy naevi remaining unaffected in alopecia universalis.

Differential diagnosis

The diagnosis of AA is usually a straightforward clinical diagnosis. The differential diagnosis of an atypical solitary

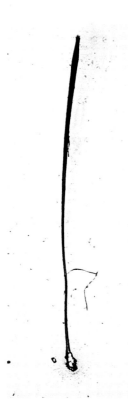

Fig. 6.3 An exclamation mark hair.

patch of AA on the scalp includes tinea capitis, lupus erythematosus, trichotillomania and a subtle scarring alopecia. If doubt about the diagnosis exists Wood's light examination, fungal culture of skin scrapings or a biopsy will enable the correct diagnosis to be made. Secondary syphilis resembles multiple patches of AA and can be distinguished on serology. Congenital triangular alopecia (p. 132) and post operative occipital alopecia (p. 90) also sometimes cause difficulty.

Pathology

A scalp biopsy can be used to confirm the clinical diagnosis in difficult cases. It is especially useful for diffuse AA. The histological findings will be influenced by the disease activity at the biopsy site. The hallmark of this condition is a dense lymphocytic infiltrate around the anagen hair bulbs that has been likened to a swarm of bees. Lymphocytes also infiltrate the dermal papilla and the hair bulb matrix. It is most commonly seen in early lesions and in longstanding disease the infiltrate may be sparse.

A low power scanning view shows a decreased number of terminal hairs deep in the dermis (Fig. 6.14). The ratio of telogen and catagen to anagen follicles is increased and there is a sparse to moderate mononuclear cell inflammatory infiltrate in the superficial and deep dermis, as well as infiltrating the dermal papillae and the glassy membrane around the hair bulbs (Fig. 6.15). Telogen hairs are not inflamed, nor are anagen I and II hairs. The target seems to be only anagen III–VI hairs.

In general hair follicles are not destroyed and the potential for recovery is retained in spite of total hair loss for many years. However, in longstanding disease there may be a reduction in follicle numbers associated with perifollicular fibrosis.

Associated features

Nail changes occur in about 50% of children, but are less common in adults (around 20%). The most common finding is pitting in several fingernails (Fig. 6.16). Only exceptionally are the toenails involved. Other potential changes include red lunulae, Beau's lines and onychomadesis, trachyonychia, onychorrhexis, thinning or thickening of nails and cross fissures. Twenty nail dystrophy, or trachyonychia of all 20 nails may occur in children and precede the onset of the AA by a number of years. It can also be associated with the later development of psoriasis or lichen planus and as such is not specific for AA.

The incidence of thyroid disease is increased from 2% in the general population to 8% in AA, while vitiligo occurs in 4% compared to 1% in the general population. Routine investigation for subclinical thyroid disease is not indicated, as it does not alter the management. Investigations are only required for symptomatic disease.

Prognosis

Alopecia areata is an enigmatic disorder and for no individual is a confident prognosis possible. Regrowth from the first episode occurs within 6 months in about one-third of cases and within a year in about two-thirds. Thirty-three per cent of patients never recover from their initial patch, some of whom rapidly progress to alopecia totalis.

The outcome from an episode of AA is influenced by a number of factors shown in Table 6.1. Overall about 30% of patients go on to develop alopecia totalis, and almost all patients will develop other patches of AA at some stage in their life.

Treatment

Psychological

No treatment is available that modifies the natural history of AA and there is no universally successful method of produc-

Table 6.1 Factors that adversely affect the prognosis of alopecia areata.

Childhood onset
Personal history of atopy
Down's syndrome
Coincident endocrinopathy
Oophiasis pattern of alopecia
Alopecia totalis or universalis
Poor response to treatment

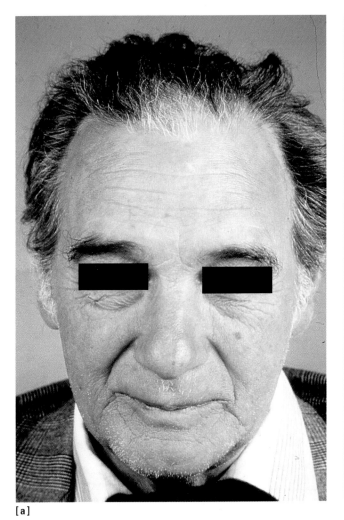

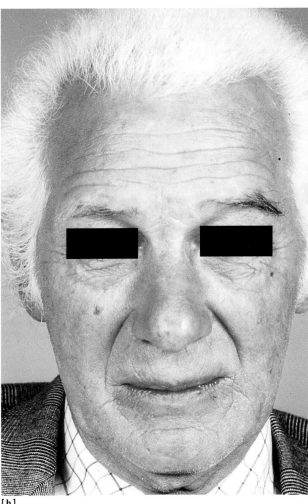

[a]   [b]

Fig. 6.4 Overnight greying of the hair due to rapid onset of alopecia totalis. (Courtesy of Dr D. Fenton, London.)

ing a temporary regrowth. The best available therapies produce regrowth in more patients than placebo, but the duration of any subsequent remission is unaltered. Partial regrowth is unlikely to be cosmetically acceptable to the

patient and this should be taken into account when considering the various treatment options.

Many different treatments have been proposed for AA, but because of the uncertain natural history and tendency to spontaneous remission, only those agents that have been verified in placebo-controlled blinded trial should be considered. There is no place for the prolonged use of expensive placebos, that only delay the patient from coming to terms with his or her disability.

Alopecia areata produces considerable distress. People stare and sufferers of AA feel self-conscious. On the whole children learn to cope with the alopecia quicker than their parents or their adult counterparts.

Doctors need to give patients considerable time to voice their fears and their difficulties. Patient support groups can provide a wealth of information regarding hair styling and cosmetics to minimize the impact of the hair loss. The reassurance of knowing they are not alone and others are affected too is also of considerable benefit.

Fig. 6.5 Regrowth of white hairs during resolution of alopecia areata.

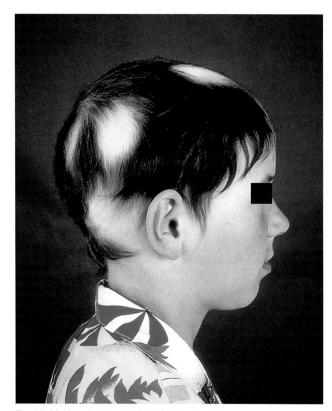

Fig. 6.6 Multiple discrete patches of alopecia areata.

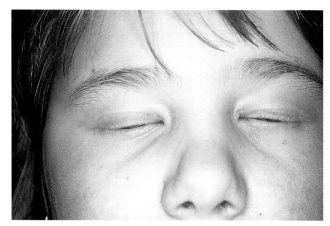

Fig. 6.8 Alopecia areata of the eyelashes. (Courtesy of Dr M. Haskett, Melbourne.)

First line pharmacological therapy

Fluorinated topical steroids applied twice daily with or without occlusion at night produce regrowth in a significant proportion of patients. Alopecia of recent onset and young children below the age of 10 years appear to be the most responsive.

A 3 month trial is required before deeming the treatment unsuccessful. If hair growth occurs the treatment can be cautiously continued, observing the patient at regular intervals for early signs of scalp atrophy.

Intralesional steroids are useful for the eyebrows and for isolated small patches. This is painful and if large areas are injected there can be systemic effects. Response occurs in about two-thirds of patients as an all or nothing phenomenon. Initially the response is localized to injection sites (Fig. 6.17), but a more general improvement may follow. Hairs first appear at around 2 weeks and satisfactory regrowth has usually occurred within 6 weeks. Remissions are in the order of 6–9 months. The injection must be delivered very superficially in the dermis as the target telogen hair follicles lie superficially. Repeated injections eventually produce atrophy (Fig. 6.18) and periocular injections can induce glaucoma and cataracts. Relapse eventually occurs even with continued injections. The steroid atrophy partially reverses on the scalp over 6–9 months.

Second line pharmacological therapy

For patients who fail first line therapy, progression to second line therapy is not automatic and it might be better for the patient to simply change their hair style or to get a wig. For

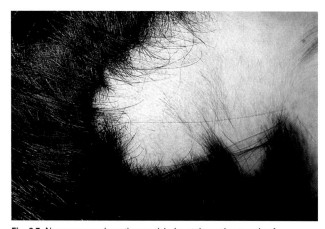

Fig. 6.7 Numerous exclamation mark hairs at the active margin of a patch of alopecia areata.

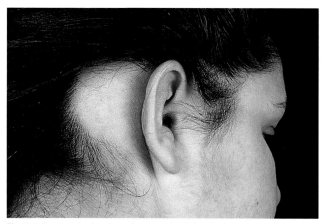

Fig. 6.9 Retroauricular alopecia areata involving the hair margin.

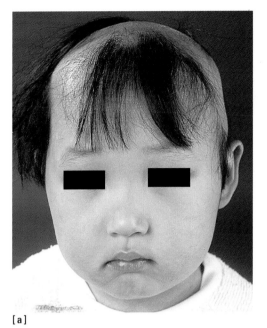
[a]

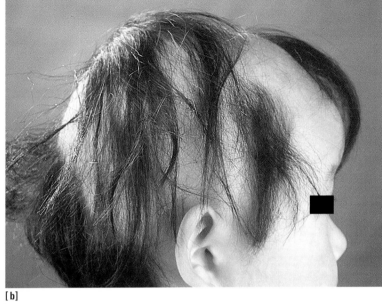
[b]

Fig. 6.10 Reticular pattern of alopecia areata.

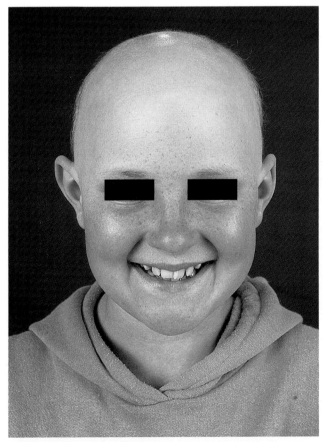

Fig. 6.11 Alopecia totalis. Note the preservation of the eyebrows.

those patients who proceed, therapeutic options include systemic immunosuppression with either prednisolone or PUVA; contact irritants and sensitizers such as dithranol and diphencyprone (DCP) or minoxidil. None is universally successful and each has its drawbacks.

Prednisolone used in a dose of 50 mg daily causes partial regrowth in three-quarters of patients treated after 3–6 weeks. It has been suggested that the threshold dose for response is 0.8 mg/kg. However, complete regrowth is less common and prolonged remissions are exceptional. Many patients relapse on cessation of therapy or dose reduction, while some relapse

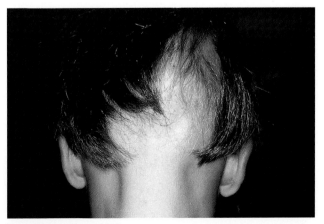

Fig. 6.12 Alopecia oophiasis.

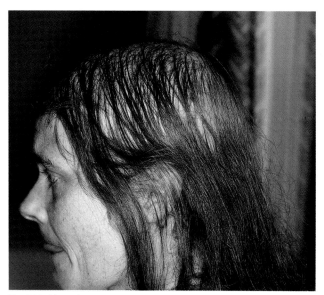

Fig. 6.13 Alopecia areata presenting as diffuse hair loss.

despite continued full dose therapy. Not all patients respond to steroids and even with daily intravenous pulses of methyl-prednisolone (500 mg) some remain refractory. The main value of oral prednisolone is in early, rapidly progressive disease, and once the hair loss has stabilized further treatment with either DCP or PUVA is recommended rather than long-term oral steroid therapy.

Systemic PUVA may work better than topical PUVA (Fig. 6.19). A minimum of 20–40 erythemogenic treatments are required before the treatment can be said not to have worked, and if there is a response the treatment should be continued. About 30–50% of AA patients will regrow hair, but relapse is common (50–90%) on discontinuation of therapy. Long-term risks include induction of skin cancer, particularly in children, and no patient should receive more than 200 treatments during his or her life.

Dithranol has been used as a topical irritant in the treatment of AA. The mechanism of action is unknown, but two-

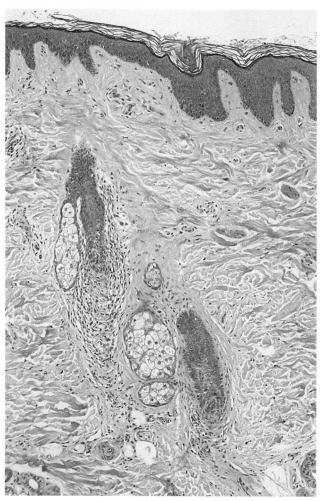

Fig. 6.14 Low power photomicrograph of alopecia areata showing an overall reduction in the number of follicles, while among those present there is an increased proportion of catagen follicles and anagen vellus follicles. The scant mononuclear cell infiltrate is better seen on high power.

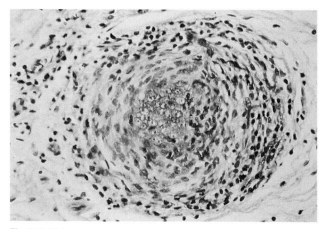

Fig. 6.15 High power photomicrograph showing perifollicular lymphocytic inflammation.

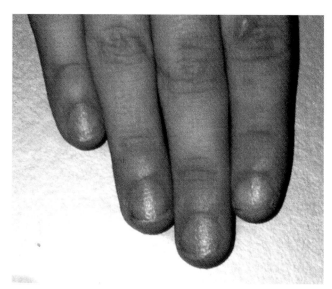

Fig. 6.16 Fingernail pitting in alopecia areata.

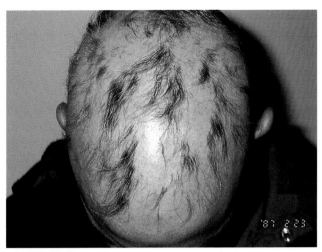

Fig. 6.17 Regrowth of alopecia areata following intralesional triamcinolone.

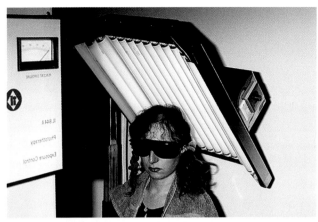

Fig. 6.19 Psoralens and ultraviolet A (PUVA) treatment.

thirds of patients treated develop some hair regrowth and in about half this is cosmetically significant. The concentration of dithranol is increased until patients experience irritation. Unless there is a response within 3 months, the treatment is abandoned. By this time there is usually significant dithranol pigmentation (Fig. 6.20), but this resolves with time.

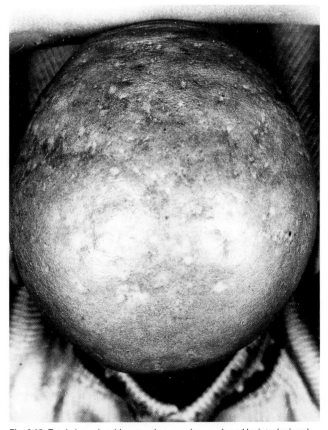

Fig. 6.18 Total alopecia with extensive scarring produced by intralesional injection of corticosteroids.

The response does not correlate with the degree of pigmentation.

Diphencyprone (DCP) has largely replaced dinitrochlorobenzene (DNCB) as the agent used to induce a contact allergic dermatitis on the scalp. DCP is photodegradable and so patients are told to wear a hat. The chemical is applied weekly after the patient has been sensitized (Fig. 6.21). The chemical needs to be in contact with the scalp for 24 hours after application (without wetting the scalp). Many patients develop severe itching, burning, blistering or urticaria in response to treatment that makes wig wearing difficult. Retroauricular lymphadenopathy is common (Fig. 6.22) and can distress patients until they are reassured it is benign. This can be reduced by commencing treatment with very low doses in the order of 0.001%. The dose is then adjusted upwards no more frequently than at monthly intervals with the aim of producing a mild dermatitis that lasts 24–48 hours. Publications quote a beneficial response rate of about 45% in patients with severe AA. There are no reliable predictive factors as to who will respond. Remissions are of variable duration, but are occasionally prolonged. Sometimes contact sensitivity is lost during therapy and can

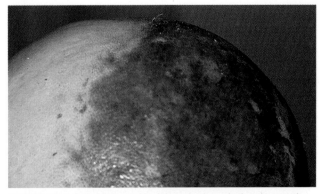

Fig. 6.20 Alopecia totalis treated by dithranol only producing pigmentation and dermatitis but no regrowth. In this patient the dithranol was applied only to one half of the scalp.

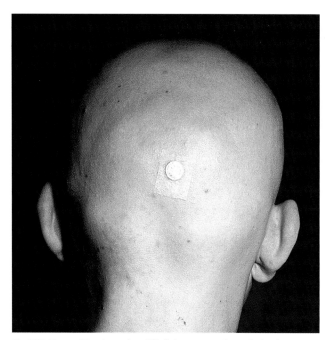

Fig. 6.21 To sensitize the patient, 2% diphencyprone is applied to the occiput for 24 hours in a Finn chamber.

be restored with oral cimetidine in a dose of 300 mg three times daily.

Some physicians allow the patients to apply the DCP themselves at home, while others, fearing the consequences of incautious handling, apply the DCP themselves. Sensitization of medical staff is also a hazard. Potential side-effects include pruritis, blistering, secondary infection, vitiligo and urticaria. DCP has not been shown to be mutagenic. Patients should be warned that tender postauricular lymphadenopathy is the norm.

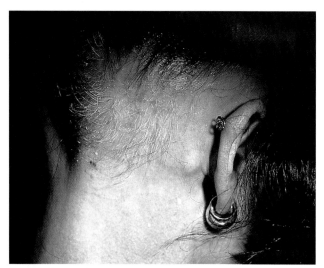

Fig. 6.22 Contact allergic dermatitis to diphencyprone associated with retroauricular lymphadenopathy.

The treatment should be continued for 6 months before it is judged to have failed. Patients who fail to respond to contact sensitization tend to fail to respond to all other available treatments, suggesting there is a subgroup of AA patients who are resistant to all available therapy. Unfortunately it is not possible to identify these nonresponders in advance.

Minoxidil 2% lotion is primarily used for androgenetic alopecia, but has also been used for AA. Initial results were promising, however they were not sustained in later trials, even when the concentration was increased to 5%. Patients with alopecia totalis do not seem to respond to minoxidil and few develop cosmetically significant regrowth.

Third line pharmacological therapy

This consists of a variety of unproved therapies that have at one time or another been reported as successful in small series. In general those patients with widespread AA who have not responded to any of the first or second line treatments are doomed to remain bald.

Such treatments including cryotherapy (two freeze–thaw cycles); azathioprine in a dose of 100 mg daily; topical nitrogen mustard 0.2 mg/ml daily over the entire scalp; oral zinc supplementation with 600 mg zinc sulphate daily and cyclosporin A have all been reported in open trials.

Cyclosporin A is not currently available in any effective topical formulations. Oral cyclosporin in a dose of 3.5 mg/kg has to date produced cosmetically acceptable regrowth in only a few patients. As it is nephrotoxic and can induce cancer after long-term use, it is not considered suitable for the routine treatment of AA unresponsive to other therapy. There are also reports in the literature of patients whose AA developed or progressed while on high-dose cyclosporin for the prevention of transplant rejection

The natural history of AA, and in particular the tendency to spontaneous remission should not be forgotten when evaluating treatment modalities.

Physical therapies

Some patients with extensive AA shave their head and walk about bald (hopefully with sunscreen!). Others wear a hat or a scarf. Many choose to wear a wig. Wigs are discussed in greater detail on p. 55.

Patients are often apprehensive about wearing a wig and either speaking to another patient who has a good wig or the advice of a quality wigmaker is invaluable. Patient support organizations can usually suggest a good wigmaker and give useful advice on styling and wig maintenance.

Hair transplantation has been used for long-standing fixed patches, without ongoing inflammation on biopsy, but in active disease the grafted hairs generally fall out due to continued immunological attack.

Chapter 7

Nonscarring traumatic alopecia

7.1 Trichotillomania

Definition

Trichotillomania (TTM) is a habit tic, often unrecognized by presenting patients, where individuals so-inclined repeatedly play with and pluck their hair. It is classified in the Diagnostic and Statistical Manual of Mental Disorders (DSM-IV) as an impulse disorder not elsewhere classified. The diagnostic criteria are listed in Table 7.1

Epidemiology

It is thought that as many as 2 million people in the United States are affected by TTM. Most are women and adolescent girls who recognize their habit of pulling their hair out and do not seek medical attention. Such cases are akin to nail biting.

Children account for almost 90% of cases of TTM seen by dermatologists, and males are affected slightly more frequently than females in this age group.

Aetiology

The hair loss in TTM is self-inflicted. The inability to resist the desire to pluck in children has been linked to child–mother disharmony, however, treatable disorders are rarely found and psychiatric referral is only required in a minority of children. Nevertheless it is pertinent to inquire regarding any psychological stress around the onset of TTM.

In adults anxiety disorders have been demonstrated in up to 75% of sufferers and depression in 65%. Less common associations include substance abuse, schizoaffective disorders and eating disorders.

Pathogenesis

Telogen hairs are removed cleanly, while anagen hairs are twisted and broken at various lengths. A stubble of hair uniformly 2.5–3 mm long is characteristic: this length being dictated by the difficulty of manually plucking the shorter remaining and regrowing hairs.

Clinical features

Trichotillomania presents as nonscarring ill-defined patches of alopecia. Patients may complain that the hair never grows long in an affected area. Close examination reveals a normal scalp on which the hairs are twisted and broken at various lengths (Fig. 7.1). Hair other than on the scalp can be affected (Fig. 7.2). Pulling from two sites is the norm. The commonest sites are the scalp, eyebrows and upper eyelashes (lower eyelashes are too difficult to grasp) and only rarely are the hairs pulled from the trunk or pubic regions. Occasionally the hair is cut rather than pulled (trichotemnomania) or extracted with tweezers.

The hair pulling develops gradually and unconsciously, but is not usually denied by the patient when confronted (Fig. 7.3). The hair pulling is usually secretive and patients hide their plucked hair and some conceal their hair loss with creative hair styles or even wigs. Plucking often occurs while the patient is relaxing watching television, talking on the phone, lying in bed or reading a book. It may be exacerbated during times of stress, and there may be plucking binges. There is often a ritual to the plucking with the desired hairs carefully identified and each hair removed using an identical technique.

This habit tic may be precipitated by eczema of the scalp or may occur following alopecia areata (AA) (Fig. 7.4). Hair is

Table 7.1 Diagnostic criteria for trichotillomania.

1. Recurrent pulling out of one's own hair resulting in noticeable hair loss.
2. An increasing sense of tension immediately prior to pulling out the hair or when attempting to resist the impulse.
3. Pleasure, gratification or relief when the hair has been pulled out.
4. The disorder is not explained by a coexistent mental illness.

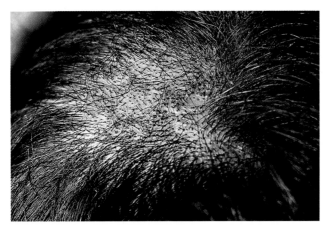

Fig. 7.1 Trichotillomania of the scalp in a young boy, showing the broken hair shafts. (Courtesy of Dr J. Brenan, Melbourne.)

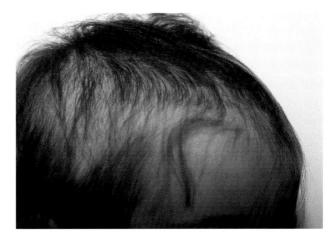

Fig. 7.3 Bizzare angular hair loss due to trichotillomania in a girl with associated loose anagen syndrome. The ability to pluck hair painlessly helped to exaggerate her habit tic.

plucked most frequently from the frontoparietal region. The loss can be dramatic (Fig. 7.5). Some children also suck and eat the hair (trichophagy) and tangled hairs are occasionally found in their mouth.

Parents of affected young children frequently fail to recognize the cause of their child's hair loss, while some postadolescent women deny participation in their hair disorder. These two small subgroups are more likely to present to the dermatologist and thereby influence medical perceptions of this relatively common condition.

There are a number of differences between the presentation of TTM pre- and postadolescence. Postadolescence TTM is much more likely to reflect a refractory underlying personal-

ity or anxiety disorder. Females are almost exclusively affected and may vigorously deny any interference with their hair. An inappropriate lack of concern or *la belle indifférence* may be a clue to the diagnosis.

Extensive areas of the scalp may be plucked although the hair margin is usually inexplicably left alone (Fig. 7.6) producing a characteristic tonsure alopecia, which is pathognomonic. Tonsure alopecia (Fig. 7.7) has an appalling prognosis and after many years of plucking scarring can be produced.

Diagnosis

The main differential diagnosis is tinea capitis where broken hairs invariably occur on an inflamed scalp. Examination with a Wood's lamp and skin scrapings for fungal microscopy and culture are necessary in some cases. Hair shaft disorders tend to be diffuse rather than patchy, although monilethrix may be deceiving. Loose anagen syndrome may be a contributory factor in this condition as the hairs are extracted painlessly (Fig. 7.3). Traction alopecia may need to

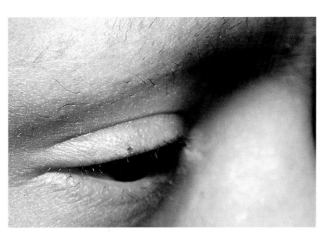

Fig. 7.2 Trichotillomania of the eyebrows.

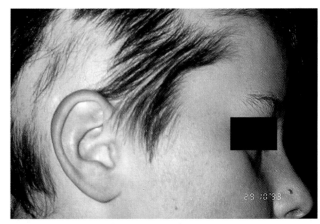

Fig. 7.4 Trichotillomania following alopecia areata.

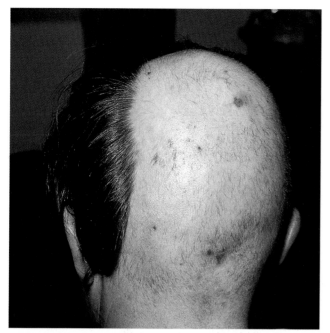

Fig. 7.5 Extensive bizarre hair loss, in a man, due to trichotillomania. (Courtesy of Dr A. Callen, Melbourne.)

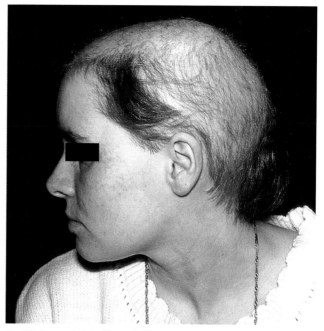

Fig. 7.7 Tonsural trichotillomania. (Courtesy of Dr Munro, Glasgow.)

be considered and it is useful to know how the patient styles his or her hair. Alopecia areata is distinguished by the fact that affected patches are predominantly bald with only a few fractured exclamation mark hairs (which are easily extracted). Scalp biopsy is rarely required for diagnosis.

Investigations

Hair shafts should be examined to exclude tinea capitis and hair shaft disorders. A hair pluck will be required, and patients are often more than willing to do this themselves. In the face of vigorous denial by the patient a biopsy of an affected area can be useful to verify the diagnosis. Coexistent morbid psychopathology has already been discussed.

Pathology

The pathology is diagnostic. Numerous empty hair canals are seen, and some dilated follicular infundibula contain horny plugs. Many follicles are in catagen and some in early anagen. There are few in telogen. There is practically no perifollicular inflammation, and this distinguishes TTM from AA (Fig. 7.8). Some follicles are severely damaged and show perifollicular haemorrhage, separation of the follicular epithelium from the connective tissue sheath, pigmented casts in the isthmus of infundibular region of the follicle (Fig. 7.9) and trichomalacia, consisting of injured follicles producing clumped, soft, twisted corkscrew hairs.

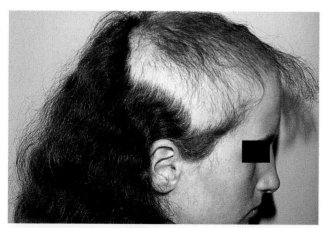

Fig. 7.6 Trichotillomania, in a woman, sparing the scalp margin. (Courtesy of Dr A. Callen, Melbourne.)

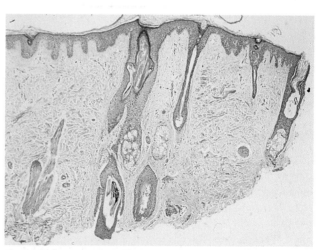

Fig. 7.8 Low power scanning photomicrograph of trichotillomania. Numerous catagen hairs are seen. (Courtesy of Dorovitch Pathology, Melbourne.)

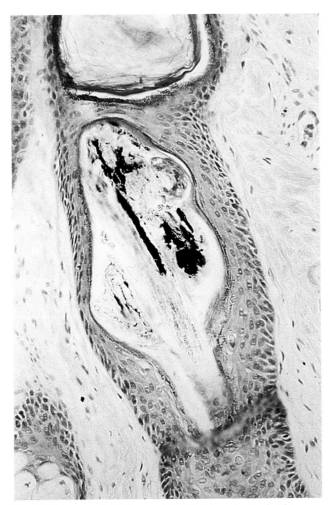

Fig. 7.9 High power photomicrograph of trichotillomania showing the diagnostic pigmented casts. (Courtesy of Dorovitch Pathology, Melbourne.)

Associated features

Nail biting is said to be more common in patients with TTM.

Prognosis

Trichotillomania is a nonscarring alopecia and if patients stop pulling their hair out it will grow back normally. Children tend to pluck their hair episodically, with complete remissions occurring 2–3 times a year, before they ultimately grow out of it. In the adolescent and adult groups the condition tends to be chronic, with few periods of remission.

Tonsure alopecia has an appalling prognosis despite psychoanalysis, psychotherapy, behaviour modification therapy and the use of both major and minor tranquillizers.

Treatment

Children often respond to a frank explanation of the condition and advice not to play with their hair. A soft, woolly, whiskery toy may be employed as a substitute.

Behavioural therapy is useful, and the main habit reversal techniques involve awareness training followed by relaxation therapy, and aversion therapy. Cognitive therapy employing thought stopping, correcting faulty self-talk and enhancing the patient's self-esteem are also useful, particularly if one has access to a psychologist with an interest in TTM.

Even if the child continues to pluck his or her hair, the parents can be reassured this is not a serious disorder, that the child will grow out of it and that the hair will eventually grow normally. Parents who have not observed their child playing with his or her hair can have difficulty accepting the diagnosis at first. A video of the child at play may help to convince them.

Clomipramine at doses of 100–250 mg per day and fluoxetine (Prozac) at between 40 and 80 mg per day are the most efficacious of the antidepressants tried. A response usually takes 8 weeks but may be seen as soon as 2 weeks. Some sufferers may initially respond to low doses, but later require higher doses to maintain remissions. Relapse on cessation of the medications is usual.

Key points

A compulsive disorder where patients pull sufficient hairs out to produce patches of alopecia. Plucking as a cause of circumscribed patches in childhood is usually initially unrecognized by the parents, eventually accepted after explanation, not associated with underlying psychopathology and has a good prognosis. In diffuse tonsural alopecia in an adolescent or young adult plucking is usually denied, not accepted after detailed explanation, associated with a personality disorder or major psychiatric illness, has a poor prognosis and is best considered a variant of dermatitis artefacta. In TTM, if and when the patient ceases to pluck hairs the alopecia resolves.

7.2 Traction alopecia

Definition

Traction alopecia is a mechanical alopecia, where unlike TTM the hairs are traumatized unintentionally and usually slowly by prolonged traction which is a consequence of certain hair styles.

Epidemiology

Traction alopecia is largely a disease of black females. Currently it is common in the United States, less common in the United Kingdom and rare in Australia.

Aetiology

Prolonged traction, particularly in childhood with the hair styled into tight braids or ponytails places great stress particularly on the scalp margins and the outermost hairs of the braid. These hairs are lost first producing receding hair lines and widening of the parts.

While commonly to blame, hair styling is not the only cause of traction alopecia. It may follow vigorous combing or brushing (especially when using a nit comb following an attack of head lice).

Pathogenesis

Hair, sometimes weakened by chemical applications, can be broken by friction or tension. Negroid hair is fragile and more likely to fracture. Prolonged tension leads to inflammation of the follicle that may ultimately produce scarring. Traction eases telogen hairs out of the follicle and patients with incipient androgenetic alopecia are more prone to traction alopecia, as they have more telogen hairs.

Clinical features and investigation

The dictates of religion, fashion and custom have produced an immense variety of hair styles, each producing a different stress on hair. Pony tails produce frontal or parietal alopecia (Fig. 7.10); tight braiding in 'corn-rows' produces marginal or central alopecia with widening of the parts (Fig. 7.11); twisting hair into a bun on top of the head produces frontal and parietal alopecia (Fig. 7.12); brush rollers applied too tightly produce an irregular alopecia; and vigorous brushing or over-enthusiastic massage produce a diffuse alopecia. Future hair styles will undoubtedly produce new patterns of traction alopecia.

The essential changes on examination are short broken hairs, folliculitis, and some mild scarring in circumscribed patches. This condition can resemble, but is distinct from,

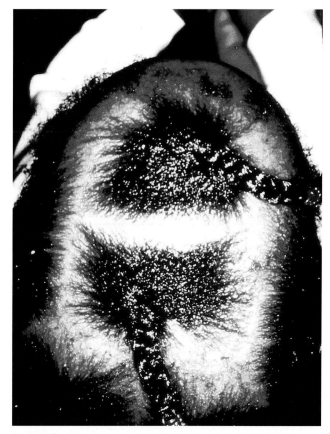

Fig. 7.11 Traction alopecia produced by tight braiding of the hair.

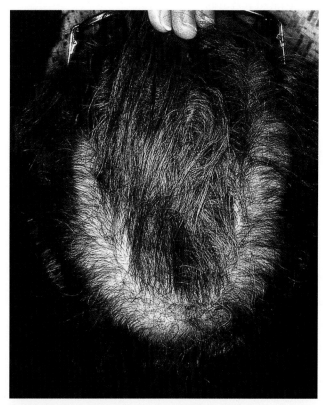

Fig. 7.12 Traction alopecia produced by twisting the hair into a tight bun on top of the head.

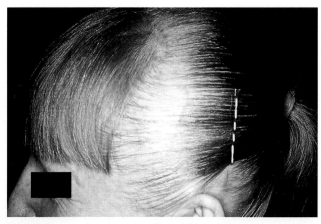

Fig. 7.10 Traction alopecia produced by a tight ponytail.

the hot-comb alopecia or follicular degeneration syndrome of black men and women in which scarring is more prominent.

Diagnosis

The important differential diagnoses are tinea capitis, hair shaft disorders and TTM. All can produce patches of hair loss covered by a stubble of short hairs. Other causes of scarring alopecia will need to be excluded in advanced cases.

Investigation

Wood's light examination, hair plucks for fungal microscopy and culture and examination of hair shafts by light microscopy will exclude most other diagnoses. Many cases will require a biopsy for prognostic reasons as well as to exclude other causes of scarring alopecia and TTM.

Pathology

Histologically early traction alopecia is similar to TTM, with an increase in terminal catagen and telogen hairs, a mild reduction in the total number of terminal hairs and, in occasional cases, trichomalacia. Late disease is characterized by a marked decrease in the total number of terminal hairs, fibrous tracts and scarring without significant inflammation.

Associated features

Usually none.

Treatment

Patients are often surprisingly resistant to changing their hair style. Many have long suspected the cause of their hair loss and seek consultation to find a treatment that allows them to continue styling their hair the same way.

Unfortunately the only measure that halts progression and allows regrowth of traction alopecia is redistributing the tension in the hair. A return to normal is not possible for those who have coincident androgenetic alopecia or for those who have developed scarring from prolonged traction.

Key points

A potentially scarring circumscribed alopecia with an unusual distribution that corresponds to the patient's hair style.

7.3 Postoperative occipital alopecia

Definition

Postoperative occipital alopecia is a nonscarring occipital alopecia that follows prolonged surgery.

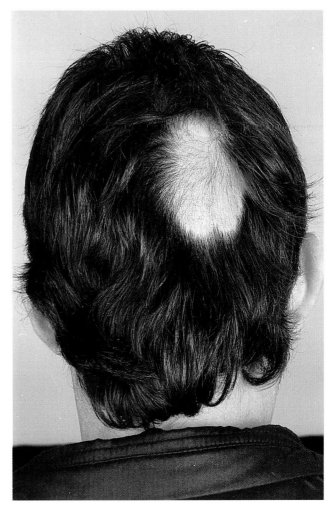

Fig. 7.13 Post cardiac surgery occipital alopecia. (Courtesy of Dr J. Kelly, Melbourne.)

Aetiology

Cardiac surgery with hypothermia and prolonged obstetric surgery with the patient in the lithotomy position are the most common antecedent operations.

Pathogenesis

It is due to a localized anagen effluvium secondary to pressure ischaemia of the scalp. This induces a temporary arrest of mitosis in the matrix, that narrows the hairs to breaking point.

Clinical features

The hair loss begins a few days postoperatively. All the anagen hair on the occiput (about 85% of the total) is rapidly shed (Fig. 7.13). The hairs do not come out with the bulb, but rather fracture of the base of the partially keratinized hair shaft. The hair loss may be preceded by redness and swelling and even crusting and ulceration in severe cases.

Diagnosis

The main differential diagnosis is AA, and a biopsy may be required to distinguish these two conditions.

Investigation

Microscopy of extracted occipital hairs shows mainly fractured hairs with a tapered proximal end and a few hairs with dystrophic roots. This is characteristic of the condition.

Pathology

Biopsy shortly after the hair loss begins shows intravascular thrombosis, oedema, hair follicle necrosis, and a perivascular infiltrate. Numerous catagen hairs are seen in the more severe cases if a localized telogen effluvium has also been precipitated. Later the histology may only show dermal fibrosis and inflammation.

Associated features

None.

Prognosis

Complete spontaneous recovery generally occurs quickly as most of the occipital hairs have merely fractured proximally and are still in anagen. Occasional cases with permanent hair loss in the centre of the patches have been reported.

Treatment

Postsurgery anagen effluvium can be prevented by frequently moving the patient's head during the surgery. Inflatable rings have been used to redistribute the pressure during surgery, but tend to only redistribute the alopecia.

Key points

A localized occipital anagen effluvium may be precipitated by prolonged cardiac or obstetric surgery and is believed to be due to the combination of pressure ischaemia exacerbated by hypothermia.

Section D
Scarring alopecia

Chapter 8

Acquired cicatricial alopecia

8.1 Definition, diagnosis and classification of cicatricial alopecia

Cicatricial or scarring alopecia are general terms applied interchangeably to areas of permanent hair loss associated with destruction of the hair follicles. There are numerous possible causes for scarring alopecia, both congenital or acquired. Destruction of stem cells in the bulge region of the hair follicle is responsible for the permanency of the hair loss.

Scarring in an area of alopecia is not always easy to recognize. The skin is characteristically smooth and shiny due to atrophy (Fig. 8.1), with a few single hairs emerging where isolated follicles have escaped destruction. A hand lens or a dermatoscope may allow the loss of follicular pores to be seen (see Fig. 1.36) and enable nonscarring alopecias such as alopecia areata to be distinguished. A helpful confirmatory sign is the presence of pili multigemini or tufting of hairs (multiple hairs arising from a single follicular opening) within a patch of cicatricial alopecia (Fig. 8.1). This is produced by distortion of the follicles and is not seen in nonscarring alopecias. Light microscopic examination of these hairs may reveal irregular twisting, but true pili torti does not occur.

Additional features that should be noted include inflammation of the scalp, pustules, perifollicular hyperkeratosis, pigmentation alterations, perifollicular erythema and broken hairs. These signs may help determine the cause of the scarring alopecia, however, no one sign in isolation is pathognomonic for a particular disease, and a correlation of clinical and histological features is usually needed to make a specific diagnosis.

When scarring is the only physical sign, examination of the entire skin surface may provide a clue to the diagnosis. Up to 40% of patients with scalp lichen planus and 30% with discoid lupus of the scalp will have cutaneous disease elsewhere on the body.

When the cause of the scarring alopecia is uncertain, hairs from the edge of a bald patch should be plucked for mycology and the scalp examined with a Wood's lamp. Any pustules should be swabbed and the fluid cultured. Serology for antinuclear antibodies is recommended for suspected cases of lupus.

Most cases will require a diagnostic biopsy to confirm the presence of scarring and to determine its aetiology. Two or more 4 mm punch biopsies give the most useful information. They should be taken from the active edge of a lesion and immunofluorescence should be performed. The biopsies should be sectioned both horizontally and transversely by the pathologist, as this enables numerous follicles to be examined (Figs 8.2 & 8.3). Half of the vertically sectioned specimen can be used for direct immunofluorescence. Even if the cicatricial alopecia seems to have burnt out, useful prognostic information may be gained by biopsy.

Despite these investigations a specific diagnosis is not always possible, and a generic diagnosis such as scarring alopecia may be appropriate. In such cases a trial of oral steroids or antimalarials may be considered to assess the potential for regrowth.

Surgical correction of small areas of cicatricial alopecia can be performed once the underlying disorder has burnt out. This is done by either hair transplantation (Fig. 8.4) or by excision of the area. Larger areas of scarring alopecia may require the prior use of tissue expanders.

The commonest causes of acquired cicatricial alopecia are lichen planus, discoid lupus erythematosus, folliculitis decalvans, pseudopelade of Brocq, traumatic or postinfectious

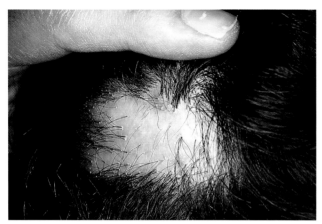

Fig. 8.1 Multiple hairs arising from a single follicle at the edge of scarring alopecia (tufted folliculitis).

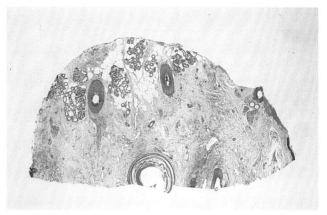

Fig. 8.3 Horizontally sectioned scalp biopsy from the edge of a patch of cicatricial alopecia showing a reduction in follicles and perifollicular inflammation. (Courtesy of Dr C.W. Chow, Melbourne.)

cicatricial alopecia morphoea and erosive pustular dermatosis of the scalp. All other causes are rare and a schematic classification is presented in Table 8.1.

Congenital alopecia and hypotrichosis is discussed separately in Chapter 9 and infections causing scarring alopecia are dealt with in Chapter 11. Tumours, in particular metastatic nodules from renal, breast and lung carcinomas should not be forgotten as a possible cause of scarring alopecia and are described in Chapter 12.

8.2 Lichen planus and lichen planopilaris

Definition

Lichen planus is an inflammatory dermatosis that may affect the skin, nails, mucous membranes and the scalp. There are a number of cutaneous variants of lichen planus. On the scalp it tends to produce a scarring alopecia. The scalp may be affected alone or in conjunction with lichen planus elsewhere.

Epidemiology

Lichen planus occurs worldwide and affects both sexes equally. It accounts for 1% of people seen in dermatology clinics. Over 80% of cases affect people aged between 30 and 70 years. Lichen planus accounts for about 40% of cases of cicatricial alopecia caused by inflammatory dermatoses.

Aetiology

Lichen planus is most commonly idiopathic, but is occasionally drug-induced.

Pathogenesis

The pathogenesis of the scarring alopecia involves inflammation of the hair stem cells in the bulge region of the follicle.

Clinical features

Recent lesions of lichen planus show violaceous flat topped polygonal papules, erythema and scaling. These papules quickly resolve and are replaced by follicular plugs and scar-

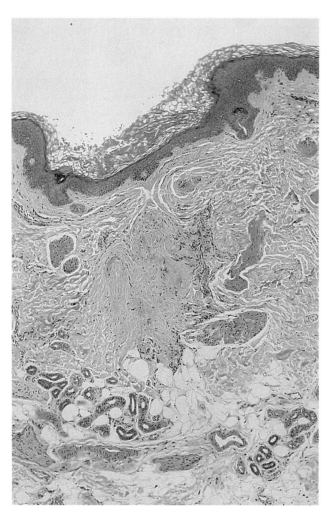

Fig. 8.2 Longitudinal scalp biopsy showing loss of hair follicle, scarring, lone arrector pili muscles and streamers. (Courtesy of Dr C.W. Chow, Melbourne.)

Table 8.1 Causes of acquired scarring alopecia.

INFLAMMATORY		
Lichenoid	Lichen planus	Graham-Little syndrome
	Frontal fibrosing alopecia	cGVHD
	Pseudopelade of Brocq	Porokeratosis of Mibelli
Connective tissue disease	Discoid lupus erythematosus	Dermatomyositis
	Morphoea	Systemic sclerosis
	Lichen sclerosis	Acne keloidalis nuchae
Bullous	Cicatricial pemphigoid	Epidermolysis bullosa
Neutrophilic	Folliculitis decalvans	Tufted folliculitis
	Erosive pustular dermatosis	Dissecting cellulitis
	Sweet's syndrome	Pyoderma gangrenosum
Granulomatous	Sarcoidosis	Necrobiosis lipoidica
	Granuloma annulare	Temporal arteritis
Other	Alopecia parvimacularis	Mastocytosis
	Follicular degeneration syndrome	Follicular mucinosis
	Amyloid	Lipoid proteinosis
TRAUMATIC		
	Radiodermatitis	Mechanical trauma
	Post surgical (flap necrosis)	Burns
	Accidental alopecia	Dermatitis artefacta
	Traction alopecia	Hot comb alopecia
INFECTIOUS		
Bacterial	Acne necrotica	Carbuncle
	Folliculitis	Furuncle
	Tuberculosis	Syphilis
Fungal	Kerion	Favus
	Tinea capitis (rarely scarring)	
Viral	Shingles	Varicella
	HIV	
Protozoal	Leishmania	
NEOPLASTIC		
Benign	Syringoma	Cylindroma
	Other adnexal tumours	
Malignant 1°	Basal cell carcinoma	Squamous cell carcinoma
	Mycosis fungoides	Sezary syndrome
	Reticulosis	
2°	Renal	Breast
	Lung	Gastrointestinal
	Lymphoma	Leukaemia

cGVHD, chronic graft vs. host disease.

ring (Fig. 8.5). Eventually the follicular plugs are shed from the scarred area which remains atrophic, white and smooth. When postinflammatory pigmentation is prominent, the scalp may show reticulate pigmentation (Fig. 8.6). No follicular orifices can be found within the scarred area. If the patch is extending there may be follicular plugs and perifollicular erythema at the margin of the lesion. The hair pull test may be positive with anagen hairs extracted by gentle traction. Occasionally hypertrophic lichen planus occurs on the scalp (Fig. 8.7).

Patients commonly present with established pseudopelade-like patches of scarring that are nonspecific.

A recently described variant of lichen planopilaris is frontal fibrosing alopecia. Clinically this condition resembles androgenetic alopecia with frontal recession (Fig. 8.8), however, on close inspection there is subtle evidence of scarring and perifollicular erythema within the marginal hairline. With time the alopecia extends and causes the hair line to recede. Nonscarring frontal recession is common in women and in one study, 37% of normal women had frontal recession of their

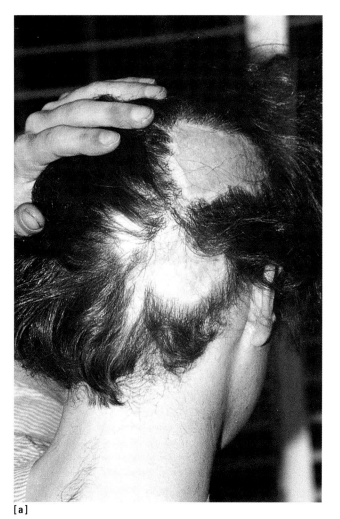

[a]

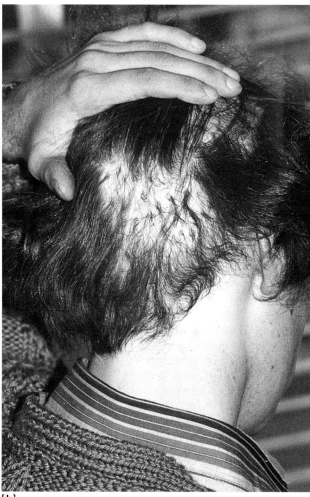

[b]

Fig. 8.4 Post-traumatic scarring alopecia, (a) before and (b) after punch grafting. (Courtesy of Dr Richard Sheils, Melbourne.)

hairline, in the absence of virilization. Nevertheless a scarring frontal alopecia is very rare.

The natural history of frontal fibrosing alopecia is for the alopecia to be slowly progressive. To date no treatment has proved effective. Systemic agents tried include prednisolone, isotretinoin and hormone replacement therapy. Topical steroids, tretinoin lotion, minoxidil lotion and dithranol cream have also failed to halt the progression of this alopecia.

Pathology

In the absence of cutaneous or mucosal lichen planus, a biopsy offers the only hope of establishing the diagnosis conclusively. Unfortunately the histological features are often nondiagnostic, particularly in burnt-out cases. The biopsy only rarely reveals classical lichen planus with a perifollicular and upper dermal band-like infiltrate consisting predominantly of lymphocytes, associated initially with epidermal hyperplasia and later atrophy, V-shaped hypergranulosis, colloid body formation and flattening of the rete ridges with a saw tooth pattern.

Usually the process predominantly involves the perifollicular region and the intrafollicular infiltrate is sparse (Figs 8.9 & 8.10). Occasionally the inflammation involves the hair follicles exclusively. The infiltrate initially surrounds the follicles, the hairs are replaced by keratin plugs and ultimately the follicle is destroyed leaving behind only fibrosis and a lone arrector pili muscle within the scar tissue. The perifollicular fibrosis appears bluish due to the presence of mucin. While perifollicular fibrosis is not specific to lichen planus, clefts between perifollicular fibrosis and narrowed infundibula suggest a diagnosis of lichen planus rather than discoid lupus. Wedge shaped hypergranulosis within follicular infundibula and acrosyringia also suggests lichen planus.

Direct immunofluorescence may reveal globular staining with IgM (Fig. 8.11) at the follicular–dermal interface (compared with linear staining with C3, IgM or IgG of the basement membrane in discoid lupus), but is not diagnostic. While linear C3 or IgM staining of the basement membrane may be an incidental finding in sun-damaged skin. IgG deposition is highly suggestive of lupus, but is not particularly sensitive, with many false negatives.

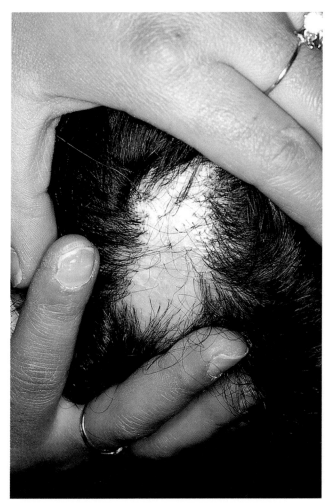

Fig. 8.5 Lichen planopilaris showing perifollicular inflammation.

Investigation

In endemic areas, hepatitis C serology should be considered when there are associated cutaneous lesions; however, the association of hepatitis C and pure lichen planopilaris has not been established.

Differential diagnosis

While lichen planus accounts for about 40% of cases of cicatricial alopecia caused by inflammatory dermatoses, discoid lupus accounts for a further 30–40% and is therefore one of the main clinical and histological differential diagnoses. As the treatment of these two conditions is potentially different, their distinction, where possible, is desirable. In general, the clinical presentation is more useful than the histology.

Associated features

Scalp involvement occurs in less than 5% of people affected with classical cutaneous lichen planus, but affects over 40% with the lichen planopilaris or bullous lichen planus variants. Scalp involvement may occur without other cutaneous involvement.

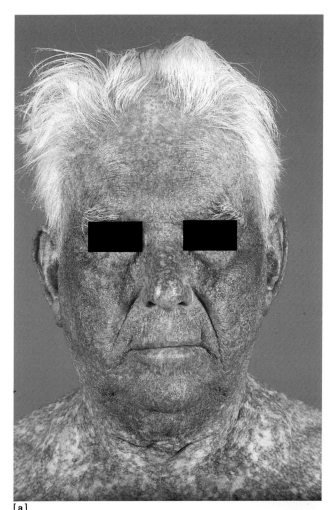

[a]

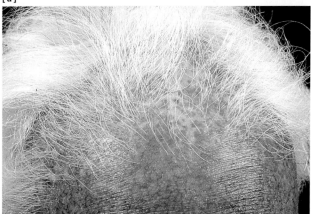

[b]

Fig. 8.6 Severe extensive lichen planus showing postinflammatory pigmentation (a) of the head and neck and (b) of the scalp.

Prognosis

The natural history of lichen planus is variable. It may run either a slowly progressive course with only a few new patches appearing every year or two, or it may be aggressive from the outset rapidly producing extensive baldness.

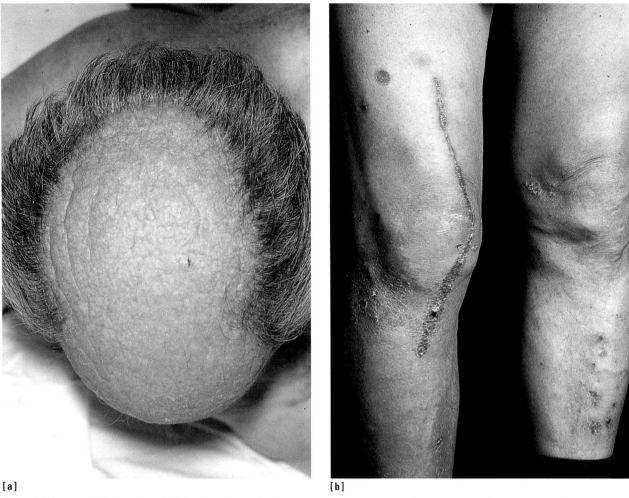

[a]   **[b]**

Fig. 8.7 (a) Hypertrophic lichen planus. (b) This patient also had Koebnerized lichen planus on his leg. (Courtesy of Dr A. Callen, Melbourne.)

Treatment

Drugs or other chemicals known to produce lichen planus (Table 8.2) should be diligently sought on history and if found stopped.

Intralesional triamcinolone or topical clobetasol propionate are helpful when there is active inflammation. A trial of systemic steroids should be considered for rapidly progressive disease. Antimalarials such as hydroxychloroquine may be considered, although their main place is in the treatment of discoid lupus erythematosus (DLE), and they have been reported to cause cutaneous lichen planus. PUVA and etretinate may have a place in maintenance therapy, and even griseofulvin has some anecdotal support. Oral cyclosporin A should theoretically be helpful, however, there is limited clinical experience with this agent. Minomycine and azathioprine have also been advocated for this condition.

The vast array of potential systemic therapies serves as testimony to the difficulty experienced in controlling this disease. In a number of cases, inexorable progression of the lichen planopilaris defies all treatment.

Once the inflammatory process has burnt out, which may take many years, corrective surgery may be possible.

Key points

Cicatricial alopecia possibly occurring in the presence of lichen planus elsewhere or demonstrating lichenoid papules or follicular plugging in the active margin. Histology and direct immunofluorescence may be diagnostic, suggestive or nonspecific.

8.3 Graham-Little syndrome

Definition

This is a distinctive condition that resembles lichen planopilaris. It has been suggested that Graham-Little syndrome is a variant of lichen planus, however, the absence of typical lichen planus elsewhere, the ill-defined histology and the lack of response to therapy suggest a valid distinction between these two conditions.

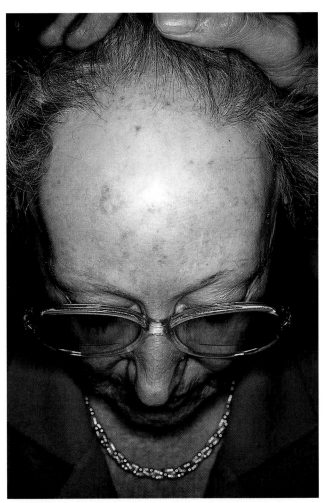

Fig. 8.8 Frontal fibrosing alopecia. Scarring and perifollicular erythema can be seen on the front margin of the hairline, associated with bitemporal recession in this postmenopausal woman.

Epidemiology

The condition is rare. Most patients are women between the ages of 30 and 70.

Pathogenesis

Unknown.

Clinical features

The essential features of the condition are progressive cicatricial alopecia of the scalp occasionally with prominent follicular plugging (Fig. 8.12), loss of pubic and axillary hair without scarring and the rapid development of keratosis pilaris. The keratosis pilaris is dramatic with horny papules developing into conspicuous spines resembling lichen spinulosus. It occurs in plaques, often on the trunk and limbs, occasionally involving the eyebrows and cheeks.

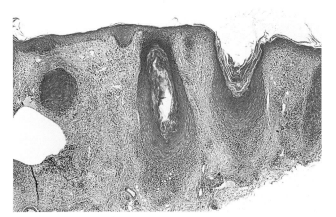

Fig. 8.9 Low power scanning photomicrograph showing lichen planopilaris. There is follicular plugging and a periappendageal inflammatory infiltrate.

Pathology

Histology shows a dilated follicular orifice filled with a keratin plug. The follicles beneath the plugs are progressively destroyed and eventually an atrophic epidermis covers a sclerotic dermis. The biopsy is remarkable for the lack of inflammation.

Investigation

Scalp biopsy.

Differential diagnosis

The condition needs to be distinguished from lichen planopilaris.

Associated features

None.

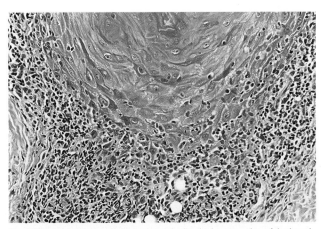

Fig. 8.10 Base of the hair follicle shows hydropic degeneration of the basal layer and a lichenoid mononuclear cell infiltrate.

Table 8.2 Drugs reported to cause cutaneous lichen planus and which may theoretically cause lichen planopilaris.

Antihypertensive medications	Methyldopa β-blockers Captopril Thiazide diuretics Loop diuretics Spironolactone
Antiinflammatory medications	Gold Penicillamine Phenylbutazone
Antituberculous medications	Isoniazid PAS Ethambutol Streptomycin
Antimalarials	Chloroquine Quinine Quinidine Mepacrine
Antiepileptic medications	Phenytoin Carbamazepine
Antipsychotic medications	Phenothiazines Lithium
Antibiotics	Sulphonamides Tetracyclines Penicillins
Miscellaneous	Arsenic Bismuth Griseofulvin Sulfonylureas Acyclovir
Topical agents	Colour film developers (rare on the scalp)

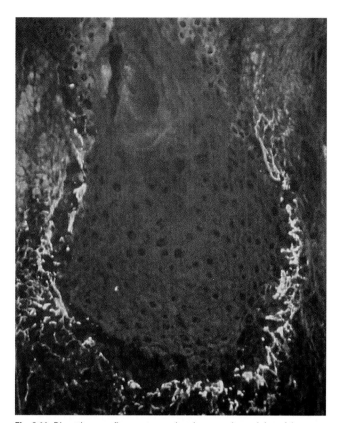

Fig. 8.11 Direct immunofluorescence showing granular staining of the dermoepidermal junction.

Prognosis

Poor. The condition tends to be progressive.

Treatment

Many agents have been tried, but none is effective.

Key points

The triad of cicatricial alopecia, loss of pubic and axillary hair, and widespread plaques of keratosis pilaris constitutes this characteristic syndrome.

8.4 Lupus erythematosus

Definition

Lupus erythematosus (LE) is an autoimmune connective tissue disease characterized by the presence of circulating nonorgan-specific autoantibodies to cell nuclear antigens.

Three different forms of LE are described, namely systemic (SLE), subacute and discoid (DLE) lupus.

Epidemiology

Lupus erythematosus occurs most commonly in women (the women:men ratios being 8:1 for SLE and 2:1 for DLE) and is about three times more common in black than in white people. The incidence is around 1 in 2000. Familial cases occur in about 10%. The peak age of onset is around 40 years.

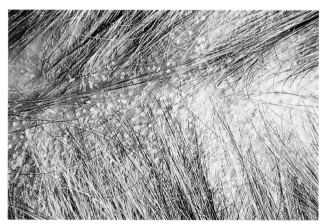

Fig. 8.12 Graham-Little syndrome.

Pathogenesis

Inflammation of the infundibular region of the hair follicle is thought to be the basis of the scarring alopecia that occurs in DLE. The diffuse hair shedding that accompanies SLE is believed to be an acute telogen effluvium.

Clinical features

Systemic lupus erythematosus is a multisystem disorder with circulating antinuclear antibodies (ANA) and antibodies to double stranded DNA. Skin manifestations include a malar erythema, photosensitivity, diffuse hair loss, mouth ulcers, vasculitis and occasionally urticarial lesions. Systemic lupus erythematosus may be primary or secondary to ingested drugs.

Diffuse nonscarring hair loss as the result of a telogen effluvium occurs in 50% of patients with SLE (Fig. 8.13), especially in the active phase of the disease. There is diffuse shedding and some scalp erythema (Fig. 8.14). The hair is dry, fragile and easily broken. Short, unruly 'lupus' hairs are seen in 30% particularly at the frontal margin. The lost hair regrows as the disease becomes inactive, but lupus hairs persist somewhat longer. If discoid lesions coexist, then a cicatricial alopecia may also occur. Antibodies against PNCA/cyclin are associated with a higher incidence of alopecia, however, these antibodies are only present in about 3% of lupus patients.

Subacute LE comprises about 10% of patients with lupus and is characterized by an annular polycyclic rash, photosensitivity and circulating antibodies to Ro, which is an extractable nuclear antigen. During pregnancy, this autoantibody may cross the placenta and be passed to the fetus. Affected babies develop neonatal LE comprising an annular rash and congenital heart block.

Diffuse nonscarring alopecia occurs in about half the patients affected with subacute LE. Localized scarring alopecia also occurs and is occasionally the presenting complaint. The annular rash of neonatal subacute LE may involve the scalp (Fig. 8.15). It resolves within 4–6 months without scarring.

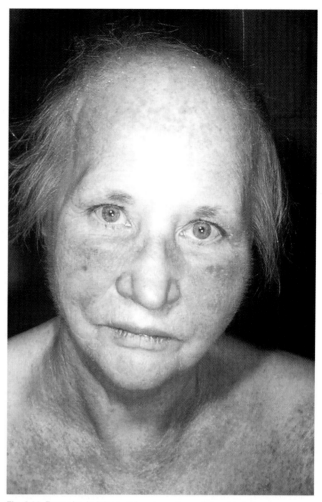

Fig. 8.14 Extensive hair loss and scalp erythema in systemic lupus erythematosus. (Courtesy of Dr J. Kelly, Melbourne.)

Cutaneous DLE presents with well-defined erythematous patches with an adherent scale and follicular plugs, that can occur on any part of the body, but are most common on the head and neck. The lesions heal with atrophy, scarring and

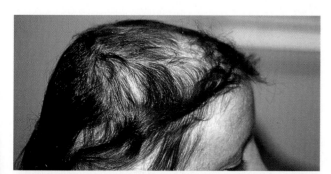

Fig. 8.13 Diffuse nonscarring hair loss in association with systemic lupus erythematosus.

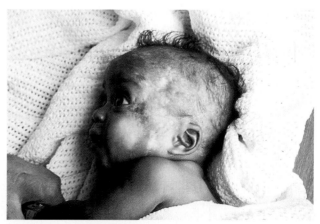

Fig. 8.15 Neonatal subacute lupus erythematosus.

pigmentary changes. Scarring alopecia occurs in 33% of patients affected with DLE (Fig. 8.16).

Scalp lesions occur in 20% of men and 50% of women with DLE, and DLE accounts for about 30–40% of all cases of cicatricial alopecia. Patches on the scalp are often itchy. Areas of erythema and scaling with follicular plugging extend irregularly across the scalp and produce scarring (Fig. 8.17). Sometimes patches of scarring alopecia develop with little in the way of preceding inflammation and resemble alopecia of Brocq. Ultimately large areas of alopecia may form. Pigmentary disturbance, particularly in dark-skinned people is common. Rarely, calcification occurs in the patches and squamous cell carcinoma has been reported in chronic cicatricial LE of the scalp.

Very occasionally lupus profundus occurs on the scalp and produces a scarring alopecia (Fig. 8.18). Lupus profundus is an unusual variant of lupus in which the inflammatory infiltrate is focused in the panniculus, with only minimal epidermal changes. In one series it was found in 6 out of 228 patients with DLE. This condition was once thought to be sarcoid, but it is now accepted as a variant of lupus

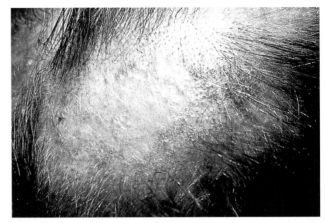

Fig. 8.17 Discoid lupus erythematosus producing cicatricial alopecia.

Pathology

The histology is indistinguishable in the three forms of LE and the characteristic findings are:
- hyperkeratosis with follicular plugging (Fig. 8.19);
- a patchy, deep and superficial, perivascular and periadnexal lymphoid infiltrate that may be sparse, moderate or heavy (Fig. 8.20);
- focal basal layer vacuolar degeneration, which is the essential feature. This may be associated with colloid body formation, pigmentary incontinence, papillary dermal oedema, thickening of the basement membrane zone and exocytosis of lymphocytes into the epidermis and follicular epithelium (Fig. 8.21).

Mucin can be seen in the dermis as a faint blue tinge between widely separated collagen bundles. Scarring manifests as homogenized collagen fibres running parallel to the surface, a loss of appendages and lone arrector pili muscles. Elastic fibres are absent from the scar.

Hypergranulosis, saw-toothing of the rete ridges, perifollicular fibrosis and clefts are not seen in lupus and help to dis-

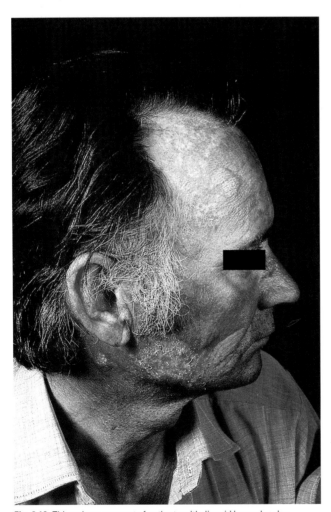

Fig. 8.16 Thirty-three per cent of patients with discoid lupus develop scarring alopecia on the scalp.

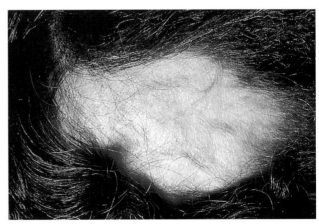

Fig. 8.18 Scarring alopecia secondary to lupus profundus.

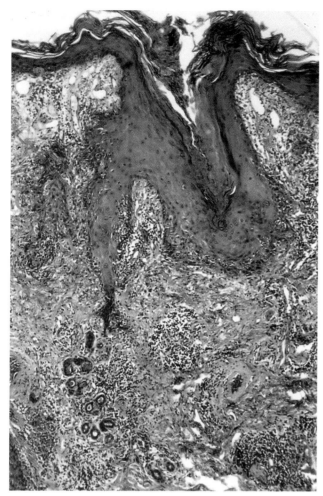

Fig. 8.19 Low power photomicrograph showing follicular plugging, superficial and deep, perivascular and periappendageal lymphocytic infiltrate. (Courtesy of Dr G. Mason, Melbourne.)

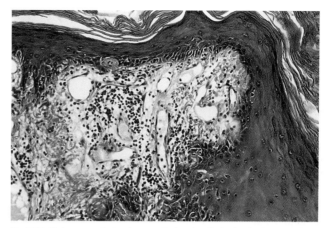

Fig. 8.20 High power photomicrograph showing the hydropic degeneration of the basal layer and the mononuclear cell infiltrate. (Courtesy of Dr G. Mason, Melbourne.)

Investigation

The diagnosis of LE usually requires serology and histology with direct immunofluorescence. Antinuclear antibodies are positive in over 80% of patients with SLE, around 35% with DLE, and in 60% with subacute LE. Anti-Ro antibodies are found in 30% of patients with SLE, 10% with DLE, and 60% with subacute LE. A positive ANA also occurs in up to 5% of the normal population and this figure increases with age.

Differential diagnosis

It is not uncommon to have cases with a negative ANA, non-specific clinical features, negative direct immunofluorescence and equivocal pathology. In such cases the diagnosis may only become clear after many years when characteristic cutaneous lesions of lupus appear.

tinguish lichen planus. A deep inflammatory infiltrate never occurs in lichen planus, but it is not always present in LE. Frequently it is not possible to separate these two conditions on routine histology and in such cases immunofluorescence may be decisive. Deposits of complement (C3), IgM and IgG stain linearly the basement membrane in more than 80% of cases of LE but not lichen planus. Direct immunofluorescence is also positive in nonlesional skin in about 50–75% of cases of SLE, depending on whether sun-exposed or nonexposed skin is chosen. Only about 20% of cases of DLE will have positive immunofluorescence of uninvolved skin. A weak false positive immunofluorescence to IgM can occur on the head and neck and is a source of confusion. Only positivity to IgG or very strong positivity to IgM (Fig. 8.22) should be used as supportive evidence of lupus on the scalp since this only rarely occurs in the absence of lupus.

In old, burnt out lesions the histology and immunofluorescence may be inconclusive and in such cases a nonspecific diagnosis such as scarring alopecia is all that can be made.

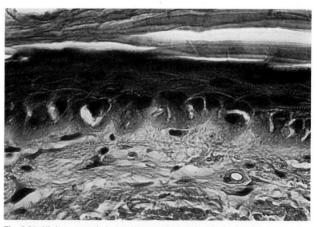

Fig. 8.21 High powered photomicrograph showing the hydropic degeneration of the basal layer. (Courtesy of Dr G. Mason, Melbourne.)

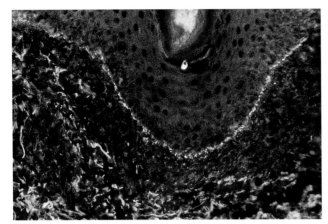

Fig. 8.22 Positive linear immunofluorescence to IgG: the lupus band test. (Courtesy of Dr G. Mason, Melbourne.)

Associated features

Discoid lupus erythematosus may occur on its own or as a part of SLE. Systemic lupus erythematosus first presents with DLE in 10% of cases and DLE can be found at some stage during the course of SLE in 33%. Conversely most patients with DLE do not go on to develop SLE. If the initial DLE is confined to the head and neck the risk is 1–2%, whereas if the lesions are generalized the risk is 22%.

Prognosis

The prognosis is variable. Some cases burn out after 1–2 years, while others continue to progress for many years.

Treatment

Drug-induced lupus needs to be excluded and a list of drugs that may cause lupus is included in Table 8.3. Potent topical corticosteroids, intralesional triamcinolone and systemic prednisolone (1 mg/kg) may halt progression of active DLE. Antimalarials form the mainstay of treatment in chronic cases refractory to topical steroids. Hydroxychloroquine in a dose of 200–400 mg daily produces a remission within 3 months in the majority and the dose can then be tapered gradually. Non-responders should be changed to chloroquine for a further 3 month trial before considering other treatments. (Scarring is of course permanent.)

Retinoids, dapsone, thalidomide or a combination of these medications may be useful in refractory cases. Cyclophosphamide, methotrexate and cyclosporin A have also been used in severe, rapidly progressive cases where all other treatments have failed.

Key points

Lesions of discoid lupus produce a scarring alopecia. Early lesions are erythematous, scaly with follicular plugs and have diagnostic histology and immunofluorescence. Late, burnt-out lesions are clinically and histologically indistinguishable from lichen planus and alopecia of Brocq. Systemic lupus produces a telogen effluvium and lupus hairs but only rarely scarring alopecia.

8.5 Pseudopelade of Brocq

Definition

Pseudopelade of Brocq is an idiopathic, chronic, slowly progressive, patchy cicatricial alopecia, that occurs without any evidence of inflammation. It is primarily an atrophy rather than an inflammatory folliculitis.

The term pseudopelade was first used by Brocq to distinguish this condition from the 'pelade' of alopecia areata. The French term pelade had been in use at that time for more than 200 years and is derived from *pelage*: the fur, hair, wool, etc., of a mammal. The term pseudopelade merely refers to scarring alopecia, and is a generic diagnosis. Confusion has arisen through the use of 'pseudopelade' and 'pseudopelade of Brocq' interchangeably.

Epidemiology

Alopecia of Brocq may occur in either sex at any age. Most commonly women over 40 years are affected, while childhood cases are rare.

Table 8.3 Drug induced lupus erythematosus.

Discoid lupus erythematosus	Systemic lupus erythematosus	
Isoniazid	Antihypertensives	Hydralazine
		Prazosin
Griseofulvin		Clonidine
		Methyldopa
Penicillamine		β-blockers
		ACE inhibitors
Dapsone		Thiazide diuretics
	Antiepileptics	Phenytoin
		Carbamazepine
	Antiarthritics	Penicillamine
		Allopurinol
		Gold
	Antibiotics	Griseofulvin
		Sulphonamides
		Tetracyclines
		Penicillins
		Isoniazid
		Streptomycin
	Miscellaneous	Lithium
		Quinidine
		Chlorpromazine
		Procainamide
		Oral contraceptives

Aetiology

The aetiology is unknown. The condition is almost always sporadic, however, the reported occurrence in two brothers suggests a genetic factor may be important.

Pathogenesis

Unknown.

Clinical features

The alopecia is asymptomatic and is often discovered by chance. It always remains confined to the scalp. The initial patch is often on the vertex but may occur anywhere (Fig. 8.23). At first there may be a brief period when perifollicular erythema can be seen at the edge.

The course is extremely variable. Most often there is slow development, over many years, of small round patches of alopecia that ultimately converge to produce larger irregular areas of hair loss. The hair in the uninvolved scalp is normal and the progression is sufficiently slow that even after 15–20 years patients may still be able to arrange their hair in such a way as to conceal the bald areas. The entire process can burn out spontaneously at any stage leaving behind only relatively small areas of alopecia.

Pathology

Early lesions may have a light lymphocytic infiltrate around the upper two-thirds of the hair follicle (including the hair bulge) that spares the epidermis and eccrine glands. This infiltrate invades the walls of the follicles and sebaceous glands and eventually destroys the entire pilosebaceous unit (Fig. 8.24). Single hairs may survive within a patch for many years.

Later patches are smooth, soft and slightly depressed and histology reveals only a thin atrophic epidermis overlying a

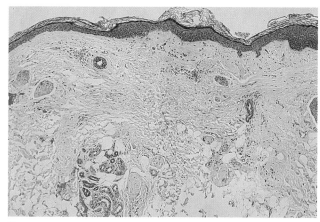

Fig. 8.24 Low power photomicrograph of pseudopelade of Brocq showing a decreased number of follicles and sebaceous glands and scarring. There is minimal inflammation. (Courtesy of Dr C.W. Chow, Melbourne.)

sclerotic dermis containing fibrotic streams extending into the subcutis. There are no inflammatory changes at this stage. These fibrotic streams are follicular 'ghosts'. Arrector pili muscles may be seen inserting into this fibrous remnant of the hair follicle. Elastic stains have been reported to be useful in differentiating alopecia of Brocq from lichen planus, discoid lupus and other scarring alopecias (pseudopelades). With an acid alcohol orcein stain elastic fibres are seen around the lower part of the follicle, while in all the other scarring alopecias the scar tissue consists of collagen devoid of elastin.

Investigation

Lichen planus or DLE can produce a similar picture and evidence of these two conditions, including a biopsy should be sought as there are specific treatments for these conditions.

Differential diagnosis

There is no doubt that lichen planus and DLE can produce very similar and sometimes identical clinical pictures. However, the histological criteria proposed by Pinkus can be used to exclude these and differentiates a group of patients who never display any clinical, serological or histological evidence of either of these conditions. This group of patients have a separate, distinct disease entity as was first described by Brocq in 1885. The diagnostic criteria of Braun-Falco, shown in Table 8.4 and based on the histological criteria of Pinkus should be fulfilled before this specific diagnosis is made. Cases that do not fulfil these criteria should be diagnosed generically as scarring alopecia

Associated features

None reported.

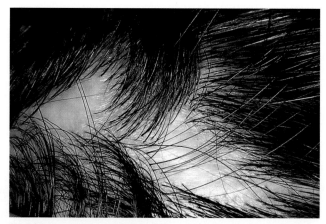

Fig. 8.23 Pseudopelade of Brocq on the vertex of the scalp.

Table 8.4 Diagnostic criteria for pseudopelade of Brocq (after Braun-Falco, 1986).

Clinical criteria
Irregularly defined and confluent patches of alopecia
Moderate atrophy (late stage)
Mild perifollicular erythema (early stage)
Female to male ratio, 3·1
Long course (more than 2 years)
Slow progression with spontaneous termination possible

Direct immunofluorescence
Negative (or only weak IgM on sun exposed skin)

Histological criteria
Absence of marked inflammation
Absence of widespread scarring (best seen with elastin stain)
Absence of significant follicular plugging
Absence, or at least a decrease of sebaceous glands
Presence of normal epidermis (only occasional atrophy)
Fibrotic streams into the dermis

Prognosis

The prognosis is extremely variable. Some patients develop only three or four patches that appear suddenly, and rapidly reach full size over a few months and do not enlarge further. New patches may appear over the next year or so and then the condition 'burns out'. Other patients may develop patches that continue to enlarge and ultimately coalesce into a large area of alopecia.

Treatment

Alopecia of Brocq does not respond to either topical or intralesional steroids and no treatment is known that halts progression of this condition. Once it has spontaneously burnt out corrective surgery may be possible.

Key points

The development of small patches of cicatricial alopecia in the absence of any clinical inflammation other than transient erythema.

8.6 Folliculitis decalvans and tufted folliculitis

Definition

A scarring alopecia, associated with pustules.

Epidemiology

Men may be affected from adolescence onwards, while women tend not to get this condition until their thirties.

Aetiology

Bacterial folliculitis, associated with inflammation that destroys the hair bulge. *Staphylococcus aureus* is commonly isolated from the follicular pustules.

Pathogenesis

Many people develop a bacterial pustular folliculitis of the scalp at some stage. In the vast majority it is transient, resolves with antibiotics and heals without scarring. In some people the folliculitis is more persistent, tends to recur after apparently successful treatment with antibiotics and produces a scarring alopecia. An abnormal host response to *Staphylococcus aureus* is postulated which may be the result of a defect in cell-mediated immunity.

Clinical features

Following a pustular folliculitis of the scalp, multiple rounded patches of alopecia develop, each patch surrounded by a few follicular pustules. Successive crops of pustules appear and are followed by progressive destruction of the affected follicles (Fig. 8.25). In some cases the folliculitis spreads along the scalp margin in a coronal pattern, or along the edge of an androgenetic alopecia (Fig. 8.26). The scalp may be the only site affected or there may be involvement of virtually any hairy region of the body.

Tufted folliculitis is a variant of folliculitis decalvans where circumscribed areas of scalp inflammation heal with scarring characterized by tufts of up to 15 hairs emerging from a single follicular orifice (Fig. 8.27). *Staphylococcus aureus* can be cultured from affected scalps and the histology of these two conditions is similar. The tufts consist of a central anagen hair surrounded by telogen hairs, each arising from independent follicles, converging towards a common dilated follicular infundibulum. Cases in which the tufts comprised only anagen hairs have also been described. Based on an animal model, it is suggested that erythema and scaling are the initial events and the tufting is a consequence of the emergence of hairs from beneath the free edge of the scales.

Pathology

Histology reveals follicular abscesses with a dense perifollicular polymorphonuclear infiltrate and scattered eosinophils and plasma cells (Figs 8.28 & 8.29). Foreign body granulomas occur in response to follicular disruption, which is followed by scarring. Eventually all that remains of the follicle is extensive fibrosis. An elastin stain is useful for demonstrating scarring.

Investigation

A scalp biopsy is required to confirm the diagnosis and swabs should be taken of any pustules. Investigation for an underly-

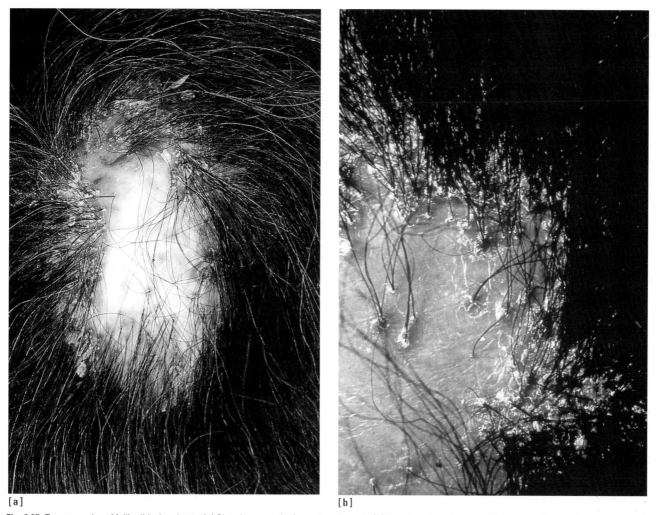

[a]   [b]

Fig. 8.25 Two examples of folliculitis decalvans. (a) Showing a patch of scarring alopecia; (b) the edge of a patch magnified to show the crusting, pustules and tufting of the hairs.

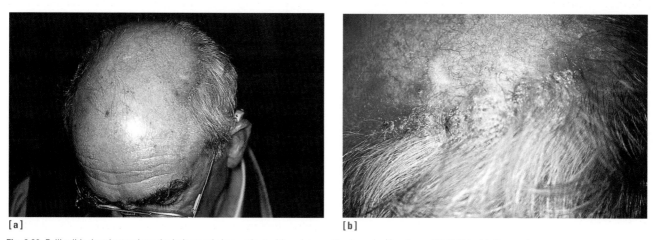

[a]   [b]

Fig. 8.26 Folliculitis decalvans along the hair margin in a patient with androgenetic alopecia. (Courtesy of Dr B. Tate, Melbourne.)

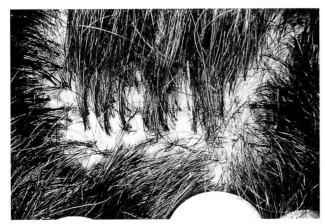

Fig. 8.27 Tufted folliculitis.

ing defect in cell mediated immunity is generally unrewarding, but is indicated in certain cases.

Differential diagnosis

A fungal kerion may mimic folliculitis decalvans. Hairs should be plucked for fungal culture and a periodic-

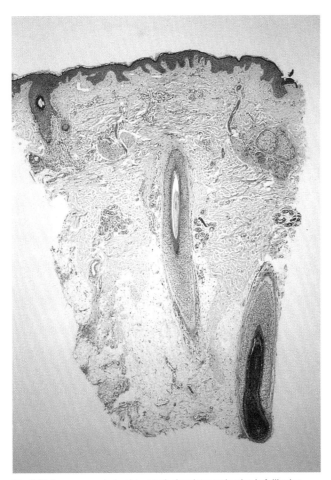

Fig. 8.28 Low power photomicrograph showing a reduction in follicular density and perifollicular inflammation.

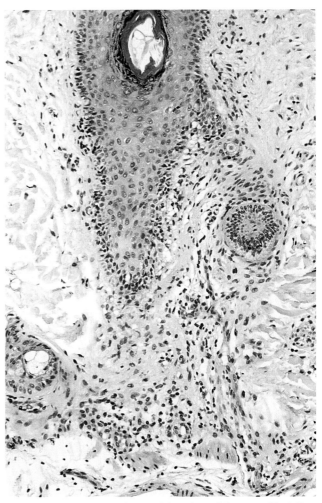

Fig. 8.29 High power photomicrograph from the top left corner of Fig. 8.28 demonstrating the mixed mononuclear and polymorphonuclear perifollicular inflammatory infiltrate.

acid–Schiff (PAS) stain should be performed on the scalp biopsy.

Associated features

Seborrhoeic dermatitis commonly coexists.

Prognosis

Most cases follow a chronic and relapsing course. Eventually the condition burns out, however, this may take many years.

Treatment

The essential treatment is eradication of *Staphylococcus aureus* from the scalp. Prolonged courses of flucloxacillin induce remission, but relapse occurs when the antibiotics are stopped. Rifampicin eradicates staphylococcal nasal carriage and may produce prolonged remissions. Isotretinoin has been used to alter the follicular environment to make it less suitable for staphylococcus colonization, but may increase cutaneous staphylococcus carriage and make the condition worse. Tufting may be reduced by measures directed at reducing the scale, such as the use of tar shampoos and topical keratolytics.

Key points

The cardinal feature of folliculitis decalvans is a scarring alopecia with pustules either at the active margin of the patch or elsewhere in the scalp where new areas are evolving. An abnormal host response to *Staphylococcus aureus* is postulated as most people with folliculitis do not develop a scarring alopecia.

8.7 Erosive pustular dermatosis of the scalp

Definition

An inflammatory scarring alopecia confined exclusively to the scalp.

Epidemiology

Erosive pustular dermatosis of the scalp is not as uncommon as was first thought. It occurs in the elderly, especially in partly bald, sun-damaged scalps (Fig. 8.30).

Aetiology

The aetiology is unknown. The role of bacterial infection in the causation of this condition has been controversial; however, it appears that the bacteria is a secondary colonizer rather than a primary pathogen.

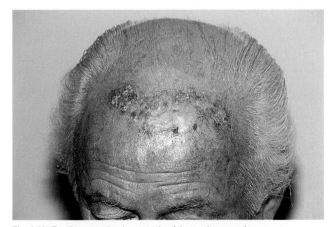

Fig. 8.30 Erosive pustular dermatosis of the scalp occurring on a sun-exposed bald scalp.

Pathogenesis

Unknown.

Clinical features

It is characterized by a large crusted erosion of the scalp. Beneath the crust is a boggy mass containing discrete pustules. The initial lesion can be precipitated by trauma and consists of pustules, erosions and crusts that slowly expand over the scalp and produce a scarring alopecia.

Pathology

Histology from the base of the lesion shows an eroded epidermis, a dense lymphohistiocytic infiltrate in the papillary dermis with scattered plasma cells, foreign body giant cells and replacement of hair follicles by scar tissue.

Investigation

Culture from affected areas often grows *Staphylococcus aureus*, but other organisms have been also been isolated. A scalp biopsy for routine histology and direct immunofluorescence will exclude other causes of scarring alopecia.

Differential diagnosis

Differential diagnoses include pustular psoriasis, temporal arteritis and cicatricial pemphigoid.

Associated features

Androgenetic alopecia and solar elastosis are normally seen in the affected areas.

Prognosis

There is no tendency to spontaneous resolution and the condition may have been present many years before the patient consults. Scarring is permanent and the condition tends to relapse on cessation of treatment.

Treatment

Potent topical steroids produce a rapid and dramatic response while antibiotics alone fail to make an impact on the condition. It is prudent to use a combination of potent topical steroids and antibiotics. A remission is usually induced in about 2–3 weeks. An astringent such as Burow's solution may be used in the initial stages is there is excessive weeping.

Key points

The hallmarks of erosive pustular dermatosis are a boggy mass of pus, with superficial crusting on the scalp of an elderly, partly bald, sun-damaged man or woman that responds to potent topical steroids. It is easily mistaken for an ulcerated skin cancer.

8.8 Dissecting cellulitis of the scalp

Definition

This rare condition is also known as perifolliculitis capitis abscedens et suffodiens. It manifests with a perifolliculitis of the scalp with deep and superficial abscesses in the dermis, sinus tract formation and extensive scarring.

Epidemiology

Dissecting cellulitis of the scalp is rare, occurs predominantly in males aged between 18 and 40 years, and is seen most commonly in dark-skinned races. Familial cases are exceptional, as is childhood onset.

Aetiology

The aetiology of this inflammatory condition is unknown, and while staphylococci, streptococci and pseudomonas may be cultured from various lesions, no specific organism has been incriminated.

Pathogenesis

The condition is of unknown origin, but occurs with hidradenitis suppurativa and acne conglobata as part of the follicular occlusion triad. This suggests that apocrine gland dysfunction is involved in the pathogenesis of this disorder.

Clinical features

Painful, firm, skin-coloured nodules develop near the vertex of the scalp and later become softer and fluctuant (Fig. 8.31). Confluent nodules form tubular ridges with an irregular cerebriform pattern, on a red and oedematous background (Fig. 8.32). Thin blood-stained pus exudes from crusted sinuses, and pressure on one region of the scalp may cause discharge of pus from a neighbouring intercommunicating ridge. Cervical adenitis is present in some cases, but is more remarkable for its absence in many others. Progressive scarring and permanent alopecia occur. Characteristically hair is lost from the summits of these inflammatory lesions and retained in the valleys. Fatal squamous cell carcinoma (SCC) has developed within the areas of scarring after many years.

Pathology

Histology shows a perifolliculitis with a heavy infiltrate of lymphocytes, histiocytes and polymorphonuclear cells.

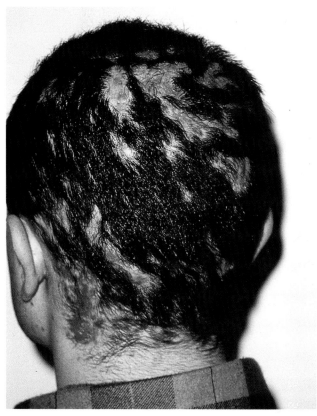

Fig. 8.31 Dissecting cellulitis of the scalp. (Courtesy of Dr Dyall-Smith and the *Australasian Journal of Dermatology* (1993) **34**, 81–2.)

Abscess formation results, and leads to destruction initially of the pilosebaceous follicles and eventually the other cutaneous appendages. Keratin fragments induce a granulomatous reaction with foreign body giant cells, lymphoid and plasma cells. Special stains for bacteria, fungi and mycobacteria are negative.

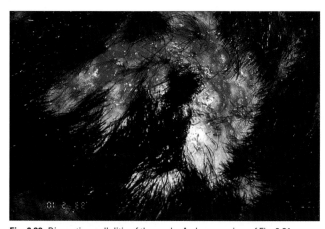

Fig. 8.32 Dissecting cellulitis of the scalp. A close-up view of Fig. 8.31 showing the tubular ridges and irregular cerebriform pattern. (Courtesy of Dr Dyall-Smith and the *Australasian Journal of Dermatology* (1993) **34**, 81–2.)

Investigation

Culture from affected areas often grows bacterial organisms. Fungal cultures and a scalp biopsy for routine histology and direct immunofluorescence will exclude other causes of scarring alopecia.

Differential diagnosis

Clinical differential diagnoses include kerion, pyoderma gangrenosum and erosive pustular dermatosis of the scalp.

Associated features

Other disorders of the follicular occlusion triad may be present and there may be an associated pilonodal sinus (the follicular occlusion tetrad) or spondyloarthropathy. An asymmetrical peripheral and axial arthritis occurs with sacro-ileitis in 73%. The activity of the arthritis parallels the activity of the skin.

Prognosis

The condition is chronic with frequent acute exacerbations.

Treatment

Although systemic antibiotics and topical or intralesional corticosteroids are sometimes helpful, relapses are frequent and the course is usually protracted. Isotretinoin in full dosage (1 mg/kg) in combination with prednisolone (1 mg/kg) and erythromycin 500 mg qid may induce a rapid remission and significant hair growth in areas not yet irreversibly damaged. Because the inflammation is predominantly perifollicular, a surprising amount of regrowth may occur. The antibiotics can be stopped after 4 weeks and the prednisolone gradually weaned and replaced by topical steroids. The isotretinoin should be continued for at least 6 months and reintroduced if the condition relapses. In recalcitrant cases widespread excision and grafting may be considered, or alternatively in older patients, epilating doses of radiotherapy have been used with success.

Key points

A rare chronic suppurative disease of the scalp producing widespread areas of cicatricial alopecia. It is idiopathic and usually occurs alone, but may be associated with acne conglobata and hidradenitis suppurativa as part of the follicular occlusion triad.

8.9 Morphoea, chronic graft vs. host disease and lichen sclerosis

Definition

Morphoea, chronic graft vs. host disease (sclerodermatous phase) and lichen sclerosis are distinct autoimmune connective tissue disorders characterized by hardening of the skin (scleroderma). There is minimal inflammation and hair follicles disappear from affected areas by apoptosis.

Epidemiology

Circumscribed morphoea is rare in the scalp. It is more common in females than in males (3 : 1) and generally occurs between the ages of 10 and 30.

Lichen sclerosus is a relatively uncommon disease that affects females 10 times more commonly than males and usually involves the vulva. Scalp involvement is rare.

Aetiology

Unknown.

Pathogenesis

Unknown.

Clinical features

When circumscribed morphoea occurs on the scalp the centrifugally expanding lilac border seen in early cutaneous macules is disguised by the hair. Only well established ivory white, smooth plaques that have shed their hair tend to be seen. The skin is thickened and feels hard due to dermal sclerosis and there may be hyperpigmentation. Any hair loss tends to be permanent. The lesions may be single or multiple and often there are no distinguishing features (Fig. 8.33). Without morphoea elsewhere on the body, the diagnosis can only be established on biopsy.

Linear morphoea on the frontal scalp (also known as *en coup de sabre*), produces a slowly progressive noninflammatory linear alopecia extending upwards from the forehead (Fig. 8.34). The line of morphoea may extend inferiorly into the cheek, nose and upper lip and involve the mouth and tongue.

Generalized morphoea with widespread sclerosis of the skin may also involve the scalp and produce a scarring alopecia. In some cases the entire body from head to toe is involved.

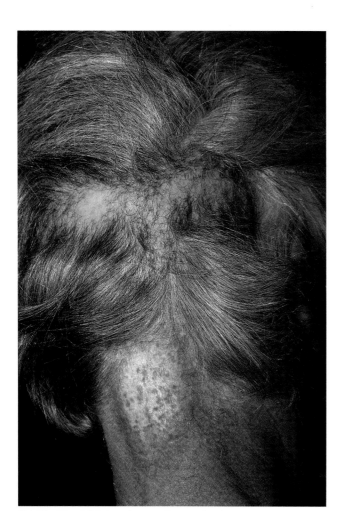

Fig. 8.33 Cicatricial alopecia secondary to scleroderma.

The sclerodermatous phase of chronic graft vs. host disease (cGVHD), which usually follows acute graft vs. host disease from organ transplantation, may also involve the scalp to produce a cicatricial alopecia (Fig. 8.35). Porphyria cutanea tarda may also produce scleroderma on the scalp (Fig. 8.36).

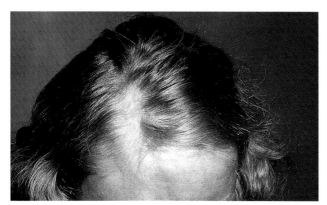

Fig. 8.34 Linear morphoea (*en coup de sabre*). Having had this lesion since adolescence this woman recently developed biopsy proven lichen sclerosis of the vulva.

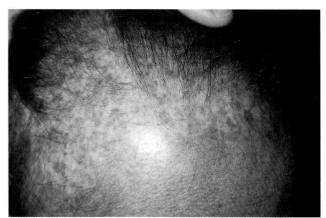

Fig. 8.35 Cicatricial alopecia due to chronic graft vs. host disease. (Courtesy of Dr T. O'Brien, Geelong.)

Lichen sclerosis is closely related to but distinct from morphoea, although the two conditions may coexist. Lichen sclerosis may involve the scalp and produce a scarring alopecia with few distinctive features (Fig. 8.37). The diagnosis is suggested by finding typical cutaneous and mucosal lesions elsewhere, and requires histological confirmation.

Pathology

The histology of morphea shows collagen fibrosis, associated with the disappearance by apoptosis of cutaneous appendages. Unlike scar tissue elastin is not lost and can be demonstrated by special stains. A clue to the diagnosis of early lesions is the loss of the perieccrine fat pad.

The histology of lichen sclerosis shows a characteristic hyalinized band of dermal collagen beneath an atrophic but hyperkeratotic epidermis, and above a linear band of lymphocytes.

Investigation

Scalp biopsy is required to establish the diagnosis.

Differential diagnosis

The clinical features of the hair loss are not distinctive and all other causes of scarring alopecia may need to be considered. Systemic sclerosis is a multisystem disorder characterized by vascular abnormalities, connective tissue sclerosis, and circulating autoantibodies. It may produce a diffuse telogen hair loss, similar to SLE, but it does not cause a scarring alopecia.

Associated features

Scleroderma and lichen sclerosus of the skin and mucous membranes may accompany the scalp changes. In linear morphoea the alopecia may be preceded by greying of the hair

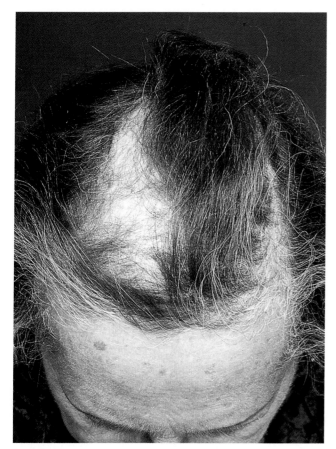

Fig. 8.36 Cicatricial alopecia occurring in porphyria cutanea tarda with sclerodermoid change.

and the condition is occasionally accompanied by facial hemiatrophy (Romberg's syndrome).

Prognosis

All of these conditions are progressive without treatment.

Treatment

Potent topical steroids such as clobetasol propionate or intralesional triamcinolone may stop progression of morphoea and lichen sclerosis, but systemic therapy is often required. Oral corticosteroids, penicillamine, salazopyrin and chloroquine have all been used with varying success. Surgical excision of *en coup de sabre* may provide definitive treatment, although recurrences occur especially if the lesion is enlarging at the time of excision. Physiotherapy is important to prevent joint contractures in associated involved limbs.

For cGVHD high-dose cyclosporin A combined with prednisolone is required. PUVA may also be of benefit. Nevertheless up to 40% of patients with cGVHD die within 10 years either due to the disease or the immunosuppression.

Key points

Scleroderma, meaning hard skin, can result from a number of localized or generalized connective tissue disorders. These may rarely affect the scalp and produce a noninflammatory scarring alopecia that requires a biopsy to establish the exact diagnosis.

8.10 Traumatic and cosmetic causes of scarring alopecia

Definition

Permanent hair loss due to mechanical destruction of the follicles.

Epidemiology

Probably the most common cause of scarring alopecia; however, most patients do not present to dermatologists. Radiodermatitis of the scalp following treatment of tinea capitis is fortunately now rare.

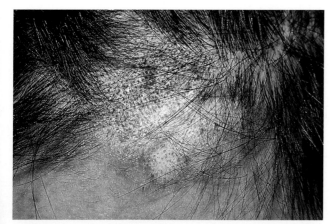

Fig. 8.37 Lichen sclerosis of the scalp.

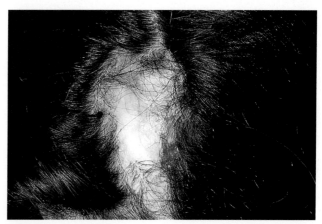

Fig. 8.38 Traumatic alopecia.

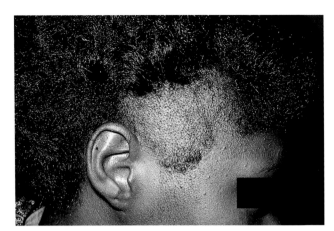

Fig. 8.39 Hot comb alopecia, or the follicular degeneration syndrome.

Aetiology

Common insults include burns, accidental mechanical injury (Fig. 8.38), and hot combs used to straighten hair (Fig. 8.39). Exceptionally, self-inflicted, artefactual injuries may involve the scalp and produce scarring (Fig. 8.40).

Pathogenesis

Any process that damages hair stem cells may produce a scarring alopecia.

Hot-comb alopecia is a permanent alopecia attributed to the use of hot combs and hair cosmetics to straighten Negroid hair. Scarring alopecia may result from severe thermal burns especially if the hot oil is allowed to run back along the hair onto the scalp. Alternatively the oils may produce a chemical folliculitis. Because hot comb straightening relaxes in the rain, it has largely been superseded by chemical straightening techniques using sodium hydroxide or ammonium thioglycollate-based products. These agents can also produce a chemical folliculitis or chemical burns resulting in a scarring alopecia.

Radiotherapy is still used to treat skin neoplasms and intracerebral tumours. A single dose of 3–4 Gy will induce temporary alopecia while single doses exceeding 10 Gy (or multiple tumour doses) will produce permanent alopecia. Superficial Grenz ray therapy may be preferable since it does not penetrate deep enough to damage follicles and produce alopecia.

Clinical features

Most often patients present with a circumscribed patch of scarring alopecia (Fig. 8.38).

Hair straightening is very widely practised amongst black people, who have fragile tightly curled hairs, but fortunately complications are relatively rare. The scarring alopecia that may develop as a consequence of hot-combs begins at the vertex and slowly extends centrifugally. Cumulative damage over many years may produce extensive alopecia. Black women may develop a similar pattern of alopecia without having used hot combs. The exact pathogenesis of this disorder is unknown and the terms follicular degeneration syndrome or unclassified alopecia in black women have been variously applied to women (or occasionally men) with a similar clinical presentation who give no history of having used hot-combs.

The follicular degeneration syndrome (Fig. 8.41) usually presents with a scarring alopecia over the crown that spreads centrifugally. It resembles very closely hot comb alopecia but occurs in black people who have used neither hot combs nor chemical hair straightening techniques. The histology resembles that of lichen planopilaris, but is distinguished by the characteristic premature degeneration of the inner root sheath. The alopecia slowly extends outward, with relative sparing of the periphery. Patients may complain of an itch, tenderness or pins and needles in the affected areas during periods of activity. The possibility that there is a relationship between follicular degeneration syndrome and dissecting cellulitis of the scalp is suggested by the occasional coexistence of these two conditions.

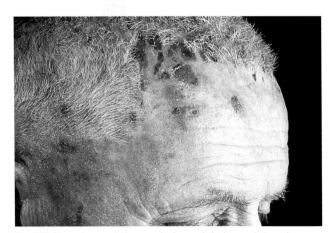

Fig. 8.40 Neurotic excoriations producing scalp lesions and alopecia. (Courtesy of Dr J. Kelly, Melbourne.)

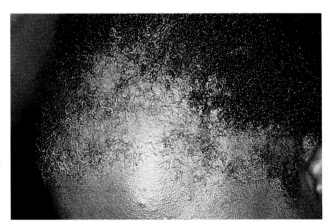

Fig. 8.41 Follicular degeneration syndrome.

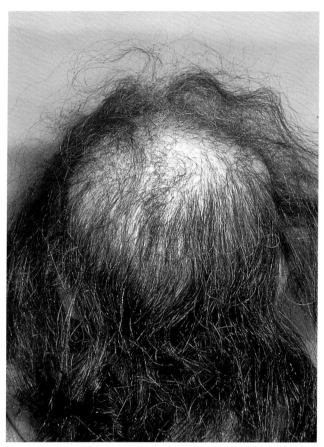

Fig. 8.42 Diffuse scarring following X-ray epilation for childhood tinea capitis 30 years previously.

Radiotherapy epilation was used to treat tinea capitis until the 1960s when griseofulvin (discovered in 1958) became available. Chronic radiodermatitis with cicatricial alopecia of the scalp is still seen as a late complication of this treatment (Fig. 8.42) and degenerative changes of sun-exposure and ageing may be superimposed on those due to the radiotherapy. Atrophy, telangiectasia and cicatricial alopecia may be combined with multiple neoplasms. Radiation necrosis may resemble a primary or recurrent skin neoplasm and a punch biopsy is useful for diagnosis.

Pathology

Scar tissue without inflammation is the commonest finding. Hair follicles are absent. Follicular stellae may be seen.

Investigation

Scalp biopsy may be required in certain cases for prognostic information and to exclude coexistant inflammatory disorders.

Differential diagnosis

Trauma of this severity is usually recognized by the patient,

but occasionally patients do not associate the injury with the alopecia, or deny the injury. Conversely a scarring alopecia may be falsely attributed to trauma, for example aplasia cutis congenita.

Associated features

None.

Prognosis

The hair loss is nonprogressive and permanent.

Treatment

Small areas of scarring alopecia can be excised and larger ones treated by hair transplantation or excision following the use of tissue expanders.

Radiation damage can be minimized by protective shielding of areas outside the field of treatment. Surgical excision is suitable for small areas, however, healing may be impaired. Hair transplantation requires caution and the grafts need to be widely spaced as the vascular supply is reduced in chronic radiodermatitis.

Key points

Traumatic alopecia presents as a localized area of scarring alopecia corresponding to the site of an injury. Cosmetic alopecia may result from cumulative damage over a number of years and is more common in black people. The aetiology is frequently unrecognized by the patient.

8.11 Other causes of scarring alopecia

Cicatricial pemphigoid

Cicatricial pemphigoid (CP) is an autoimmune blistering disease with circulating antibodies to epitopes on the 180 kD bullous pemphigoid antigen found within the lower portion

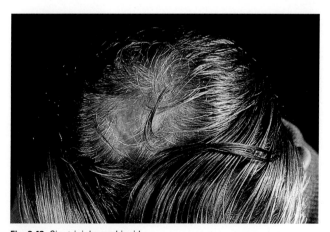

Fig. 8.43 Cicatricial pemphigoid.

of the lamina lucida. These circulating antibodies are only detectable in a minority of patients using currently available techniques.

It predominantly affects the elderly and occurs more frequently in women than in men. It targets the mucous membranes particularly the ocular and genital mucosa and involves the skin in only 40–50% of cases. Favoured sites are the face and scalp (Fig. 8.43). The skin lesions are usually confined to a limited area within which bullae repeatedly recur and heal with a thickened scar. The bullae and the associated mucosal lesions differentiate CP from other forms of cicatricial alopecia; however, the skin lesions may precede the mucosal lesions by months or years and occasionally there is no history of blisters. In such cases the diagnosis relies on the biopsy revealing the subepidermal split and direct immunofluorescence showing positive staining with IgG and C3.

Topical clobetasol propionate is often insufficient to control the blistering. Oral prednisolone, azathioprine or cyclosporin A may be required if there is significant mucosal involvement, especially if vision is threatened. Excision and grafting of a localized area of recurrent blister formation may be helpful in some circumstances.

Epidermolysis bullosa

Epidermolysis bullosa (EB) comprises a group of hereditary mechanobullous disorders characterized by traumatic blistering of the skin and mucosa. It is subclassified according to the pattern of inheritance and the level of the split in the skin. The recessive dystrophic type is the one most commonly associated with cicatricial alopecia, however, permanent alopecia may also occur in cicatricial junctional EB and very

rarely in EB simplex. Epidermolysis bullosa acquisita is an acquired autoimmune disorder with circulating antibody to type VII collagen in the anchoring filaments (270 kDa antigens), mimicking EB dystrophica.

Dystrophic EB presents with bullae at birth. The defect is within the anchoring fibrils and is due to an alteration of type VII collagen that results in separation of the dermis and epidermis with the split forming in the upper dermis. Blisters heal with atrophic scars and occasionally leave a localized absence of skin. The recessive form of dystrophic EB is a particularly devastating disease (Fig. 8.44) producing fusion of the digits, oesophageal strictures, blindness and premature death due to neoplasia (SCC) of the skin, mouth and oesophagus. Cicatricial alopecia occurs and may be associated with hair that is generally fine and sparse. Sclerosis of the skin may develop and contribute to the alopecia.

Cicatricial junctional EB is an autosomal recessive condition. The split occurs in the lamina lucida and generalized blistering begins at birth in response to trauma and heals with atrophy. Patches of cicatricial alopecia of the scalp, eyebrows, axillary and pubic regions may occur. The blistering is sufficiently dramatic to cause few diagnostic difficulties, although electron microscopy is required to distinguish this form of EB from dystrophic EB.

Generalized atrophic benign junctional EB is an autosomal dominant condition that produces widespread blistering at birth that improves with age. Dystrophic nails, dental enamel defects and oral involvement occur. There is a multifocal scarring alopecia (Fig. 8.45). The clinical features are less reliable than electron microscopy in determining the subtype of inherited EB.

Epidermolysis bullosa acquisita (EBA) is an acquired autoimmune blistering disease that may mimic bullous pem-

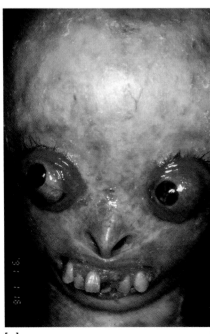

[a]

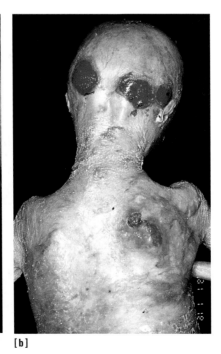

[b]

Fig. 8.44 Recessive dystrophic epidermolysis bullosa. (Courtesy of O. Ishikawa, S. Wanta, K. Ohnishi and Y. Miyachi and the *British Journal of Dermatology* (1993) **129**, 602.)

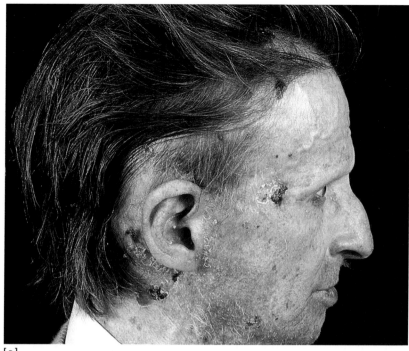
[a]

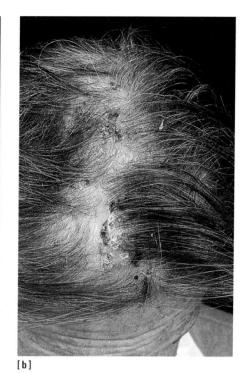
[b]

Fig. 8.45 Benign atrophic junctional epidermolysis bullosa.

phigoid (BP). Acral blisters may occur and EBA is notoriously unresponsive to treatment. Scarring alopecia may occur. Immunofluorescence of salt-split skin, or immunoblotting of a circulating antibody help to differentiate EBA from BP.

Treatment of the scarring forms of EB is generally unsatisfactory and revolves around supportive care and genetic counselling for the hereditary forms.

Alopecia parvimacularis

Outbreaks of alopecia areata-like lesions rapidly develop on the scalps of children in this mysterious condition. Numerous patches occur on affected scalps and are characteristically irregularly angular in shape. Epidemics in either schools or asylums occur and up to 60 children in one school were affected simultaneously. The alopecia in most children regrows completely, however, around 10% of affected individuals are left with scarring.

Pathology resembling that of pseudopelade of Brocq has been seen in some cases with a moderate lymphocytic infiltrate surrounding the upper two-thirds of the follicle, but sparing the epidermis. Only some follicles are involved and the degree of scarring depends on the number of contiguous follicles destroyed. Mycotic infections, multiple insect bites, secondary syphilis and AA all need to be excluded and a biopsy may be necessary.

Pyoderma gangrenosum

Pyoderma gangrenosum is a destructive, necrotizing, nonin-

fective ulceration of the skin that forms part of the spectrum of neutrophilic dermatoses. It most commonly occurs in association with a systemic disease such as inflammatory bowel disease, inflammatory arthritis, malignancy, autoimmune disease, monoclonal gammopathy and blood dyscrasias. The exact mechanisms involved in the development of this condition is unknown.

It occurs equally in men and women and may develop at any age. Lesions are usually solitary. It most commonly occurs on the lower extremities, but can develop anywhere on the body. Scalp lesions are unusual. Köebnerization is said to occur in 20%. Lesions may present as furuncle-like nodules, pustules or haemorrhagic bullae. The characteristic lesion is a rapidly developing tender erythematous nodule, first red, then becoming blue in the centre before ulceration occurs. Ulcers have a distinctive blue border, surrounded by a zone of dusky erythema when active. Untreated, the lesions run a chronic course over many months. Ulceration may extend rapidly and extension in one part may occur at the same time as healing in another. Healing produces scarring which on the scalp manifests with alopecia.

Histology of established lesions is nonspecific, however, the active margin may show a lymphocytic vasculitis with numerous polymorphs and leucocytoclasis that is suggestive of the diagnosis.

Activity of the pyoderma correlates with activity of an associated underlying disease, and treatment of the underlying disease, if possible, frequently leads to resolution of the pyoderma. Small, stable lesions may respond to intralesional

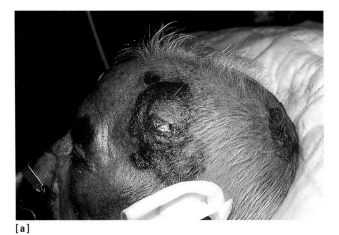

[a]

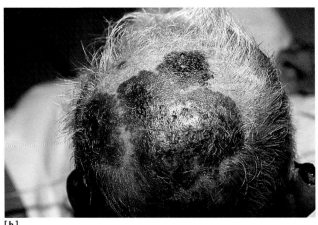

[b]

Fig. 8.46 Sweet's syndrome affecting the scalp.

steroids, however, the majority will require high-dose oral steroids for disease control. Dapsone, clofazamine, azathioprine and cyclosporin are used in resistant cases.

Sweet's syndrome

Sweet's syndrome is a nonulcerating variant of pyoderma gangrenosum that may occur as a paraneoplastic phenomenon. The skin lesions consist of one or more plum-coloured painful nodules or plaques accompanied by fever, leucocytosis and malaise. The nodules may be studded with pustules and blisters may form. However, ulceration does not tend to occur and this distinguishes Sweet's syndrome from pyoderma gangrenosum. Central clearing may result in annular lesions. Scalp involvement is unusual (Fig. 8.46), but produces scarring alopecia. Women are much more commonly affected than men and Sweet's syndrome is most common in the fourth and fifth decades.

Sweet's syndrome may occur following an upper respiratory tract infection, as an idiopathic phenomenon or in association with malignancy or a myeloproliferative disorder in up to 50% of patients. The vesicular pustular form is particularly associated with myeloproliferative disorders.

The histology shows a heavy diffuse infiltrate of neutrophils with leucocytoclasis in the mid and upper dermis, without significant vascular damage. The lack of significant vascular damage allows Sweet's syndrome to be distinguished from vasculitis, and a negative Gram stain helps to exclude cellulitis.

Sweet's syndrome may respond to nonsteroidal anti-inflammatory agents such as indomethacin, however, steroids are commonly required and tend to be dramatically effective. A daily dose of 30 mg of prednisolone is usually sufficient and should be tapered over 3–4 weeks. Relapse is common, especially with ongoing activity of the underlying condition.

Temporal arteritis

Temporal (or giant cell) arteritis is a giant cell granulomatous arteritis predominantly affecting large and medium sized arteries which preferentially affects the temporal artery. It is commonly associated with polymyalgia rheumatica. An autoimmune aetiology has been hypothesized. It is a disease of the elderly. Headaches are the usual initial manifestation and a very high erythrocyte sedimentation rate (ESR) (>100 mm/hour) strongly supports the diagnosis which is then confirmed by a temporal artery biopsy. Rapid progression with involvement of the retinal arteries may lead to sudden blindness without warning.

The scalp over affected arteries may be red, tender and pigmented with localized loss of hair that may be linear or generalized and either unilateral or bilateral. Bullae, ulceration and necrosis can occur (Fig. 8.47). Necrosis produces scarring alopecia that can be very extensive. Scalp necrosis is strongly associated with blindness and a higher mortality rate.

The arteritis is patchy but biopsy of a 1 cm strip of the tem-

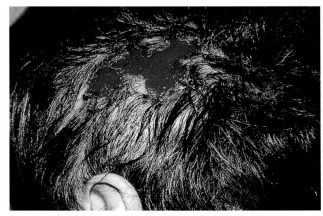

Fig. 8.47 Temporal arteritis of the scalp.

poral artery detects 94% of cases. Involved arteries show inflammation extending through the entire thickness of the arterial wall composed of lymphocytes, macrophages and multinucleate giant cells. Scalp necrosis and follicular destruction heals with fibrosis. Damage to the internal elastic lamina can be demonstrated with an elastin stain. In contrast to polyarteritis nodosa there is no frank necrosis of the arterial wall.

High-dose systemic steroids (60–100 mg of prednisolone) induce a rapid remission and a low maintenance dose (5–10 mg alternate days of prednisolone) is subsequently required to prevent relapse.

Dermatomyositis

Dermatomyositis is a rare autoimmune connective tissue disorder that primarily affects skin and muscle. It frequently occurs as a paraneoplastic phenomenon.

Diffuse alopecia of the scalp is present in 50%, and in the acute stages, this may be associated with hypertrichosis of the face and limbs. Later in the illness poikilodermatous changes with marked atrophy replace the acute inflammatory lesions. When this occurs on the scalp, scarring alopecia develops (Fig. 8.48).

The histological changes may be quite subtle with mild basal layer vacuolar change and colloid bodies in the dermis. There is a sparse superficial perivascular infiltrate and a variable amount of oedema and mucinous change in the dermis. Distinction of dermatomyositis from cutaneous lupus is difficult, although in the latter there is usually thickening of the PAS positive basement membrane zone, positive direct immunofluorescence and occasionally a deep and superficial perivascular infiltrate.

With the possible exception of children, all patients should be investigated thoroughly for a primary malignancy. If the investigations are all negative, the patient should be clinically reevaluated periodically.

High-dose corticosteroids may induce a remission of the cutaneous and muscular manifestations. Methotrexate is a useful steroid-sparing agent. Antimalarials may also be useful for the cutaneous eruption, but do not improve the myositis. If malignancy has been confidently excluded, cyclosporin A can be used and is helpful. Effective treatment of an underlying malignancy may effect a cure.

Necrobiosis lipoidica and granuloma annulare

Necrobiosis lipoidica is a degenerative disorder of collagen that occurs in 0.3% of diabetics. Seventy per cent of patients with necrobiosis have diabetes. Granuloma annulare is an idiopathic, possibly reactive process that may be localized or generalized. Localized lesions tend to occur on acral sites, while generalized lesions may develop anywhere on the skin.

Plaques of necrobiosis lipoidica usually occur on the shins, but may be found on other parts of the body including the scalp (Fig. 8.49). Lesions have a characteristic clinical appearance, presenting as sharply demarcated plaques of atrophic yellowish skin, which may or may not ulcerate. The atrophic centre has a glazed appearance often with prominent telangiectases. Scarring is a prominent feature.

On the scalp necrobiosis lipoidica may produce large areas of cicatricial alopecia, or multiple small areas of scarring resembling pseudopelade of Broq. Some lesions may have a slightly raised border and resemble sarcoidosis.

Histology is characteristic and demonstrates collagen necrosis. The process is characterized by blurring and a loss

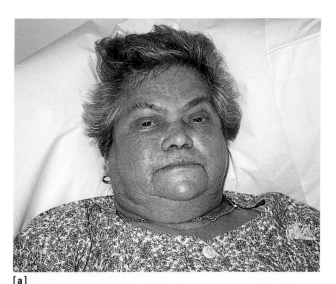

[a]

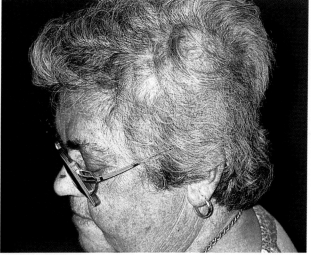

[b]

Fig. 8.48 Dermatomyositis of the scalp producing scarring alopecia. (a) Patient with heliotrope rash and second degree Cushing's syndrome. (b) Patchy and scarring alopecia.

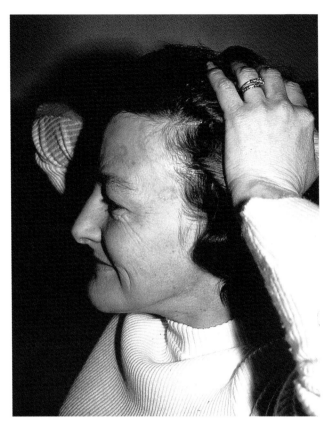

Fig. 8.49 Necrobiosis lipoidica of the forehead and anterior scalp margin.

of definition of collagen fibres, a loss of fibroblasts and increased eosinophilia. The area is surrounded by epithelioid histiocytes and giant cells, with a few associated plasma cells and the occasional eosinophil. Lipid may be demonstrated within the areas of 'necrobiosis' with Sudan stains and there may also be small amounts of mucin.

This histological picture resembles that of granuloma annulare; however, that condition in general has more mucin, more defined areas of necrobiosis, less lipid, no plasma cells and a neat palisade of histiocytes around the areas of necrobiosis. Granuloma annulare can also mimic necrobiosis lipoidica clinically and in a series of 100 patients with generalized granuloma annulare, nine had scalp or face involvement. On the scalp, distinction between these two conditions may rest on the morphology of associated lesions elsewhere on the skin.

The course of necrobiosis lipoidica is unrelated to the duration of the diabetes or to diabetic control, but it may coexist with other complications of diabetes. In 14% of cases it precedes the onset of diabetes, sometimes by as much as 2 years, so those patients not known to be diabetic should be investigated with a fasting blood glucose.

Local injections of triamcinolone or potent topical steroids under occlusion can improve the appearance of the lesions of necrobiosis lipoidica, however, the atrophy and scarring remain. Local excision and grafting of lesions may produce a

cure, although the necrobiosis lipoidica can recur. Once a site is stable it can be removed and hair bearing flaps swung in to restore the defect. Alternatively hair transplantation into the affected area can be performed.

Generalized granuloma annulare tends not to remit spontaneously, but may respond to a number of treatments. Topical and intralesional steroids may halt extension of this type of scarring alopecia. Oral steroids are effective and low dose systemic chlorambucil is useful for (widespread) unresponsive disease. Cryotherapy has been used, however, overzealous freezing may itself produce a permanent alopecia. Oxpentifylline, dapsone and antimalarials have also been used with varying success.

Sarcoidosis

Sarcoidosis is a multisystem disease characterized by the formation of noncaseating epithelioid granulomas in affected organs. Sarcoidosis only rarely occurs in the scalp. Most cases involve black women. Occasionally cicatricial alopecia is the first manifestation of sarcoidosis.

The lesions may initially be papular or nodular (Fig. 8.50)

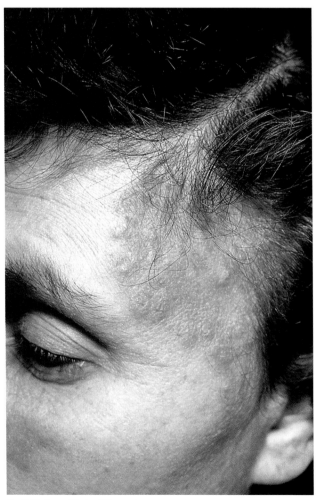

Fig. 8.50 Sarcoidosis of the scalp.

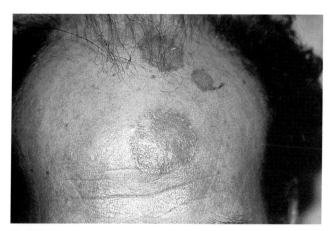

Fig. 8.51 Annular sarcoidosis of the scalp.

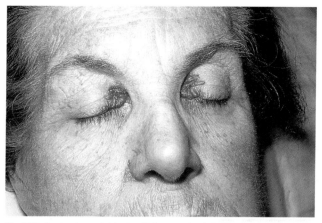

Fig. 8.53 Systemic amyloidosis with haemorrhagic lesions around the eyelids.

and coalesce to form plaques, which flatten to leave areas of cicatricial alopecia showing variable degrees of erythema and scaling. These plaques may have a slightly raised annular border, but are otherwise nondescript (Fig. 8.51). In the absence of characteristic lesions elsewhere on the skin or a known diagnosis of sarcoid, the diagnosis is made by demonstrating the characteristic naked, noncaseating epithelioid granulomas on biopsy. Special stains for acid-fast bacilli and fungi are negative. The Kveim test is no longer routinely used to confirm the diagnosis of sarcoid.

Topical or intralesional steroids should be tried first. Resistant cases will require systemic steroid to control the alopecia. Long-term maintenance therapy with low dose methotrexate as a steroid sparing agent is usually successful. The prognosis is variable, but treatment is required for at least 6 months in the vast majority.

Amyloidosis

Amyloid is a proteinaceous material that is deposited in tissues in a wide variety of conditions. The β-structure of the amyloid fibrils is resistant to proteolysis and so once deposited in tissues the amyloid persists indefinitely The different proteins that make up the fibrils in different disorders account for the various clinical manifestations.

Systemic amyloidosis occurs when a serum acute phase protein is synthesized in excess in response to continued inflammation; or an immunoglobulin light chain component is produced in excess as a result of paraproteinaemia. The protein precipitates and is deposited perivascularly in a number of tissues and produces disease.

Cutaneous amyloid (Fig. 8.52) develops when an as yet unidentified protein derived from filamentous degeneration of the epidermis is deposited in the papillary dermis; however, there is no involvement of internal organs.

In myeloma (or paraproteinaemia) related amyloidosis, the most characteristic lesions are yellow, waxy papules, which may be haemorrhagic. They occur on the face, particularly around the eyelids (Fig. 8.53), and on the scalp. Nodules and plaques may also occur in systemic amyloidosis, but these are rare on the scalp. Diffuse infiltrates may mimic scleroderma (Fig. 8.54).

Alopecia may be a conspicuous feature of systemic amyloidosis. Both a diffuse loss and a patchy loss of scalp hair can occur. Body hair may also be lost. Diffuse hair loss is associated with a loss of hair pigment and caused by cycling

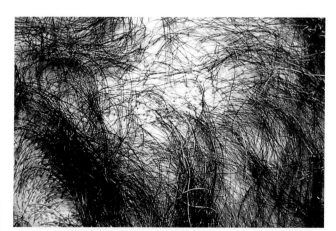

Fig. 8.52 Lichen amyloidosis of the scalp.

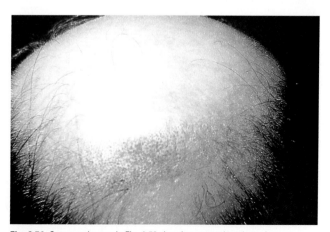

Fig. 8.54 Same patient as in Fig. 8.53 showing extensive alopecia.

hairs failing to re-enter anagen (a prolonged latent phase). Alopecia universalis has been described as a manifestation of occult systemic amyloidosis. Patchy loss is due to destruction of the pilosebaceous units by periappendageal deposition of amyloid. The proteinaceous material surrounds and compresses the hair follicle inducing atrophy and early loss of the hair.

Histology is diagnostic. In systemic amyloid there is deposition of amorphous masses of material perivascularly, periappendageally and in the subcutaneous fat (amyloid rings). In cutaneous amyloid, deposits are found either in the subepidermal region (macular and lichen amyloidosis), or diffusely throughout the entire dermis and subcutis (nodular amyloid). The amyloid protein stains red with congo red, and there is green birefringence when viewed with a polarized light.

Potent topical steroids are used for the lesions of cutaneous amyloid, but there is no treatment known to be effective for systemic amyloid other than treatment of the underlying disorder.

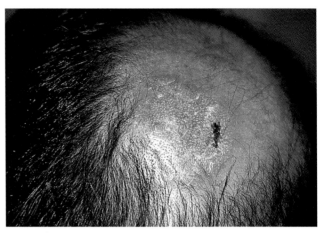

Fig. 8.56 Follicular mucinosis of the scalp.

Follicular mucinosis

Follicular mucinosis occurs in two forms: a primary idiopathic form and a secondary form. The secondary form is most commonly associated with lymphoma, especially mycosis fungoides, but it has also been associated with chronic DLE, angiolymphoid hyperplasia with eosinophilia and verruca vulgaris. The clinical features of primary and secondary cases are indistinguishable.

Primary follicular mucinosis can occur at any age from early childhood onwards, but is most common between the ages of 10 and 40 years. Secondary follicular mucinosis tends to occur in an older age group.

Follicular mucinosis consists of grouped, sometimes itchy, follicular papules and erythematous, boggy plaques that occur mainly on the head and face (Figs 8.55 & 8.56), but they can occur anywhere. Some may ulcerate. Characteristically the plaques are devoid of hair and patulous follicular openings are visible to the naked eye. The follicles are sometimes studded with horny plugs, and mucin can be expressed from the affected follicles. Hair loss is not obligatory and for this reason the name follicular mucinosis is preferred to the original name alopecia mucinosa. Linear lesions following Blaschko's lines have been described.

In the secondary group the lesions may be widely disseminated on the trunk and limbs. Untreated the plaques often resolve spontaneously within 2 months to 2 years, but in older patients they may be more persistent. Some 15–20% of these chronic cases are associated with mycosis fungoides.

All cases require a biopsy to confirm the diagnosis and to look for histological evidence of mycosis fungoides. The histology is characteristic and demonstrates reticular degeneration of hair follicles and sebaceous glands associated with copious mucin (hyaluronic acid), especially in the outer root sheath of the hair follicle (Fig. 8.57). A variable dermal inflammatory infiltrate is present and should be studied carefully for evidence of mycosis fungoides. In many cases the

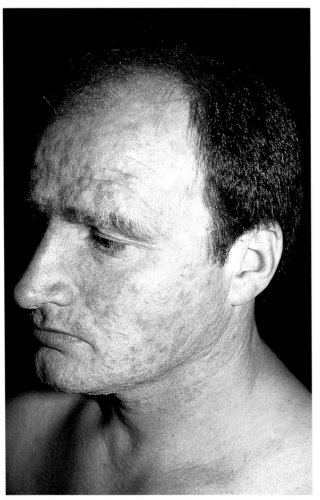

Fig. 8.55 Follicular mucinosis of the face.

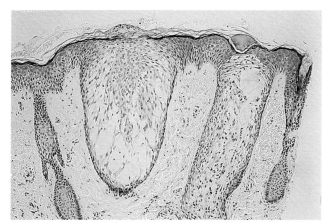

Fig. 8.57 Photomicrograph showing clear cell degeneration of the hair follicles. (Courtesy of Dorovitch Pathology, Melbourne.)

features of mycosis fungoides are subtle. In such cases only regular follow-up of the patient will distinguish primary from secondary causes of follicular mucinosis.

Many cases spontaneously improve and topical or intralesional steroids may hasten this. Superficial radiotherapy helps cases secondary to mycosis fungoides. Widespread pruritic lesions may benefit from PUVA, low-dose systemic steroids or occasionally dapsone. Unresponsive patients for whom radiotherapy is undesirable are very difficult to treat and follicular mucinosis can run a prolonged course.

Porokeratosis of Mibelli

Porokeratosis of Mibelli presents as a distinctive, irregular, annular lesion with a bald, atrophic centre and a raised hyperkeratotic border. The hands and feet are the most frequent sites followed by the limbs, neck, shoulders, face and scalp. The border is the clinical correlate of the cornoid lamella seen on histology. Local excision is curative. Extension of the lesion can be halted with cryosurgery, however, the central alopecia does not resolve.

Mastocytosis

Mastocytosis comprises a group of disorders in which mast cells are present in the skin in excessive numbers. Solitary mastocytomas may occur on the scalp and resolve with cicatricial alopecia. Telangiectasia macularis eruptiva perstans (TMEP) presents later in life with generalized telangiectasias and only rarely involves the scalp. Biopsy confirms the overabundance of mast cells.

Lipoid proteinosis

Lipoid proteinosis is a rare autosomal recessive metabolic disorder that characteristically produces a hoarse voice, beaded papules on the eyelids, cutaneous nodules, oral mucosal infiltrates and occasionally a scarring alopecia. Widespread internal involvement occurs but the condition in general runs a benign course.

Section E
Developmental disorders

Chapter 9

Hereditary and congenital alopecias and hypotrichosis

9.1 Definition and nomenclature

Hereditary and congenital alopecias and hypotrichosis are among the most complex areas of diseases of the hair and scalp. Literally hundreds of distinct clinical entities have been described. The field is akin to stamp collecting with each new condition having a distinctive characteristic that distinguishes it from syndromes previously described. In addition many new cases defy a specific diagnosis.

Different classifications have been postulated for the hereditary and congenital alopecias, but until the pathogenesis of these conditions is known, classification is usually based on morphology and as a result is cumbersome, confusing and often inadequate.

At present genetic studies seem to be increasing the complexity of inherited disorders by identifying genetic heterogeneity (phenocopies) within disease complexes. Hopefully, genetics will eventually identify unifying concepts that link apparently disparate disorders. Once this occurs, a new classification based on the genetic considerations will allow simplification of these disorders.

The classification used in Table 9.1 is based firstly on whether the hair loss is focal or diffuse, secondly on whether there are associated disorders and thirdly on whether within a multisystem disorder the hair loss is a major feature of the syndrome or an incidental finding.

Specific treatment is only discussed where appropriate. The aim of management is an accurate diagnosis for purposes of explanation, reassurance, detecting associated abnormalities, predicting the natural history and genetic counselling.

9.2 Aplasia cutis congenita and focal dermal hypoplasia

Definition

The focal absence of skin may occur anywhere on the body, but around 85% are found on the scalp. The depth of the ulcer is variable, and the defect may comprise epidermis alone, epidermis and dermis, and in some cases the cranial vault. Occasionally lesions heal completely *in utero*, and the child is born with a scar devoid of appendages.

Focal dermal hypoplasia is a hereditary ectodermal dysplasia, with a number of distinctive clinical features, while focal facial dermal hypoplasia tends to occur as an isolated abnormality.

Epidemiology

Aplasia cutis congenita (ACC) is a congenital anomaly seen in 0.03% of live births.

Aetiology

Aplasia cutis congenita can be sporadic, familial with an autosomal dominant inheritance (Fig. 9.1) or the hallmark of a syndrome (Table 9.2).

Pathogenesis

Several hypotheses have been proposed to explain ACC. Most have emphasized mechanical, vascular or developmental factors. The intrauterine development of the scalp occurs

Table 9.1 Congenital and hereditary causes of scarring alopecia and hypotrichosis.

Cause	Page reference
Isolated focal developmental alopecia	
Aplasia cutis congenita	129
Focal dermal hypoplasia	129
Sebaceous naevus	216
Epidermal naevus	216
Developmental cysts (hair collar sign)	30
Triangular alopecia	132
Occipital alopecia of the newborn	10
Porokeratosis of mibelli	125
Isolated diffuse developmental alopecia	
Atrichia congenita (AD, and AR)	133
Hereditary hypotrichosis	133
Marie Unna hypotrichosis	139
Developmental alopecia with associated disorders	
Ectodermal dysplasia	140
Keratosis pilaris decalvans	141
Ichthyosis follicularis	143
Atrichia congenita with papular cysts	135
Atrichia with mental retardation	135
Moynahan syndrome	148
Jeanselme and Rime hypotrichosis	145
Chondrodysplasia punctata (Conradi syndrome)	146
Cartilage hair hypoplasia	146
Hypomelia–hypotrichosis–facial haemangioma	148
Developmental disorders with associated alopecia	
Facial hemiatrophy	115
Epidermolysis bullosa	118
Ichthyosis	141
Premature ageing syndromes	150
Down's syndrome	152
Kleinfelter's syndrome	152
Other hereditary hypotrichosis syndromes	145
Bazex syndrome	149
Dyskeratosis congenita	148
Incontinentia pigmenti	148
Dubowitz syndrome	149
Johanson–Blizzard syndrome	149
Myotonic dystrophy	149
Cronkhite Canada syndrome	150
Mendes Da Costa syndrome	150
Baraitser's syndrome	150

AD, autosomal dominant; AR, autosomal recessive.

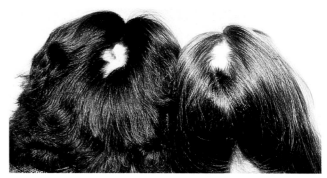

Fig. 9.1 Aplasia cutis congenita in a mother and daughter.

present as a scar. Lesions may be oval, linear, rhomboidal or stellate in shape. In up to 20% of cases the aplasia includes the dura with lysis of the underlying skull. The defect is usually 1–2 cm in diameter, but may be much larger (Fig. 9.3). The ulcer usually heals rapidly in the postnatal period to produce an atrophic, or rarely a hypertrophic scar. Most commonly the lesions are solitary (70–75% of cases), however, in 20% there are double and in 8% triple lesions. Lesions that involve the calvaria pose a risk of meningitis or haemorrhage.

Focal dermal hypoplasia (Figs 9.4 & 9.5) or Goltz syndrome is an X-linked dominant disorder of ectodermal and mesodermal tissues, lethal *in utero* in males. Sporadic cases

Table 9.2 Clinical subtypes of aplasia cutis based on associated findings.

Type 1	*T*raumatic or idiopathic ACC
Type 2	ACC with *i*ncomplete limbs (distal limb reduction abnormalities with or without persistent cutis marmorata—the Adams Oliver syndrome)
Type 3	ACC with associated epidermal or organoid *n*aevi
Type 4	ACC overlying *e*mbryonic defects such as omphalocele, myelomeningocele or encephalomeningocele or overlying occult visceral *a*bnormalities
Type 5	ACC with foetus *p*apyraceous
Type 6	ACC as a feature of *e*pidermolysis bullosa
Type 7	ACC secondary to teratogenic *d*rugs such as methimazole
Type 8	ACC secondary to intrauterine herpes zoster or simplex *i*nfection
Type 9	ACC in malformation *s*yndromes such as EEC syndrome, focal dermal hypoplasia, Hallerman–Streiff syndrome, Johanson–Blizzard syndrome, ectodermal dysplasia (ED) of Carey and ED of Tufti

ACC, aplasia cutis congenita; EEC, ectrodactyly, ectodermal dysplasia, cleft lip and palate.
Other congenital conditions that are occasional associations of ACC include: cleft lip and palate, tracheo-oesophageal fistula, double uterus, patent ductus arteriosus, polycystic kidneys, mental retardation, cutis marmorata, and ocular abnormalities.
The letters in italic spell *Tinea pedis* which is a useful *aide mémoire* for the subtypes of ACC.

from the periphery to the vertex, where the growing islands of skin fuse. Aplasia cutis congenita occurs most commonly over the parietal whorl and usually represents a failure of skin fusion.

Clinical features

Aplasia cutis congenita may present at birth as a sharply circumscribed ulcer with a red raw base simulating a wound (Fig. 9.2) or it may have completely healed *in utero* and

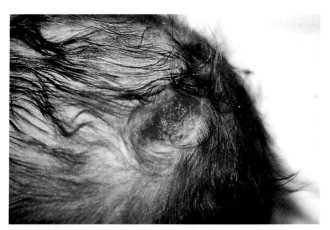

Fig. 9.2 Aplasia cutis in infancy showing a sharply circumscribed ulcer with a red base.

have occurred in males with either an XXY karyotype, a gametic half chromatid mutation or a somatic mutation early in embryogenesis. Females demonstrate Lyonization*, due to random inactivation of the X chromosome, and present with streaks of dermal hypoplasia, hypopigmentation, telangiectasia and herniations or hamartomas of fat following Blaschko's lines (Fig. 9.6). In some cases an autosomal dominant inheritance has been observed and the proposed gene for this variant mapped to chromosome 9.

Osteopathia striata is the radiological hallmark and represents Lyonization of chondroblasts. Other characteristics of this syndrome are an aged leonine facies, absent eyebrows, puckered periorbital skin, a rubbery texture to the nose and chin and congenital symmetrical scar-like defects on each temple following Blaschko's lines. These scar-like defects are seen in between 10 and 50% of cases and are hairless, pigmented, puckered areas above the eyebrows, that extend upwards and outwards.

* The Lyon hypothesis states that:
1 In the somatic cells of female mammals, only one X chromosome is active. The second X chromosome is condensed and inactive and appears in interphase cells as the sex chromatin (Barr body).
2 Inactivation occurs early in embryonic life (12th to 16th day post-fertilization).
3 The inactive X can be either the paternal or the maternal X (X^P or X^M) in different cells of the same individual; but after the decision as to which X will be inactivated has been made in a particular cell, all the clonal descendants of that cell will abide by that decision and will have the same inactive X. Thus inactivation is random but fixed. The relative proportions of X^P to X^M vary from female to female even in identical twins.
4 If the mutation is present only in somatic cells, all the descendants of these cells will be affected, but the abnormality will not be transmitted to subsequent generations. However, if the mutation is also present in the gametes then the abnormality is heritable.

Pathology

Histologically, there is atrophy of the dermal and subcutaneous tissues and loss of the pilosebaceous units, but the epidermis is normal. Striated muscle can be seen high in the dermis and may be responsible for the puckered appearance. Focal facial dermal hypoplasia produces very similar symmetrical temporal scar-like lesions, without any associated defects. It is inherited as an autosomal dominant trait.

Investigation

None usually required for aplasia cutis.

Associated features

Aplasia cutis most commonly occurs as an isolated defect, however, in 20–25% of cases, associated developmental defects are present. The wide spectrum of associated disorders has been classified into nine different subtypes of ACC (Table 9.2).

Prognosis

The patch of hair loss is fixed.

Treatment

Parents often suspect obstetric mismanagement to be the cause of the ACC and a detailed explanation of the condition is often required to placate them. If the lesion is deep or does not heal quickly, skin grafting is usually advocated to counter the risk of infection.

Once healed a small lesion requires no treatment. When the child is older, consideration may be given to surgical excision with primary closure to correct the alopecia. For larger areas tissue expanders may be required. Hair transplantation is a reasonable alternative.

Key points

Congenital absence of skin over the vertex usually occurs as a developmental defect, rather than as a result of obstetric trauma. Healing usually occurs spontaneously to leave a patch of alopecia that can be corrected when the child is older. Associated developmental abnormalities should be sought.

Focal dermal hypoplasia is an unrelated condition that also produces scar-like lesions, but the epidermis is intact. It is an X-linked dominant syndrome lethal in males. Focal facial dermal hypoplasia occurs as an isolated autosomal dominant defect.

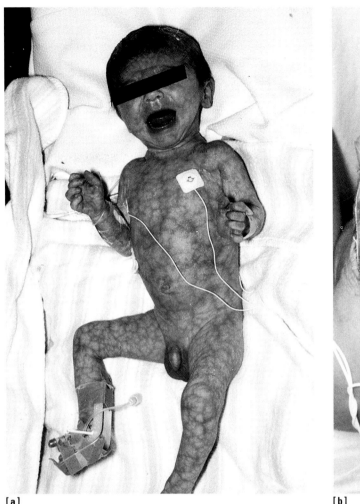

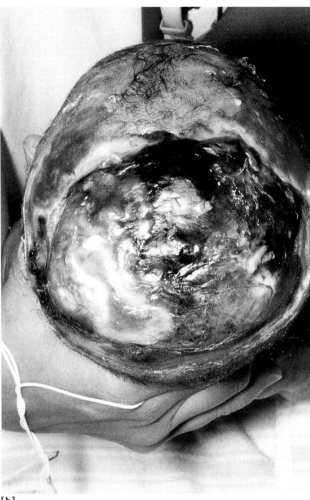

[a]   [b]

Fig. 9.3 Adams Oliver syndrome with (a) cutis mamarata telangiectasia, abnormal development of the right foot and (b) extensive aplasia cutis congenita. (Courtesy of POSSUM.)

9.3 Triangular alopecia

Definition

Congenital triangular alopecia is a nonscarring alopecia of the scalp, first described by Sabouraud in 1905. An acquired form of triangular alopecia also occurs.

Epidemiology

Relatively rare.

Aetiology

Noninherited, isolated, developmental defect.

Pathogenesis

The alopecia is produced by the replacement of terminal hairs with cosmetically insignificant vellus hairs.

Clinical features

Whilst often present at birth, congenital triangular alopecia is generally not noticed by the parents until the child is between 3 and 6 years and the surrounding hair has become pigmented and thickened. The characteristic patch of nonscarring alopecia is located above the ear overlying the frontotemporal suture and is triangular in shape with the apex of the triangle pointing towards the vertex (Fig. 9.7). The alopecia measures between 3 and 5 cm from apex to base. This distribution seems to follow Blaschko's lines and triangular alopecia may be a naevoid abnormality. While usually unilateral, triangular alopecia is occasionally bilateral.

A late onset form of this condition has been described. The site and appearance are the same as the congenital form, and it is distinguished from androgenetic alopecia by being unilateral. The postulated mechanism is a local hypersensitivity to androgens, as the biopsy shows features of androgenetic

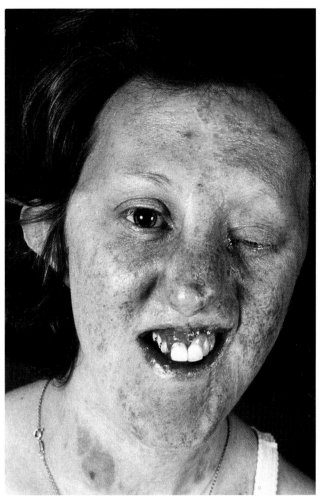

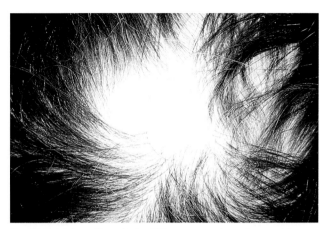

Fig. 9.5 Focal dermal hypoplasia within an area on the scalp resembling aplasia cutis congenita.

Fig. 9.4 Focal dermal hypoplasia with asymmetry, loss of the eyebrows and streaks of hyperpigmentation that follow Blaschko's lines. (Courtesy of POSSUM.)

alopecia. Acquired triangular alopecia may first appear at any age.

Pathology

Histology of affected areas shows a normal epidermis and numerous vellus hair follicles. There is no scarring.

Investigation

A scalp biopsy may be helpful.

Diagnosis

Acquired triangular alopecia needs to be distinguished from AA and androgenetic alopecia. While androgenetic alopecia usually produces bitemporal recession, it may be asymmetrical in its early phases.

Associated features

None.

Prognosis

The natural history is for congenital triangular alopecia to remain unchanged throughout life, however, some cases of acquired triangular alopecia resolve spontaneously.

Treatment

No treatment is usually required. Hair transplants can be effective, and excision and primary repair following the use of tissue expanders, has also been successfully used.

Key points

Congenital triangular alopecia is a nonscarring alopecia with a characteristic shape and location, that is due to the presence of an island of vellus hairs amidst the terminal hairs of the scalp. Acquired triangular alopecia may result from a localized hypersensitivity to androgens. It differs from androgenetic alopecia by being unilateral.

9.4 Congenital hypotrichosis and atrichia

Definition

There are several apparently distinctive genotypes, that share as a common phenotype a total and permanent absence of hair, or atrichia congenita.

Congenital hypotrichosis is a less severe form of the same process, where hair is present, but is diffusely thinned. Scarring may or may not be present. It may occur as an isolated defect or as just one manifestation of a more generalized disorder.

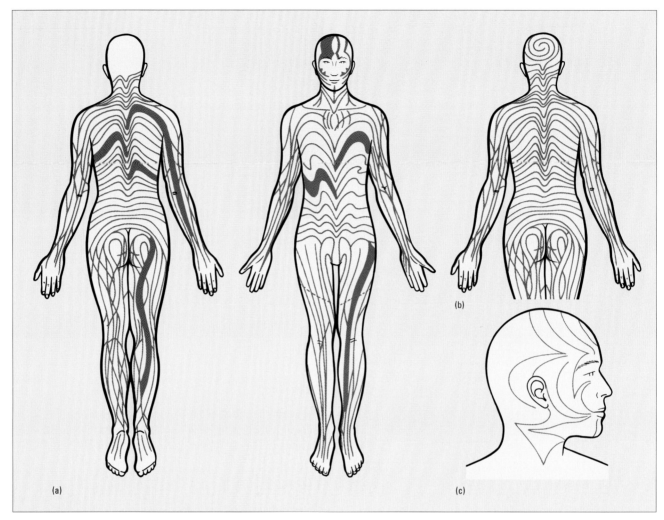

Fig. 9.6 Blaschko's lines on the body and scalp.

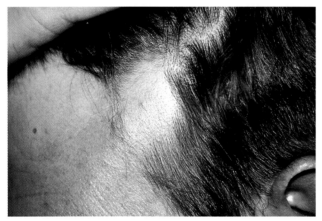

Fig. 9.7 Triangular alopecia in an adult. This occurs more laterally than the bitemporal recession in androgenetic alopecia. The alopecia is nonscarring.

Epidemiology

Rare.

Aetiology

Most cases of atrichia congenita and congenital hypotrichosis are autosomal recessive and are not associated with any other developmental abnormalities. Several autosomal dominant pedigrees have also been described in the literature with subtle differences

Pathogenesis

The hair loss is either due to follicular agenesis or programmed destruction. Loss within the first year is probably due to an abnormality that affects the unsynchronized postnatal pelage (which develops at approximately 12 months of age), but spares the first two synchronized hair moults that begin *in utero* at 26 weeks and 38 weeks gestation (and are complete by 12 weeks of age). The explanation for atrichia

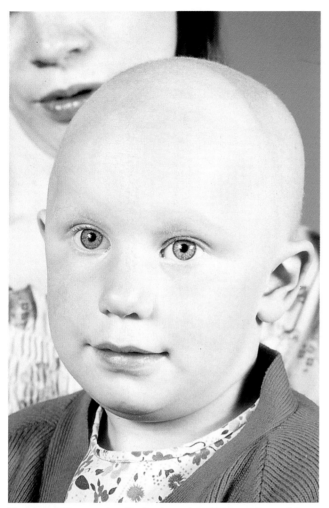

Fig. 9.8 Atrichia congenita affecting the scalp, eyebrows and most of the eyelashes. Alopecia areata can be distinguished on histology.

congenita developing later in childhood, the so called acquired form, is unclear, but may involve two (or more) successive gene mutations akin to Knudson's hypothesis for the development of retinoblastoma*.

Clinical features

In atrichia congenita (Fig. 9.8) the child may be either completely bald at birth; or the normal coat of lanugo hair may be

*In 1971 Knudson proposed an hypothesis explaining the inheritance of bilateral retinoblastoma that is now readily accepted. Development of this malignancy requires two successive gene mutations: the first is inherited as an autosomal dominant trait in the germ line and consequently is present in all somatic cells; the second is somatic, occurring in a retinal cell. Since the second change is a random one the retinoblastoma may then occur in only one eye or not at all. Sporadic cases require two mutations in the somatic cell line to initiate the tumour. As this is unlikely to happen in both eyes, such cases are always unilateral and since the germ cells are unaffected, it is not heritable.

present and then gradually lost. It may take up to 5 years before all this hair disappears.

In some of the autosomal recessive (AR) pedigrees of atrichia congenita, lanugo hair is normal at birth, but is soon shed and never replaced. Hair follicles are absent, but sebaceous glands are normal in number, albeit small. In other AR pedigrees the children are bald from birth.

Atrichia with papular cysts is a variant of autosomal recessive atrichia congenita, where in addition to scalp hair loss, numerous pin-head sized, white, smooth epidermoid cysts develop around the time of puberty on the cheeks.

In autosomal dominant (AD) atrichia congenita the hair is normal until about the age of 5 years when it is replaced by short, sparse hair of a lighter colour. Diffuse thinning of the scalp hair tends to progress, such that by the late-teens very few hairs remain on the scalp.

The related condition of Madarosis is the congenital absence of eyebrows. Inheritance is AD and within a family the scalp hair may or may not also be affected.

Atrichia congenita associated with atrophoderma vermiculata and epidermoid cysts is probably an autosomal dominant condition and histology shows scarring alopecia (Fig. 9.9).

Hereditary hypotrichosis (Fig. 9.10) may also occur as an isolated anomaly, present either from birth or first noticed around the age of three. The severity of the hypotrichosis is extremely variable. Most cases are sporadic, and scarring is not a prominent feature.

Investigation

A scalp biopsy may be useful to exclude AA and for prognostic reasons.

Diagnosis

The absence of ichthyosis and the normal nails, teeth and sweat glands seen in the various forms of atrichia congenita separates them from ectodermal dysplasias with atrichia or hypotrichosis (Table 9.3). Alopecia totalis rarely occurs in the first year of life.

Prognosis

The hair loss is usually permanent.

Treatment

Wigs are the only appropriate treatment as there is no donor hair available for transplantation, and there is no medical therapy. Psychological support of the parents initially, and later the child is important.

Key points

Total baldness, occurring either at birth or delayed for up to 10 years occurs either as part of an ectodermal dysplasia or

Table 9.3 An abbreviated list of the ectodermal dysplasias associated with abnormalities of the hair (modified from Olsen).

Ectodermal dysplasia (ED)	Inheritance	Hair (1)	Conical teeth (2)	Nail dystrophy (3)	Decreased sweating (4)	Associated features
1-2-3-4						
Anhidrotic ED (Christ, Siemens, Touraine)	XLR	Sparse, pale, fine, short, increases at puberty	+	+	+	Distinctive facies, absent nipples, recurrent URTIs
Hypohidrotic ED	AR	Sparse, pale, fine, short	+	+	+	The sweating defect is less severe than in the XLR form
RAPP–Hodgkin syndrome	AD	Sparse, pale, like steel wool	+	+	+	Distinctive facies, deafness +/– syndactyly
Ectrodactyly ED, cleft lip & palate (EEC)	AD	Sparse, light, wiry	+	+	+	Lobster-claw hand, CLP
Rosselli–Guilienetti	AR	Downy, fair, thin, woolly	+	+	+	Distinctive facies, CL2, syndactyly, abnormal genitalia
Alopecia–Onycho dysplasia-hypohidrosis-deafness	?	Bald	+	+	+	Deafness, PPK, toenails affected, but fingernails normal
Basan syndrome	AD	Hair normal until shed second decade	+	+	+	Absent dermoglyphic pattern
Greither type	AD	Bald	+	+	+	Blindness, PPK
Xeroderma-talipes-enamel defect	AR	Sparse, coarse, slow growing	+	+	+	CLP talipes, MD and EEG abnormalities
Ankyloblepharon–ED-cleft lip & palate	AD	Fine, wiry, sparse or absent	+	+	+	Syndactyly, abnormal ears, eyes and nipples
Anonychia & flexural pigmentation	AD	Coarse and sparse	+	+	+	Bizarre, mottled flexural hyperpigmentation, nails absent from birth
Tricho-odonto-dental dysplasia	DA	Curly hair that later straightens	+	+	+	Distinctive facies, taurodontic molars
Keratosis, ichthyosis, deafness (KID) syndrome	AD?	Diffuse, fine, sparse or absent; improves with time	+	+	+	Distinctive facies, blindness, ichthyosis, deafness
Pachyonychia congenita	AD	Generalized hypotrichosis in >10% and kinky hair	+	+	+	Grossly thickened nails, PPK with bullae, keratosis pilaris, leukoplakia, warts
Focal dermal hypoplasia (Goltz syndrome)	XL	Sparse, brittle hair and focal areas of aplasia cutis	+	+	+	Limb asymmetry, syndactyly, ectrodactyly, focal dermal hypoplasia, eye abnormality
Zanier-Roubicek syndrome	AD	Hypotrichosis	+	+	+	Decreased tearing, mammary hypoplasia
Carey ED	?	Thin, pale hair and focal aplasia cutis	+	+	+	Deafness, syndactyly, absent tear ducts
Tuffli ED	AD	Aplasia cutis	+	+	+	Delayed dentition, breast hypoplasia
Hypohidrosis with diabetes insipitus	?	Hypotrichosis	+	+	+	Diabetes insipitus, syndactyly, coloboma, abnormal haematopoiesis
Another syndrome	AR	Hypotrichosis and brittle hair	+	+	+	Clinodactyly, syndactyly, hypothyroidism, ephelides, CVS, respiratory & GIT abnormalities
1-2-3						
Hidrotic ED (Clouston)	AD	Sparse, fine, pale or absent	+	+	+/–	Keratoderma, patchy hyperpigmentation, cataracts, clubbing
Tricho-dento-osseous syndrome	AD	Curly scalp hair that later straightens	+	+	–	Distinctive facies, cortical bone sclerosis, clinodactyly
Trichorhinopharyngeal syndrome I & II	AD or AR	Sparse, pale, brittle hair & temporal alopecia	+	+	–	Abnormal facies, brachicphalyngeal dystosis, high arched palate, hyperextensible joints
Tricho-odonto-onychial dysplasia I	AD	Hypotrichosis & follicular papules	+	+	–	Absent nipples or mammaries, deafness, pigment anomalies, abnormal facies with linear scars
Tricho-odonto-onychial dysplasia & pili torti	?	Sparse blond hair & pili torti	+	+	–	Abnormal facies
Tricho-oculo-dermo-vertebral syndrome	AR	Hypotrichosis, dry & rough hair	+	+	–	PPK, ichthyosiform macules, kyphoscoliosis. skeletal abnormality, entropion
Tricho-odonto-onychodermal syndrome	AD	Hypotrichosis, aplasia cutis	+	+	–	Xerosis, poikiloderma, absent nipples, abnormal facies, clinodactyly, syndactyly, absent digits
Odonto-onychial dysplasia with alopecia	?AR	Total alopecia	+	+	–	Syndactyly, PPK, breast & ocular abnormalities
Odontotrichomelic syndrome (Freire–Maia)	AR?	Severe generalized hypotrichosis	+	+	–	Abnormal facies, hypoplastic areola, tetramelic aplasia, EEG abnormalities
Oculo-dental-digital syndrome	AD or AR	Hypotrichosis, dry brittle hair	+	+	–	Mild MR, CLP, deafness, polydactyly, camptodactyly, syndactyly, hypophalangy, abnormal facies, abnormal eyes

Syndrome	Inheritance	Hair			Clinical features
Oculotrichodysplasia	AR	Generalized hypotrichosis	+	+	Xerosis, retinitis pigmentosa
Dermo-odonto dysplasia	AD	Hypotrichosis, fragile hair, focal alopecia	+	+	Freckles, moles, xerosis, PPK, accessory nipples, simian creases, abnormal dermatoglyphics
Hypodontia and nail dysgenesis	AD	Fine and brittle, improves with age	+	+	Premature wrinkles, abnormal facies
Freids tooth and nail syndrome	AR	Marked hypotrichosis, twisting	+	+	Abnormal facies, cleft lip, branchial neck cyst
Schloph–Schultz–Passarge syndrome	AR	Marked hypotrichosis	+	+	Follicular hyperkeratosis, PPK, eyelid apocrine hidrocystomas
Schinzel–Giedion syndrome	AR	Generalized hypertrichosis	+	+	Telangiectasia simian creases, abnormal facies, skeletal, renal & cardiac abnormalities, MR & GR
Salamon's syndrome	AR	Wire-like, sparse hair, pili torti, weathering	+	+	Ocular abnormality, piriform nose
Chondroectodermal dysplasia	AR	Thin, brittle, fine, sparse hair	+	+	Chondrodysplasia, acromelic dwarfism, polydactyly, brachymetacarpy, cardiac abnormalities
Coffin–Siris syndrome	AD	Hypotrichosis scalp, hypertrichosis limbs, back & face	+	+	Abnormal facies, absent 5th terminal metacarpal, skeletal & cardiac abnormalities, eczema, peptic ulcer
Cranioectodermal syndrome	AR	Thin, short and very fine	+	+	Abnormal facies, hypotonia, rhizomelia, syndactyly, clinodactyly, osteoporosis, cardiac abnormalities
Incontinentia pigmenti	XLD	Hypotrichosis and linear alopecia	+	+	Infantile blisters, later linear verrucous lesions & whorled pigmentation CNS and retinal abnormality, CLP
Benign atrophic epidermolysis bullosa	AR?	Thin & lustreless hair, scarring alopecia	+	+	Traumatic blisters from birth, no secondary sexual hair, PPK, eye abnormalities
ED with pili torti and syndactyly	AR	Hypotrichosis, weathering, pili torti	+	+	Xerosis, syndactyly, lordosis, high arched palate, simian creases
ED with tetramelic disturbances	?	Hypotrichosis	+	+	Hypoplastic areola, absent clavicles, eye & CNS abnormalities
Mesomelic dwarfism-skeletal abnormalities-ED	?	Hypotrichosis	+	+	Abnormal facies, short forearms & hands, other skeletal abnormality, high arched palate
Dwarfism-alopecia-pseudoanondontia-cutis laxa	AR	Generalized atrichia	+	+	Cutis laxa, dwarfism, abnormal facies, hypoplastic breasts, ocular & skeletal abnormality, hepatosplenomegaly
Arthrogryphosis & ED	?	Congenital atrichia, hypotrichosis with pili torti	+	+	Syndactyly, clinodactyly, talipes equinovarus, arthrogryphosis all joints, easy bruising & scarring
Growth retardation, alopecia, pseudoanondontia, optic atrophy (GAPO) syndrome	AR	Progressive hair loss to produce atrichia	+.	+	Abnormal facies, optic & EEG abnormalities, hypoplastic breasts, hypogonadism & GR
1-2-4					
Congenital insensitivity to pain	AR	Hypotrichosis	+	−	Universal sensory loss, Charcot's joints, pseudo-ainhum
Regional ED with total bilateral cleft	?	Total alopecia	+	−	Ectropion, dermoid cysts scalp, CLP
ED with palatal paralysis	?	Absent frontal hair, brows & lashes	+	−	Deafness, palatal paralysis, abnormal speech
1-3-4					
Fischer syndrome	AD	Hypotrichosis	−	+	Syringomyelia, PPK, clubbing
Hayden's syndrome	?	Total alopecia, scalp infections	+	+	Follicular hyperkeratosis, PPK, deafness, conjunctivitis
Alopecia-onychodysplasia-hypohidrosis syndrome	?	Universal alopecia	+	+	Eczema, photophobia, epilepsy, nystagmus, hypospadius, MR
ED with severe mental retardation	?	Universal alopecia	−	+	Mental retardation, cataracts, absent breasts and nipples
Dermotrichic syndrome	XLR	Generalized atrichia	−	+	Ichthyosis, epilepsy, MR
Alopecia-onychodysplasia-hypohidrosis-hyperkeratosis-deafness	?	Severe generalized hypotrichosis	−	+	Deafness, PPK, photophobia, estropia

Continued on p. 138

Table 9.3 (*Continued.*)

Ectodermal dysplasia (ED)	Inheritance	Hair (1)	Conical teeth (2)	Nail dystrophy (3)	Decreased sweating (4)	Associated features
1-2						
Orofacial digital syndrome	XLD	Fine, dry, sparse	+	–	–	MR, facial, oral & skeletal abnormality, CLP, syndactyly, polydactyly, brachydactyly
Killian's syndrome	?	Hypotrichosis, weathering, frontal & parietal alopecia	+	–	–	Abnormal facies, MR, lax joints, deafness, high arched palate, hypopigmented patches
Hallerman–Streiff syndrome	AD or AR	Generalized hypotrichosis, focal alopecia, absent brows	+	–	–	MR, cataracts, focal cutaneous atrophy, cardiac abnormalities
Mikaelian's syndrome	AR	Sparse, coarse, brittle hair, late regrowth	+	–	–	MR, xerosis, arachnodactyly, deafness
Pili torti and enamel hypoplasia	AR	Pili torti & monilethrix	+	–	–	Generalized keratosis pilaris
Trichodental dysplasia	AD	Straight, fine, weathered scalp hair, sparse brows	+	–	–	Retained deciduous teeth
Acrorenal-ED-lipoatrophic diabetic syndrome	AR	Sparse, fine, slow growing hair	+	–	–	Lipoatrophic diabetes mellitus, mammary hypoplasia, skeletal abnormalities
Oculoosteocutaneous syndrome	AR?	Generalized hypotrichosis, fair thin hair	+	–	–	Ocular and skeletal abnormalities (large big toe), mammary & genital hypoplasia
Walbaum–Dehaene–Schlemmer syndrome	AR	Alopecia develops after infancy	+	–	–	Gingival hyperplasia
Agammaglobulinaemia-thymic dysplasia-ED	?	Near-universal alopecia	+	–	–	Ichthyosiform erythroderma with blisters, agammaglobulinaemia (IgG & IgA)
Wilson's syndrome	?	Near-universal alopecia	+	–	–	Unusual facies and preaxial polydactyly feet
Alopecia-anosmia-hypogonadism syndrome	AD	Severe hypotrichosis	+	–	–	Deafness, anosmia, cardiac, facial & pigmentary abnormality, hypogonadism, MR, CLP
Jeanselme and Rime hypotrichosis	AD	Congenital twisted hair progressing to total alopecia	+	–	–	Keratosis pilaris, thickened leathery scalp skin, red blotches on the face
1-3						
Palmer-plantar hyperkeratosis and alopecia	AD or AR	Sparse to absent scalp and body hair	–	+	–	PPK
Cantu's syndrome	AR	Hypotrichosis & short curly weathered hair	–	+	–	Chronic neutropenia, recurring infections, follicular hyperkeratosis
Trichoonychodysplasia with xeroderma	AR	Congenital universal alopecia with regrowth later	–	+	–	Severe xeroderma
Agammaglobulinaemia-dwarfism-ED	AR	Infantile onset atrichia	–	+	–	Ichthyosiform erythroderma, dwarfism, lymphopenia, agammaglobulinaemia, hypoplastic thymus
Skeletal anomalies-ED-growth and MR	?	Near universal alopecia	–	+	–	Skeletal abnormalities, abnormal facies, GR, MR, xerosis, syndactyly
Pili-torti and onychodysplasia	AD	Late childhood-onset hypotrichosis, pili torti	–	+	–	Nil
Sabina's brittle hair and mental deficiency	AR	Sparse, dry, coarse, weathered hair	–	+	–	Abnormal facies, MR, retinal abnormality, scalp hyperkeratosis
Cataracts-alopecia and syndactyly	AR	Universal alopecia	–	+	–	Cataracts, syndactyly, PPK, pseudo ainhum
Congenital atrichia, nail dystrophy, abnormal facies and psychomotor retardation	AR?	Kinky, sparse hair at birth progressing to total alopecia	–	+	–	Abnormal facies, MR, CL?
1-4						
Trichofacial hypohidrotic syndrome	XLR	Sparse, brittle hair	–	–	+	Abnormal facies, upper respiratory problems

AR, autosomal recessive; AD, autosomal dominant; XLR, X-linked recessive; XLD, X-linked dominant; MR, mental retardation; GR, growth retardation; CLP, cleft lip and palate; PPK, palmer-plantar keratoderma.

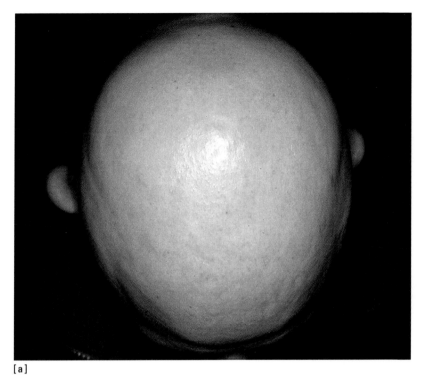
[a]

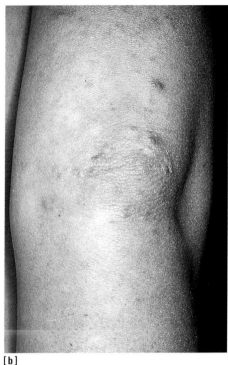
[b]

Fig. 9.9 Atrichia congenita with papular cysts. This case is different to the one previously reported where the cysts occurred on the face. In this man (a), hair was present up until the age of 5 and then it was progressively lost. He had associated atrophoderma vermiculata as well as the cysts on his elbows (b) that developed at the age of 15 and, on histology, were shown to be epidermoid cysts.

as an isolated defect not associated with nails, teeth, sweating or other developmental defects. These isolated developmental alopecias, known as atrichia congenita exist in both AD and AR forms, and may rarely be associated with papular epidermoid cysts and atrophoderma vermiculata. Body hair is generally normal, but the eyebrows may be lost in Madarosis.

Congenital hypotrichosis occurs as an isolated defect of variable severity and inheritance. Some hair remains in this condition.

9.5 Marie Unna hereditary hypotrichosis

Definition

An isolated, hereditary hypotrichosis described by Dr Marie Unna in 1925 in 27 members of one family spanning seven generations.

Epidemiology

Rare.

Aetiology

Autosomal dominant genodermatosis.

Pathogenesis

Unknown.

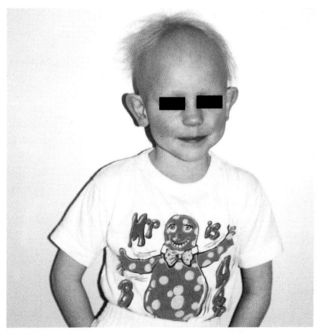

Fig. 9.10 Hereditary hypotrichosis. Hair follicle numbers were greatly diminished from birth in this child. Histology shows no inflammation and no scarring only a decreased density of follicles. This was best appreciated on a horizontal scalp biopsy.

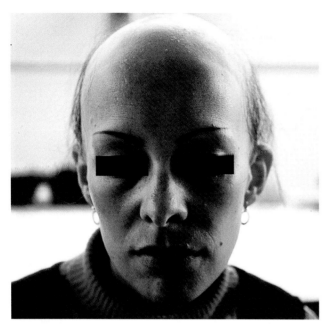

Fig. 9.11 Marie Unna hereditary hypotrichosis showing prominent alopecia over the vertex with some preservation of the marginal hairs. Hair microscopy revealed a twisting hair dystrophy, but not true pili torti.

Clinical features

The pattern of development of Marie Unna hypotrichosis is distinctive (Fig. 9.11). The hair may be normal, sparse or absent at birth. If present it remains fine and sparse for the first few years of life and during the third year it becomes coarse and twisted. If the hair was absent at birth it may regrow at this stage. The coarse, wiry hair is unruly and gives the impression that the child is wearing a second-rate wig.

At puberty, progressive loss begins at the vertex (and less so the margins) and produces a severe cicatricial alopecia. The eyebrows, eyelashes and body hair are typically absent from birth, and after puberty any axillary or pubic hair that develops is also sparse. Follicular hyperkeratosis and milia-like facial lesions may occur in association.

Pathology

Examination of the hair shafts with a scanning electron microscope shows flattening, irregular twisting and premature weathering of the hair, but the changes are not specific. In addition the hair shaft diameter is said to be thicker (100 mm) than normal (65–75 mm). Scalp biopsy shows a marked reduction in the number of follicles and evidence of scarring. There may be a granulomatous reaction around partly destroyed follicles, however, the histology is also nonspecific.

Investigation

Light and electron microscopy of hair shafts and scalp biopsies are required to make a positive diagnosis.

Diagnosis

Other causes of acquired cicatricial alopecia need to be excluded.

Associated features

Teeth, nails, skin and sweating are normal.

Prognosis

The condition tends to be slowly progressive, ultimately leading to complete hair loss.

Treatment

Minimizing hair trauma (see Table 10.2) may allow brittle hair to grow longer. No effective treatment is known for this genodermatosis. Genetic counselling is difficult due to variable expression.

Key points

An autosomal dominant hypotrichosis characterized by sparse hair at birth, that regrows curly at age 3 years, before a scarring alopecia progressively develops at the vertex and scalp margins during adolescence. Hair microscopy shows marked weathering. There are no associated abnormalities.

9.6 The ectodermal dysplasias

Ectodermal dysplasia (Figs 9.12–9.14) defines a group of inherited developmental syndromes with disorders in more than one ectoderm derived tissue. The defect presumably manifests during early embryological development some time after the third week postconception, when ectoderm can first be distinguished from mesoderm and endoderm, but before the end of the third month when ectodermal cells have become committed to differentiate into specific derivative structures.

Ectodermal cells during this period (between 3 weeks and 3 months) have the potential to develop into either neuroectoderm or surface ectoderm (Fig. 9.15).

Any developmental abnormality that damages ectodermal cells in the period prior to committed differentiation may result in abnormalities in the infant in a large number of organs. In general, those fetuses that survive to conception often manifest abnormalities of hair, nails, epidermis, teeth (Fig. 9.16) and eccrine glands. These abnormalities (Table 9.4) form the basis of classification for ectodermal dysplasias (Table 9.3).

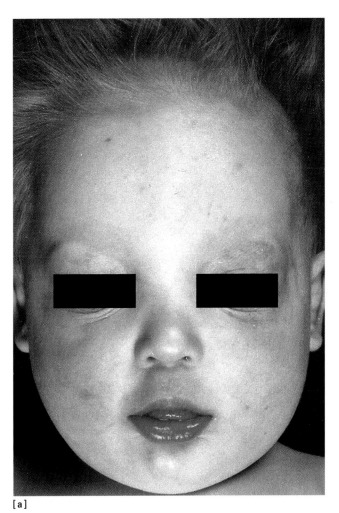

[a]

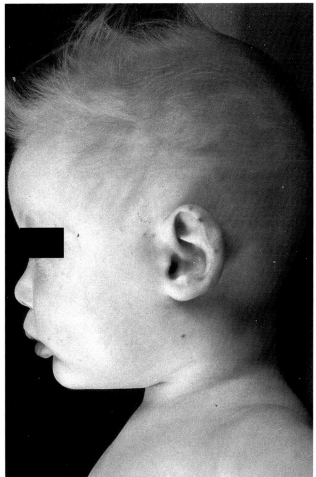

[b]

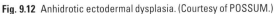

Fig. 9.12 Anhidrotic ectodermal dysplasia. (Courtesy of POSSUM.)

Other abnormalities that may occur include deafness, mental retardation, breast hypoplasia, cleft lip and palate, syndactyly, ectrodactyly (Fig. 9.17), skeletal abnormalities (Figs 9.16 & 9.17) and distinctive facies. Bony abnormalities, although reflecting an abnormality of a mesenchyme derived tissues, do not exclude a diagnosis of ectodermal dysplasia.

In order to fulfil the criteria for an ectodermal dysplasia, there must be a congenital, nonprogressive abnormality in at least two ectodermal derived tissues. For a fuller discussion, readers are referred to the parent textbook (Dawber, R. (ed.) (1997) *Diseases of the Hair and Scalp.* Blackwell Science, Oxford).

9.7 Keratosis pilaris and the follicular hyperkeratoses

Definition

Keratosis pilaris (KP) is the presence of multiple, discrete papules around follicular openings.

Epidemiology

Keratosis pilaris on its own is an exceptionally common condition, affecting up to 40% of the population. KP appears in childhood in 50%, the second decade in 35% and the third decade in a further 10–12%. Approximately half have a positive family history and a third have a personal history of atopy.

Aetiology

An AD disorder of keratinization.

Pathogenesis

Perifollicular hyperkeratosis produces the papules.

Clinical features

It is characterized by horny spines at the follicular orifices with varying degrees of perifollicular erythema (Fig. 9.18).

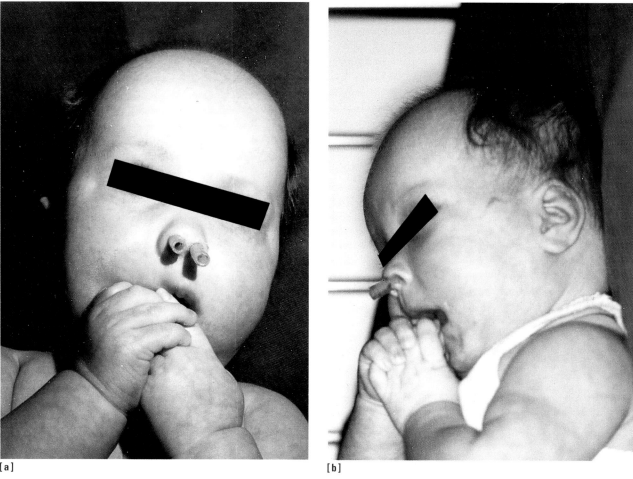

[a]   [b]

Fig. 9.13 Ectrodactyly, ectodermal dysplasia, cleft palate and lip syndrome. (Courtesy of POSSUM.)

They occur most commonly on the extensor surfaces of the upper arm, the thighs and buttocks. The condition is often asymptomatic, but can be mildly itchy. Coiled hairs may be seen (Fig. 9.19).

Pathology

Histology demonstrates follicular plugging and one or more twisted hair can be found within the plug.

Investigation

Not usually required. A biopsy may be required to distinguish keratosis pilaris decalvans from the Graham-Little syndrome or lichen planopilaris.

Diagnosis

Follicular ichthyosis, phrynoderma, Graham-Little syndrome, lichen planopilaris and lichen nitidis may all cause problems. Pityriasis rubra pilaris, Darrier's disease, lichen spinulosus and the follicular keratosis seen at amputation sites present less difficulty.

Associated features

Frequent associations include ichthyosis, xerosis or atopy, and KP is a feature of monilethrix, trichothiodystrophy, Noonan's syndrome, Down's syndrome and uraemia.

A number of conditions are been described where alopecia is associated with keratosis pilaris. The conditions where keratosis pilaris occurs with alopecia are listed in Table 9.5. The three main conditions are atrophoderma vermiculata, keratosis pilaris atrophicans facei and keratosis pilaris decalvans.

Atrophoderma vermiculata may be inherited in an autosomal dominant fashion. Although adult onset is described, it usually begins in childhood with follicular plugs, often in the preauricular area. The plugs are shed to leave a symmetrical reticulate or honeycomb atrophy of the cheeks (Fig. 9.20). The extent of the process is variable, involving on occasion the upper lip, ears or forehead. Coincidental scarring alopecia

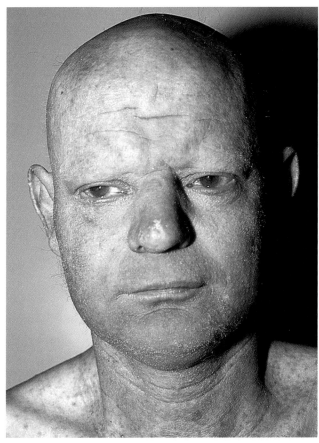

Fig. 9.14 Keratosis, ichthyosis, deafness (KID) syndrome demonstrating the alopecia and the ichthyosis. (Courtesy of Dr H. Rothstein, Melbourne.)

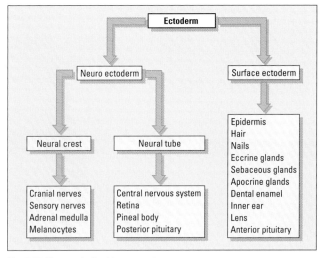

Fig. 9.15 Tissues derived from ectoderm.

Table 9.5 Conditions associated with keratosis pilaris and alopecia.

Atrophoderma vermiculata
Keratosis pilaris atrophicans facei
Keratosis pilaris decalvans
Ichthyosis follicularis with alopecia and photophobia
Atrichia with papular lesions and atrophoderma vermiculata
Alopecia, premature cataracts, widespread keratosis pilaris and psoriasis
Conradi–Hünnermann syndrome
Pili torti and enamel hypoplasia
Jeanselme and Rime hypotrichosis
Monilethrix and trichothiodystrophy are also associated with keratosis pilaris, but are not alopecias

Table 9.4 Manifestations of abnormal development of surface ectoderm-derived tissues.

Hair	Hypotrichosis, alopecia, hair shaft structural abnormalities, keratosis pilaris, follicular atrophoderma
Nails	Nonspecific dysplasia, thickening, anonychia
Epidermis	Palmar–plantar keratoderma, blisters, ichthyosis, cleft lip and palate, excessive bruising and scarring, abnormal dermatoglyphics, palmar keratoses, xerosis or poikiloderma
Apocrine glands	Supranumary nipples, mammary hypoplasia, absent nipple or areola
Eccrine glands	Defective sweating, impaired thermoregulation
Teeth	Enamel defects with premature loss, peg-shaped incisors, failure of dental eruption, abnormal dentition, gingival hyperplasia
Ears	Sensorineural deafness, prominent ears, abnormal or malformed auricles, folded or floppy ears, low-set ears
Eyes	Photophobia, corneal opacities, corneal dyskeratosis or scarring, decreased lacrimation, cataracts, glaucoma, keratoconus, entropion, nystagmus, iris atrophy

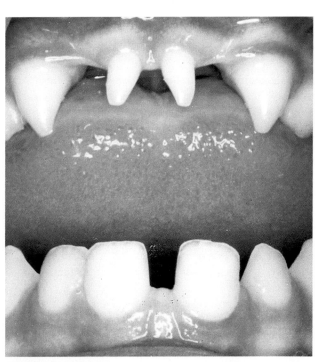

Fig. 9.16 Conical incisors.

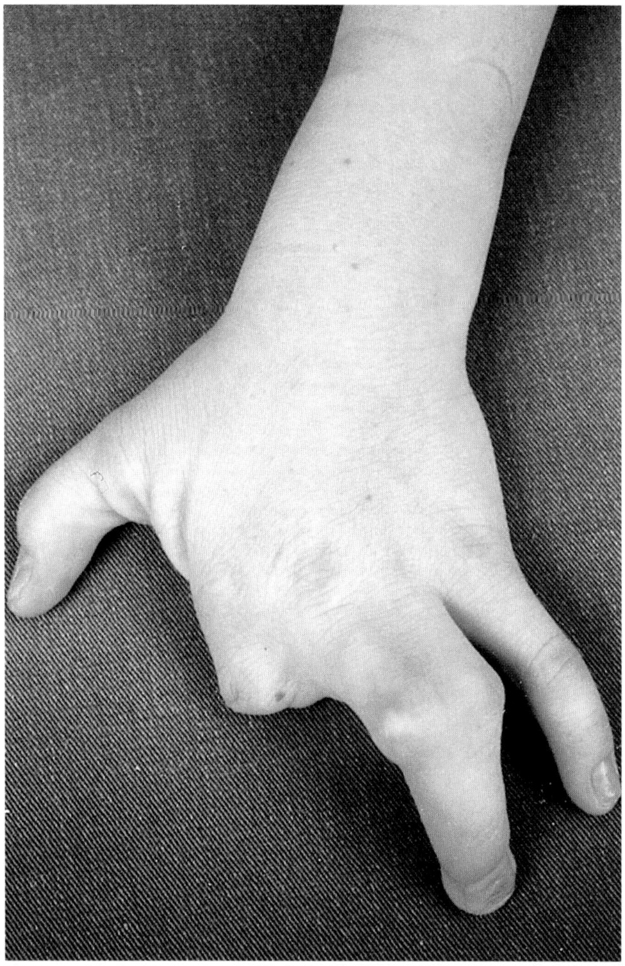

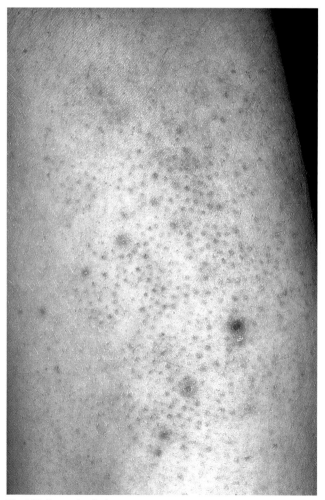

suggest there are a number of different varieties. The classic description is of inflammation and atrophy beginning on the face in infancy and progressing to scarring alopecia of the scalp (Fig. 9.23). The trunk and extremities may become involved at this stage. In the mid-teens a permanent alopecia occurs on the scalp and also the eyebrows. Both AD and X-linked dominant inheritances have been described.

Prognosis

The KP improves in summer in 40% of patients, in winter in 40% while 20% notice no seasonal variation. With time the KP improves in one-third, remains unchanged in one-half and worsens in the rest. In those that are going to improve with age, significant improvement is usually evident by the late teens.

Treatment

Only symptomatic measures are available. Keratolytics combined with a weak topical steroid may help the erythema and if used with an abrasive sponge (e.g. Buf-Puf) can remove

Fig. 9.17 Ectrodactyly.

is rare, but keratosis pilaris of the limbs is common. An association has been reported with the Rombo syndrome, Down's syndrome (trisomy 21), monosomy 18p, congenital cardiac anomalies, atrichia with papular lesions, Conradi–Hünermann syndrome (p. 146) and hypotrichosis of Jeanselme and Rime (p. 145). Chloracne produces a similar appearance.

Keratosis pilaris atrophicans facei is a cicatricial KP mainly confined to the eyebrows. It is usually sporadic but AD inheritance has been described. From early infancy the outer halves of the eyebrows are erythematous and horny follicular plugs appear laterally and progress medially destroying the follicles in the process (Fig. 9.21). Individual follicular papules are surrounded by an erythematous ring. The destruction of hair follicles may also stretch to a variable extent onto the cheeks. It is frequently seen in association with Noonan's syndrome (Fig. 9.22). The histology shows perifollicular inflammation and scarring. Distinction from atrophoderma vermiculata may be difficult as there is some overlap between these two conditions.

Keratosis pilaris decalvans is the association of KP on the face and body with a cicatricial alopecia of the scalp. Descriptions of this condition are sufficiently variable to

Fig. 9.18 Keratosis pilaris.

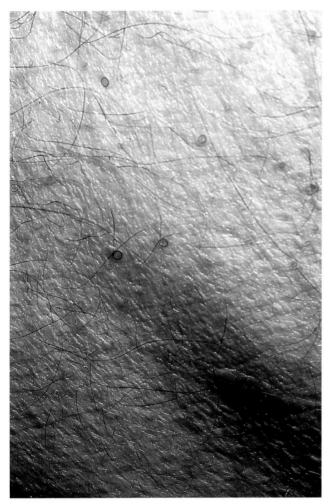

Fig. 9.19 Coiled hairs.

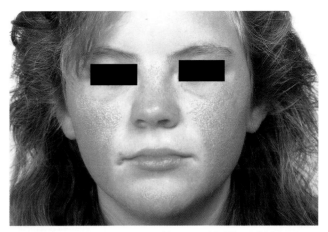

Fig. 9.20 Atrophoderma vermiculata. (Courtesy of Dr Warren Weightman, Adelaide.)

some of the follicular keratosis. Retinoic acid derivatives deserve a trial, but are rarely dramatically effective. The status of oral retinoids remains controversial, though anecdotal reports are promising. In one report of KP atrophicans facei, a 16 week course of isotretinoin (1 mg/kg) produced a marked improvement, but was followed by relapse within 6 months and a second course produced a remission of 12 months.

Key points

Keratosis pilaris is a common benign condition of extensor surfaces associated with xerosis. When it is confined to the eyebrows and resolves with atrophy and scarring it is called keratosis pilaris atrophicans. When it occurs on the cheeks and produces a honeycomb atrophy it is known as atrophoderma vermiculata, and when it begins on the face of infants, spreads then to the trunk and limbs and is associated with the development in adolescence of a cicatricial alopecia it is called keratosis pilaris decalvans.

9.8 Other developmental alopecias with associated defects

Jeanselme and Rime hypotrichosis is similar to the Marie Unna syndrome. Affected infants are born with fragile twisted hair that is lost by the age of 8 months to produce a total alopecia. Affected children have associated keratosis pilaris, a thickened leathery scalp, red blotches on their face and fragile nails. The inheritance is AD and this condition is classified as an ectodermal dysplasia.

Hallermann–Streiff syndrome is an hereditary complex of ectodermal and mesodermal defects. The scalp hair is normal at birth, but soon becomes diffusely sparse and brittle with frontal alopecia (Fig. 9.24), balding of the lateral and posterior scalp margins and a characteristic alopecia that follows the cranial sutures. Eyebrows, eyelashes, pubic and axillary hairs are sparse or absent. The scalp within the areas of the alopecia is thin and atrophic, however, histology does not reveal scarring. Associated abnormalities included a bird-like

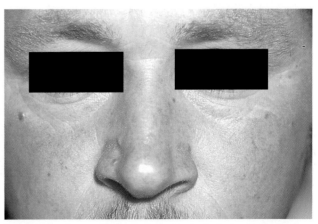

Fig. 9.21 Ulerythema ophryogenes, or keratosis pilaris atrophicans facei.

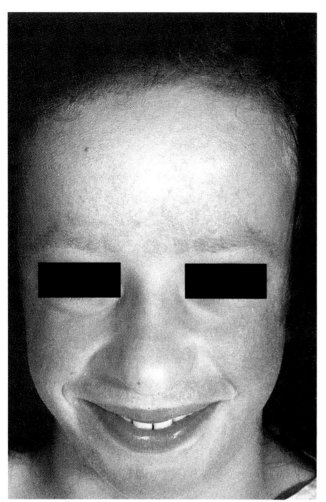

Fig. 9.22 Keratosis pilaris and ulerythema ophryogenes in Noonan's syndrome. (Courtesy of Dr K. Ward *et al.*, Birmingham and the *British Journal of Dermatology*.)

facies, physical and mental retardation, dental defects and nail changes.

Conradi–Hünermann syndrome (Fig. 9.25) consists of chondrodysplasia punctata, limb asymmetry, characteristic facies, spontaneously resolving congenital ichthyosiform erythroderma, hypotrichosis, follicular atrophoderma, keratosis pilaris, limb asymmetry, abnormal nails and cataracts.

The inheritance is X-linked dominant with lethality in hemizygous males, however, many cases are sporadic. The scalp shows coarse, lustreless and irregularly twisted hair and a patchy cicatricial alopecia. In 25% there is extensive erythema and scaling in early infancy, that resolves and is succeeded by ichthyosis. A saddle nose and a high arched palate are common and 20% have congenital cataracts. The chondrodysplasia manifests radiologically as characteristic stippling of the epiphyses, but this tends to disappear after the age of 6 years.

A *rhizomelic type of chondrodysplasia punctata* (Fig. 9.26) occurring as an autosomal recessive trait has been described and includes all of the features of Conradi–Hünermann syndrome as well as lymphoedema of the face, microcephaly and congenital cataracts in 80%. Most affected children die in infancy, while those that survive are severely handicapped.

Cartilage–hair hypoplasia is an autosomal recessive syndrome comprising scant hair and short-limbed dwarfism. Hair on the scalp and body is short, sparse, fine, light and silky. In some individuals there may be almost complete baldness. Electron microscopy of the hair is essentially normal, however, there is a reduction in the tensile strength of the hair. The limbs and digits are short due to metaphyseal dysostosis from cartilage hypoplasia. Other associated features include malabsorption and immunodeficiency with impaired cell-mediated responses.

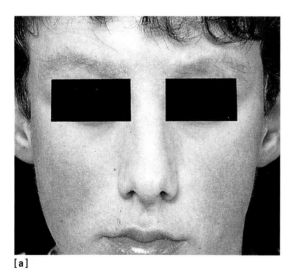

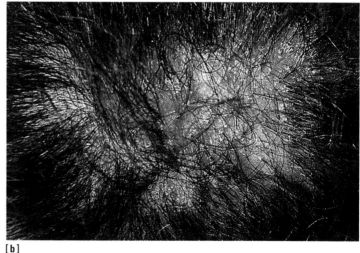

[a]   [b]

Fig. 9.23 Keratosis pilaris decalvans. The facial photograph (a) shows erythema of the patient's cheeks due to atrophoderma vermiculatum while on his scalp (b) there is a scarring alopecia. (Courtesy of R.H. Champion, J.L. Burton and F.J.G Ebling (eds) (1992) *Textbook of Dermatology*, 5th edn. Blackwell Scientific Publications, Oxford.)

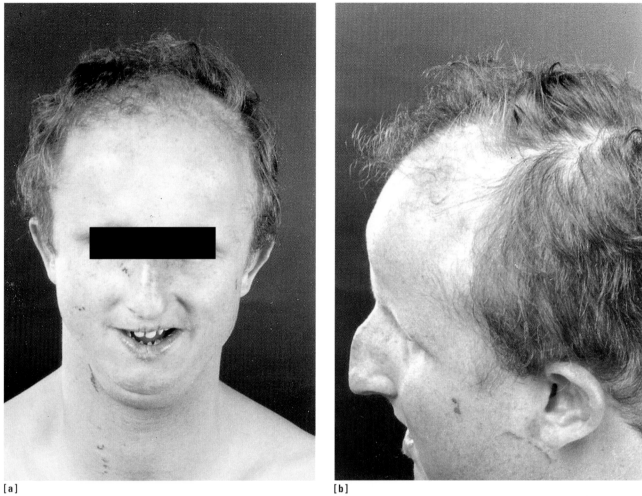

[a]   [b]

Fig. 9.24 Hallermann–Streiff syndrome. The alopecia overlying the cranial sutures is not well seen. (Courtesy of POSSUM.)

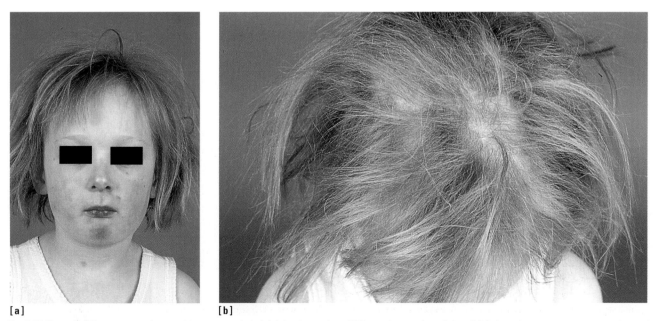

[a]   [b]

Fig. 9.25 Conradi–Hünermann syndrome with sparse scalp hair (a) that is unruly and (b) contains patches of cicatricial alopecia.

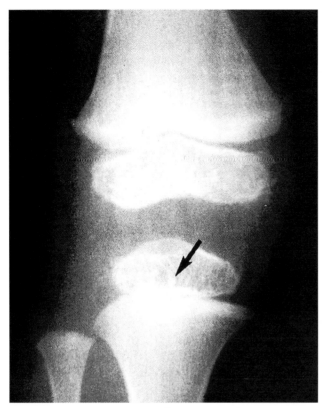

Fig. 9.26 Chondrodysplasia punctata. (Courtesy of Dr D.G. Paige *et al.* and the *British Journal of Dermatology.*)

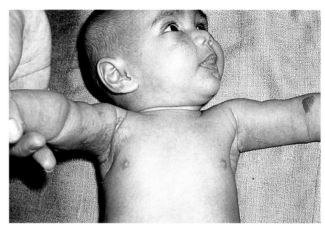

Fig. 9.27 Incontinentia pigmenti in an infant, at the early verrucous, late vesicular stage.

skin lesions that occur in three overlapping phases. First, clear, tense and often linear blisters occur mainly on the limbs (Fig. 9.27). They appear either at birth or within the first few weeks of life. They continue to occur in recurrent crops for a

Hypomelia–hypotrichosis facial haemangioma syndrome is an autosomal recessive trait with a pseudothalidomide limb deformity, a mid-facial capillary naevus and sparse silver-blond hair. Associated features include micrognathia, high nasal bridge, hypoplastic alae nasi and retroverted nares that together produce a characteristic appearance.

Moynahan's syndrome comprises mental retardation, epilepsy and total baldness of the scalp. The alopecia is present in infancy but may regrow between 2 and 4 years of age. Autosomal recessive inheritance has been postulated.

Dyskeratosis congenita is a rare syndrome that can be determined by either an autosomal or X-linked gene. Most cases are males, but females can also be affected. Affected children are generally normal until the age of 5 years when they begin to develop nail dystrophy with eventual loss, leucoplakia mainly on the oral mucosa, but also on the eyes, anorectal and urethral mucosae (eventually leading to carcinoma), reticulate pigmentation on the neck, trunk and thighs; haematological abnormalities (pancytopenia or myeloid aplasia) and macular cutaneous amyloid. The hair may be normal in this condition, but is sometimes sparse and dry. Premature canites and cicatricial alopecia have been noted in some cases. Bone marrow transplantation has been successful for the pancytopenia and etretinate is useful for the leucoplakia. Without treatment the life expectancy is short.

Incontinentia pigmenti is an X-linked inherited condition that is usually lethal in males. The diagnosis is based on the

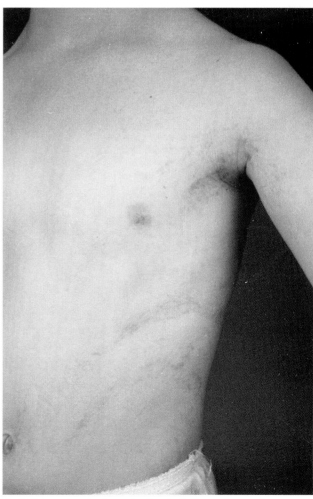

Fig. 9.28 Incontinentia pigmenti at the whorled hyperpigmented stage.

few months accompanied or followed by smooth red nodules and plaques that may ulcerate. At this stage the histology shows eosinophilic spongiosis of the epidermis. In the second phase occurring 3–5 months after the first, linear warty lesions appear on the dorsum of the hands and feet, particularly the fingers and toes. Histology shows hyperkeratosis, acanthosis, irregular papillomatosis and numerous dyskeratotic cells. The verrucous plaques persist for several months before the third phase, with whorled pigmentation following the lines of Blaschko, occurs (Fig. 9.28). Pigmentation does not only occur in sites of previous inflammation. On histology there is pigment incontinence with numerous melanophages, and hair follicles and eccrine glands are notably absent.

Occasionally hyperpigmentation is the first manifestation of the condition and such cases require a biopsy to differentiate linear and whorled hypermelanosis. The pigmentation persists for years before eventually fading, often leaving hypopigmented or atrophic streaks that resemble the hypomelanosis of Ito.

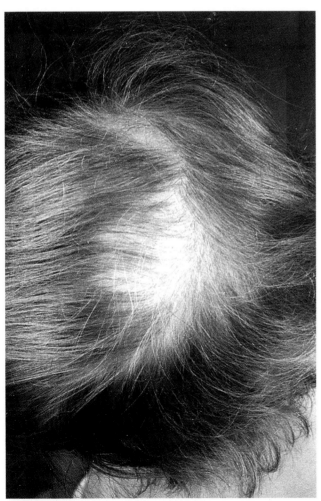

Fig. 9.29 Scalp hair loss along Blaschko's lines due to incontinentia pigmenti.

The vertex of the scalp may be affected in up to 25% of cases with hairless streaks (Fig. 9.29), although the scalp is rarely the site of blisters. Patches of cicatricial alopecia resembling the alopecia of Brocq develop in infancy along Blaschko's lines in the scalp and extend for up to 2 years. Hypoplasia of the eyebrows and eyelashes may occur and there may be a woolly hair naevus.

An eosinophilia of up to 50% is usual when the acute inflammatory lesions are present, and some patients have associated neutrophil and lymphocyte dysfunction. Other inconstant associations include dental abnormalities (peg shaped incisors), nail dystrophy, blindness, skeletal and CNS abnormalities. Incontinentia pigmenti may be considered as an ectodermal dysplasia.

Bazex's syndrome is an X-linked dominant condition with follicular atrophoderma from infancy, multiple basal cell carcinomas of the face from adolescence onwards and hypotrichosis. Males are more severely affected than females due to Lyonization. The follicular atrophoderma is mainly present on the dorsum of the hands and feet, but also occurs on the trunk. The 'ice-pick' marks characteristic of this are due to deep and lax follicular ostia rather than true atrophy. The basal cell carcinomas are often pigmented and may resemble melanocytic naevi. Hypohidrosis, comedones and pilomatrixomas may occur. The hair shafts are defective and show twisting and flattening with trichorrhexis nodes. Follicular atrophoderma is a rare and distinctive sign, that is only otherwise seen in Conradi–Hünermann syndrome and atrophoderma vermiculata; however, acne-induced perifollicular elastolysis may look similar.

Dubowitz syndrome (Fig. 9.30) is a rare autosomal recessive condition characterized by low birthweight, growth and mental retardation, a distinctive facies and eczema. The hair may be sparse and fine.

Johanson–Blizzard syndrome is an autosomal recessive disorder with aplasia cutis congenita of the scalp, sparse hair, deafness, abnormal facies, aplasia of the permanent teeth buds, microcephaly, mental retardation, malabsorption, hypothyroidism and genital abnormalities. It is an ectodermal dysplasia.

Myotonic dystrophy is a rare autosomal dominant condition with myotonia and muscle wasting developing in the third decade. Premature canites and frontoparietal balding are constant features (Figs 9.31 & 9.32). There may be a reduction in body hair, decreased sebum excretion and testicular atrophy.

Holocarboxylase synthetase deficiency and biotinidase deficiency are both autosomal recessive forms of multiple carboxylase deficiency that are associated with immunodeficiency. Alopecia may be a prominent feature of both conditions, and this has led investigators to try biotin in a diverse range of hair disorders, including uncombable hair syndrome, without success.

Griscelli's syndrome is a rare autosomal recessive immunodeficiency syndrome associated with partial albinism and an absence of cutaneous Langerhans' cells. The hair in this

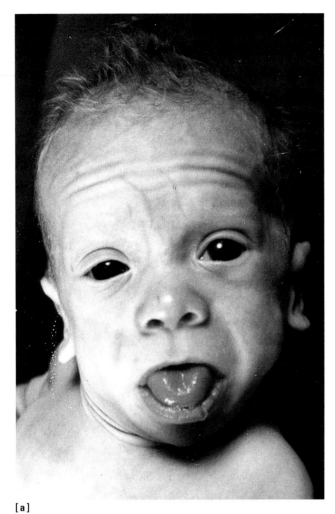

[a]

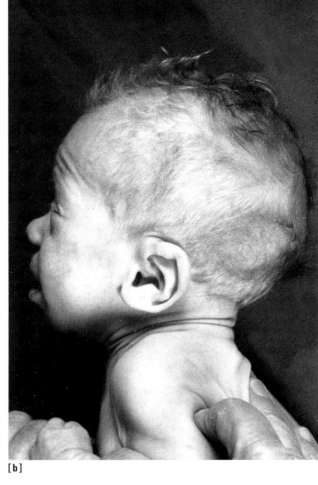

[b]

Fig. 9.30 Hypotrichosis in Dubowitz syndrome. (Courtesy of POSSUM.)

condition is silvery-grey from early childhood and electron microscopy shows clumping of pigment within the hair shafts.

Cronkhite–Canada syndrome is a rare syndrome of unknown origin associated with diffuse acral pigmentation, gastrointestinal polyposis, a protein losing enteropathy, hair changes and nail dystrophy. The pigmentation is predominantly palmar, but may be generalized. In contrast to Peutz–Jeghers syndrome there is no buccal pigmentation. A patchy alopecia initially develops, however, it becomes total after a few months.

Mendes da Costa syndrome is a sex-linked recessive blistering condition that occurs only in boys. Tense bullae, irregularly scattered on the trunk and limbs appear between the ages of 2 months and 3 years. Soon after the bullae appear the hair is lost and a reticular pigmentation develops on the face and limbs. Many are mentally and physically retarded and life expectancy is poor. This condition is probably a type of epidermolysis bullosa and should not be confused with erythrokeratoderma variabilis—Mendes da Costa's other syndrome.

Treacher Collins syndrome is an autosomal dominant condition believed to result from arrested development of structures derived from the first branchial arch. It consists of a characteristic facies, malformed ears, stenosis of the external auditory meatus, blind fistulae and skin tags between the corner of the mouth and the ears, a high arched palate and occasionally a cleft palate. There is partial or total absence of the lower eye-lashes, extension of terminal hair from the scalp onto the cheeks and circumscribed scarring alopecia of the scalp (Fig. 9.33).

Baraitser's syndrome is autosomal recessive and consists of alopecia and mental and physical retardation.

Progeria a very rare syndrome that is most likely autosomal recessive. Characteristically an apparently normal 1-year-old child develops scleroderma-like changes on the abdomen, flanks and thighs combined with mid-facial cyanosis and a glyphic nose. Growth retardation soon becomes apparent and a progressive loss of subcutaneous tissue occurs along with a total alopecia (Fig. 9.34). The eyebrows and eyelashes may also be shed. This combination makes the child look like a little old man. Associated features include insulin resistance

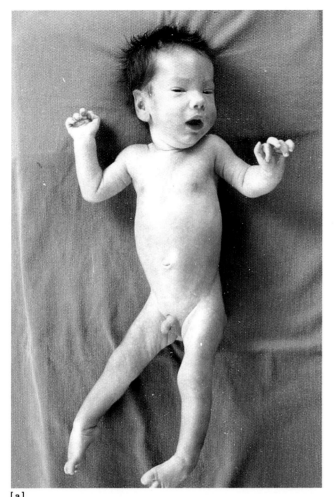
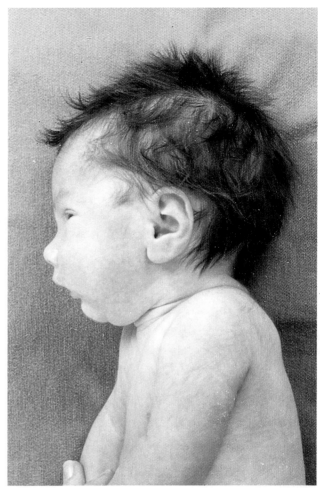

[a]   [b]

Fig. 9.31 Frontal alopecia in congenital myotonic dystrophy. (Courtesy of POSSUM.)

and early onset severe atherosclerosis that leads to an early death.

Cockayne syndrome may look very similar to progeria, but can be distinguished by the presence of photosensitivity, mental retardation, deafness, retinitis pigmentosum and dwarfism.

Metageria is an autosomal recessive condition with a loss of subcutaneous fat, a thin face with a prominent broad nose, mottled pigmentation and telangiectasia. The scalp hair is fine and sparse. Mental and physical development are normal.

Pangeria (Werner's syndrome) is a rare autosomal recessive condition that is not manifest until the age of 8–12 years. Growth ceases, premature canites begins and is complete by the age of 20 years. Progressive alopecia begins bitemporally, but soon becomes diffuse. The alopecia is associated with miniaturization of the hairs and resembles androgenetic alopecia, however, it may begin prior to puberty. Additionally these children usually have hypogonadism.

The ultimate extent of the alopecia is variable. Body hair is usually sparse. Mottled pigmentation and telangiectases

develop on the distal limbs, face and neck. Subcutaneous fat is lost and the bird like facies and spindly limbs contrast with an often obese trunk. Diabetes, cataracts, premature arteriosclerosis and malignancy are common and life expectancy is shortened.

Poikiloderma congenitale (Rothmund–Thomson syndrome) is an autosomal recessive condition that presents in early infancy with facial erythema, atrophy, telangiectasia and mottled hyper- and hypopigmentation. The hair may grey prematurely and androgenetic alopecia occurs early. Scalp, axillary and pubic hair may be sparse or lost and eyebrows and eyelashes are often scanty (Fig. 9.35). In *bird-headed dwarfism* premature canites occurs and androgenetic alopecia is well advanced by the age of 20 years.

Xeroderma pigmentosum (Fig. 9.36) is not a true premature ageing syndrome. Rather it is a group of disorders characterized by defective DNA repair and increased susceptibility to light damage. There is an early onset of pigmentary damage, cutaneous atrophy, solar keratoses and skin cancers on light exposed skin. Premature canites occurs and one patient has been reported with no hair.

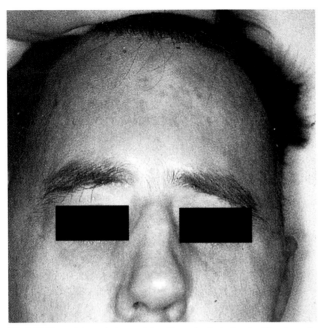

Fig. 9.32 Frontal alopecia in an adult with myotonic dystrophy. (Courtesy of R.H. Champion, J.L. Burton & F.J.G. Ebling (eds) (1992) *Textbook of Dermatology*, 5th edn. Blackwell Scientific Publications, Oxford.)

Down's syndrome (trisomy 21) is due to a chromosomal abnormality that occurs in one in 700 births. The hair in Down's syndrome is often fine, but may become sparse and dry. There is a horizontal pattern of pubic hair. A high frequency of AA (see Fig. 6.1) and keratosis pilaris is noted. Alopecia areata is generally severe when it occurs in this group and progresses to alopecia totalis/universalis in approximately 50% of cases. Premature canites and early androgenetic alopecia have also been noted.

Klinefelter's syndrome occurs in one in 400 births and the karyotype is 47,XXY. Klinefelter's syndrome is associated with hypogonadism and low fertility. There is diminished secondary sexual hair on the face, body and pubes. There is a horizontal escutcheon. Gynaecomastia is common and affected males are generally tall and obese.

In *Turner's syndrome* (45, XO) ovarian agenesis results in scanty pubic and axillary hair, however, some secondary sexual hair develops as this is initiated by adrenal androgens.

Noonan's syndrome is not a chromosomal disorder, but is nevertheless considered here because of its resemblance to Turner's syndrome. Noonan's syndrome is an autosomal dominant multisystem disorder that occurs in both sexes at a rate of approximately one in 1000 births. It has the phenotype of Turner's syndrome but a normal karyotype. Pubic hair is scanty in the male and beard growth is poor. The scalp hair is

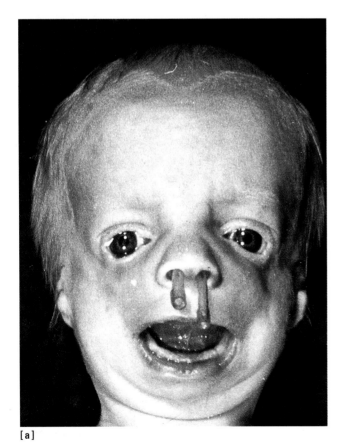

[a]

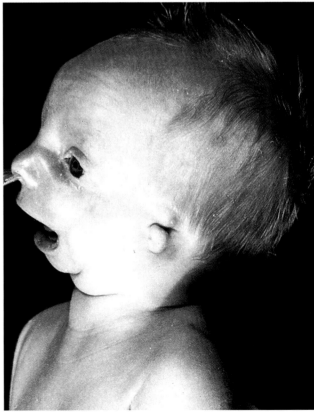

[b]

Fig. 9.33 Treacher Collin's syndrome. (Courtesy of POSSUM.)

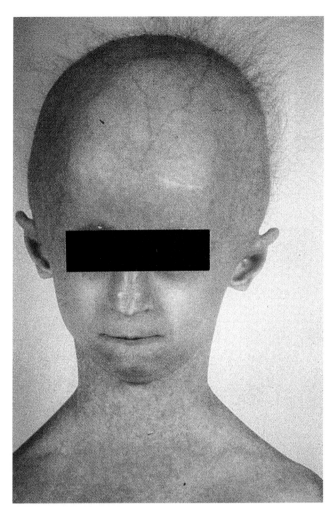

Fig. 9.34 Near total alopecia in a child with progeria. (Courtesy of Dr P. Hogan *et al.* and *Paediatric Dermatology*.)

coarse, light coloured and curly with a low posterior scalp margin (Fig. 9.37). Atrophoderma vermiculata is common and may be a cutaneous marker for Noonan's syndrome (Fig. 9.22).

The *cardio-facio-cutaneous (CFC) syndrome* is now recognized to be a variant of Noonan's syndrome. In addition to the features of Noonan's, CFC patients have coarse curly hair, ichthyosis, macrocephaly, hyperextensible skin and joints and a high arched palate. *Costello syndrome* is a variant of the CFC syndrome with the added features of loose and redundant skin, thick lips and nasal papillomata.

Cutis verticis gyrata (CVG) is a morphological description first coined by Unna for a condition characterized by hypertrophy and folding of the skin on the scalp to produce a gyrate or cerebriform appearance. The essential abnormality is an overgrowth of the scalp in relation to the underlying skull. It may occur in isolation (primary CVG) or in association with mental retardation, pachydermatoperiostosis,

acromegaly, myxoedema, Darier's disease or tuberous sclerosis. Rarely melanocytic naevi or neurofibromas may assume a cerebriform structure and mimic CVG.

Primary CVG occurs almost exclusively in males and most often appears sporadically (Fig. 9.38). Some cases have affected more than one family member and both autosomal dominant and recessive inheritance have been described. Affected individuals often have associated epilepsy and cerebral palsy. They rarely have an IQ above 35 and CVG accounts for 0.5% of the mentally retarded population. This figure may be an underestimate due to the delayed onset of CVG in many patients.

The longitudinal and irregular parallel folds of the scalp, that resemble gyri cerebri, may appear in late childhood or at puberty and slowly become more accentuated (Fig. 9.39). Biopsy shows only moderate acanthosis of the epidermis and sebaceous hyperplasia within the dermis. There is a diffuse thickening of the dermis with closely packed, broad collagen bundles. There is usually some hyalinization of the collagen.

Children with the *Lennox–Gastaut syndrome* (infantile spasms with EEG abnormalities and mental retardation) may develop CVG after the neurological manifestations. About 5–10% of children with Lennox–Gastaut syndrome have underlying tuberous sclerosis, and this figure may be higher in those with CVG.

Michelin tyre baby syndrome, so named after the effigy of the French tyre manufacturer may be a generalized variant of CVG that occurs only in females. In the original cases there was diffuse lipomatous hypertrophy within the generalized folds of redundant skin, however, this was absent in subsequent cases and the generalized folding is now thought of as a nonspecific condition that may reflect a variety of unrelated pathological processes. Hypotrichosis of the scalp may be prominent.

Pachydermoperiostosis, an autosomal dominant condition characterized by hypertrophy and thickening of the phalanges (clubbing) and long bones due to a proliferative periostitis. An acquired form of pachydermoperiostosis (also known as hypertrophic pulmonary osteoarthropathy) occurs as a paraneoplastic phenomenon. Cutis verticis gyrata occurs in both types of pachydermoperiostosis, but is more common in the hereditary form of this condition. When it occurs it is extensive, involving the scalp and often the face. The folds and furrows affecting the forehead, eyelids and cheeks produce a weary visage.

Acromegaly is frequently associated with mild CVG and occasionally patients have more pronounced forms. Cutis verticis gyrata has only rarely been described with other endocrinopathies such as hypothyroidism. An association with Darier's disease has been described but remains unexplained.

Lipoedematous scalp is a distinct disorder that is sometimes confused with CVG. In this condition there is a diffuse thickening of the subcutis (from 3.5 mm to 8 mm or more on com-

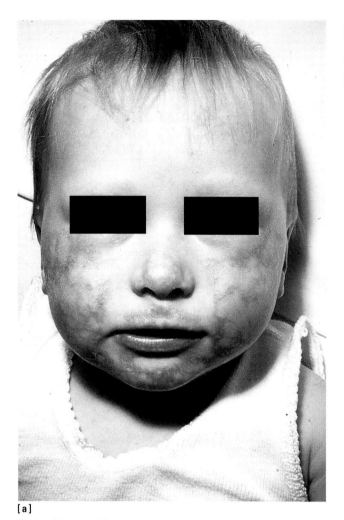

[a]

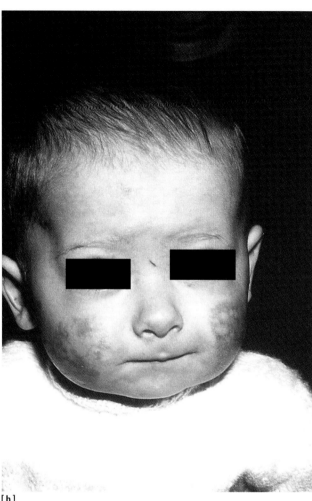

[b]

Fig. 9.35 Rothmund–Thomson syndrome in two brothers showing coarse fine hair.

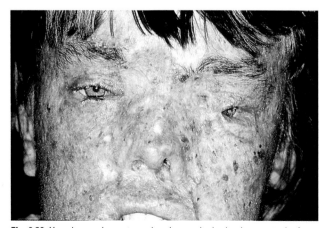

Fig. 9.36 Xeroderma pigmentosa showing marked solar damage to the face with premature greying of the hair.

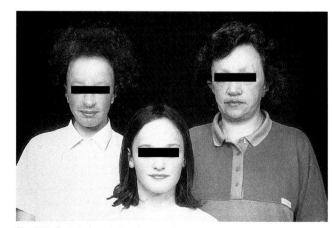

Fig. 9.37 Curly hair and ulerythema ophryogenes in a mother and daughter with Noonan's syndrome, while an unaffected daughter has straight hair. (Courtesy of Dr K Ward, Birmingham and the *British Journal of Dermatology*.)

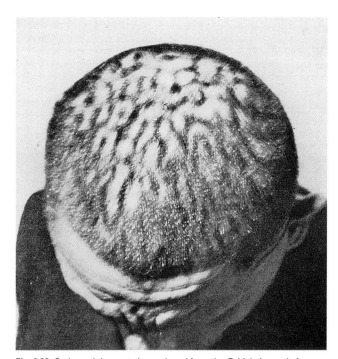

Fig. 9.38 Cutis verticis gyrata (reproduced from the *British Journal of Dermatology and Syphilis*, 1923).

puterized tomography) with or without alopecia. To date this has only been described in women, while CVG predominates in men. Itching and soreness may be described and on palpation there is a boggy or spongy consistency. *Encephalocranio-cutaneous lipomatosis*, a congenital disorder characterized by unilateral cerebral malformations and ipsilateral scalp, face and eye lesions may also be confused with CVG. Multiple soft alopecic tumours of adipose tissue are characteristic.

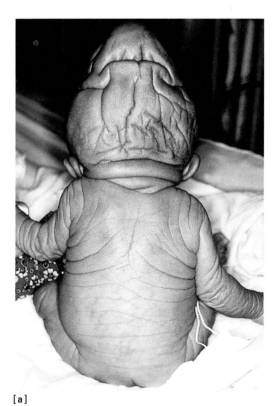

[a]

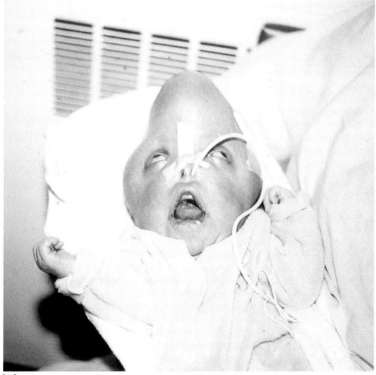

[b]

Fig. 9.39 Cutis verticis gyrata as part of the Beare–Stevenson syndrome. (Courtesy of POSSUM.)

Chapter 10

Structural abnormalities of the hair shaft

10.1 Normal hair shafts and normal weathering

On average hairs grow 1 cm per month. Thus the tip of a hair that is 35 cm long has been exposed to the environment for almost 3 years. During that period it is likely to have been washed and dried 1000 times, bleached, dyed, and permed and cut half a dozen times, and combed or brushed countless times. As a consequence the tip of the hair will show signs of deterioration.

While a normal hair will show the scars of these procedures, collectively known as weathering, it will survive this onslaught. On the other hand, a hair that has a structural weakness will not and is likely to snap off. The amount of weathering it can withstand will determine how long the hair grows before it breaks and this in turn will be determined by the nature and severity of the intrinsic structural weakness.

Many of the conditions associated with weak hair fibres are caused by single gene defects. A number of these genodermatoses will be diagnosed by examination of the fibres by light microscopy as they produce specific deformities.

If the genodermatosis not only deforms the hair but also renders is fragile, then the specific deformity will be accompanied by a constellation of environmental weathering changes. Alone these weathering changes are not specific because the changes induced by mild trauma to weak hairs are identical to those produced by severe trauma to normal hairs. When such hairs are examined microscopically, the changes occurring in the proximal few centimetres are most likely to be due to the intrinsic defect, while those only occur-

ring distally are likely to be due to weathering. Hence, any description of a hair shaft abnormality should mention the location of the defect in relation to the root of the hair.

Once the clinician is familiar with the range of nonspecific light microscopy features of weathering (pp. 14–15), and the specific features of the single gene disorders (Fig. 10.1), then the clinical features of these disorders becomes predictable.

There are only 10 recognized alterations in the hair fibre that may be seen with light and electron microscopy and are specific for a genodermatosis. They are classified into two groups on the basis of hair fragility and susceptibility to weathering (Table 10.1). Those associated with increased fragility present with hair that is fine, short, does not need cutting and does not grow long (see pp. 157–71 for full description). Hair shaft disorders without fragility are more subtle clinically and patients present with alteration of hair form, colour or texture. Their hair may be unruly, spangled or feel coarse or tacky. Occasionally they are only discovered as an incidental finding. They are discussed on pp. 171–78.

In addition to the recognized developmental hair shaft disorders discussed in this chapter, increased hair fragility can be seen in certain acquired diseases such as hypothyroidism, anaemia, malnutrition, connective tissue disorders and as a drug side-effect.

Light microscopy and electron microscopy of hair are valuable tools in the diagnosis of congenital and hereditary hair dystrophies. Patients who present with hair that is of poor quality, brittle, or fails to grow long should have a clump of around 50 hairs plucked and examined with a light micro-

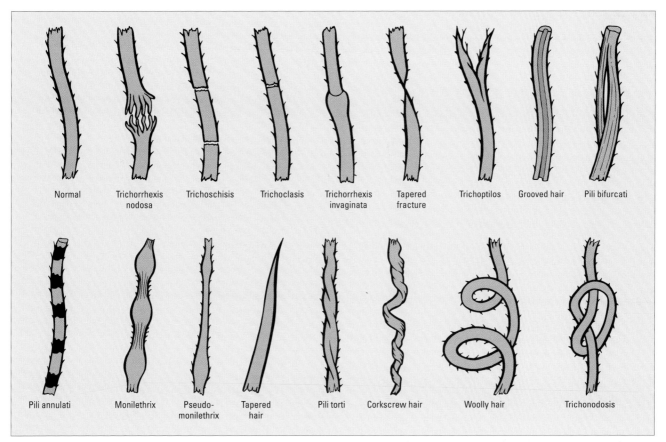

Fig. 10.1 A diagrammatic representation of the light microscopy appearances of hair in the hair shaft disorders (modified from Dr D. Whiting, Dallas, USA).

scope. This is done by examining the hair along its entire length and comparing proximal with distal abnormalities. Scanning electron microscopy is not required in all cases and the decision to do electron microscopy will be influenced by the clinical picture, the findings on light microscopy and the availability of an electron microscope. If an electron microscope is not available locally, then hairs can be mailed to a tertiary referral centre for examination.

Key points

Excessive weathering of hair is often an important diagnostic feature of congenital and inherited hair abnormalities, and while the extent of weathering may be suggestive of a partic-

Table 10.1 Weathering in congenital and hereditary hair dystrophy

Highly susceptible	Highly resistant
Monilethrix	Uncombable hair syndrome
Trichothiodystrophy	Pili annulati
Pili torti and twisting hair dystrophy	Woolly hair
Trichorrhexis nodosa	Straight hair naevus
Netherton's syndrome	Acquired progressive kinking

ular disorder, the nature of these changes is not specific and should not be over-interpreted. When describing hair shaft abnormalities it is crucial to determine the location of that abnormality in relation to the root.

10.2 Proximal trichorrhexis nodosa

Definition

Trichorrhexis nodosa is the term used to describe a localized thickening of the hair shaft due to fraying of the cortex that resembles a node (see Fig. 1.25, p. 15). Distal nodes generally indicate hair weathering. Proximal nodes, especially within 2–5 cm of the hair bulb, indicate increased hair fragility and decreased resistance to normal wear and tear.

Epidemiology

Negro hair often withstands trauma poorly and nodes are common in long hair. Vigorous attempts to straighten curly hair may cause nodes to occur closer to the root. When severe, this is described as acquired proximal trichorrhexis nodosa.

Caucasoid and Oriental hair is stronger than Negroid hair and even the most vigorous abuse tends to produce distal rather than proximal acquired trichorrhexis nodosa (Fig. 10.2).

Pathogenesis

Disruption of the hair cuticle, that normally shields the hair from the environment, permits injury to the cortex. Nodes are not a pathognomonic hair shaft defect, since they may also be a manifestation of external insult on normal hair shafts.

Clinical features

Patients with proximal trichorrhexis nodosa present with short coarse hair that fails to grow long. This may be circumscribed or diffuse and congenital or acquired.

Pathology

It appears on light microscopy as a beaded swelling associated with loss of the cuticle. At the nodes the cortex bulges and is split by longitudinal fissures. If a fracture occurs transversely through the node, the end of the hair resembles a small paintbrush. This is known as trichoclasis and the clinical correlate is a split end.

Investigation

While it can be seen in greater detail on scanning electron microscopy, this is generally not required for diagnosis.

Differential diagnosis

If the hairs are cut rather than plucked it may be impossible to determine where the nodes are in relation to the bulb.

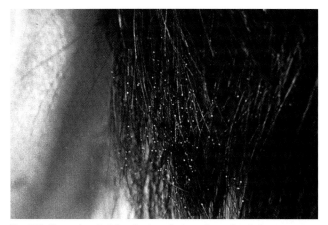

Fig. 10.2 The nodes of trichorrhexis nodosa produce a beaded appearance along the hair shaft. (Courtesy of Dr M. Rogers, Sydney.)

Table 10.2 Advice to patients with fragile or excessively weathered hair.

1 Avoid wetting the hair when showering or taking a bath.
2 Do not wash the hair more than once a week.
3 When shampooing always use a conditioner, and leave it on the scalp for at least five minutes before rinsing.
4 Use a conditioner without shampoo if the hair is clean.
5 After wetting the hair, only pat it lightly dry and do not rub it with the towel.
6 Do not blow dry the hair or use hot combs.
7 Comb the hair with a wide toothed comb no more than once a day.
8 Do not brush the hair.
9 Avoid all hairdressing procedures. In particular do not have your hair bleached, dyed, straightened, permanent waved (permed), crimped or pleated. The hair should only be cut with sharp scissors, and not a razor.
10 Protect the hair from excessive exposure to sunlight, by wearing a loose fitting hat or scarf.
11 Avoid tight hats and bathing caps.
12 Do not tie the hair back tightly in a pony tail, or in plaits.
13 Consider a satin pillow case to reduce friction whilst sleeping.

Associated features

It may be a feature of a recognized hair shaft disorder, or it may occur in isolation.

Prognosis

Improvement often follows meticulous avoidance of all unnecessary trauma (Table 10.2), however, this may be difficult to achieve and the condition may prove recalcitrant.

Treatment

Strict protection from exacerbating injury is required. These are outlined in Table 10.2.

Key points

Distal trichorrhexis nodosa is a nonspecific change seen on hair microscopy as a manifestation of weathering. If trichorrhexis nodosa occurs in the proximal 5 cm of the hair shaft, then it assumes special significance. Proximal nodes reflect an intrinsic weakness of hair structure that renders it unable to withstand trauma. This may occur as an isolated abnormality or as part of a recognized hair dystrophy.

10.3 Monilethrix

Definition

Monilethrix or necklace hair is characterized by hair fragility, baldness and distinctive beaded hairs. Keratosis pilaris is a frequent association.

Epidemiology

This is a rare disorder.

Aetiology

Monilethrix is an autosomal dominant condition with a high degree of penetrance but marked variation in expressivity. The abnormal gene is found on the long arm of chromosome 12 and is responsible for the production of type II keratin.

Pathogenesis

The gene mutation leads to the formation of abnormal hair keratins within the trichocyte cytoskeleton. This disrupts tonofilament assembly and with the electron microscope keratin tonofilament clumping and cytolysis is seen within the cells of the hair cortex and there may be a deviation of the axis of the microfibrils. The hair fragility seen in monilethrix is due to this cortical abnormality, however, the mechanism of the periodic beading seen in the hair is unknown.

The beading does not seem to be related to the hair fragility as many apparently normal hairs, that do not demonstrate the beaded appearance, also fracture at around 7 cm, despite a relatively normal cuticle. This suggests that the cortical abnormality produces the premature breakage of both beaded and unbeaded hairs, and that beading alone makes a relatively small contribution to the fragility.

Clinical features

There is marked variation in the age of onset, severity and course of this condition. While some patients have diffuse involvement of the scalp (Figs 10.3 & 10.4), in others fewer than 5% of the hairs are affected and in these patients the diagnosis is easily overlooked.

Characteristically the hair is normal at birth. After the first postnatal moult the normal hairs are replaced by horny follicular papules from which abnormal brittle beaded hairs emerge. The follicular keratosis and abnormal hairs are found most frequently on the nape and occiput (Fig. 10.5), but may affect the entire scalp. The fragile hairs easily fracture to produce a short stubble of broken hairs. Follicular distribution is abnormal and the scalp whorl (p. 17) is absent. Occasional there is no keratosis pilaris, suggesting that the follicular hyperkeratosis is not important in the genesis of the beaded hairs.

The eyebrows, eyelashes, axillary and pubic hairs may be affected, but only rarely in the absence of scalp involvement.

Investigation

Examination of the patient's scalp with an epiluminescent microscope may allow the beads to be seen and helps to locate abnormal hairs for extraction and microscopy.

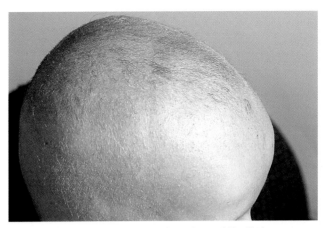

Fig. 10.3 Monilethrix in a child, producing a short stubble of hair.

Pathology

Hair microscopy is diagnostic. Elliptical nodes 0.7–1.0 mm apart are separated by narrower internodes which lack a medulla (Fig. 10.6). The width of the nodes and the distance between them is variable from hair to hair and even along the same hair. Excessive weathering of the hairs with fluting and disruption of the cuticle, best seen with scanning electron microscopy, is most marked at the internodes (Fig. 10.7). Trichorrhexis nodes form at the internodes and these tend to be the site of hair fracture.

Differential diagnosis

Unlike pili torti, which may present similarly, monilethrix hairs do not twist.

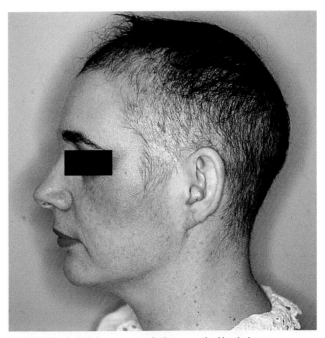

Fig. 10.4 Monilethrix in a woman who has never had her hair cut.

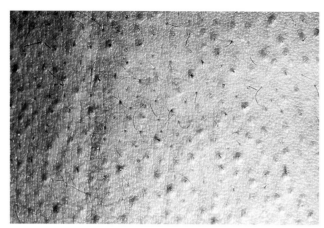

Fig. 10.5 Close-up showing keratosis pilaris and the beaded hairs emerging from the follicles.

Associated features

Associated defects such as mental and physical retardation, abnormal dentition, cataract, syndactyly and koilonychia are uncommon and may represent genetic linkage.

Prognosis

The natural history is difficult to predict as some cases improve with age, pregnancy and summer, whilst others deteriorate.

Treatment

There is no curative treatment for this condition. Reduction of hairdressing trauma may diminish the weathering and

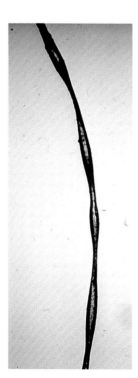

Fig. 10.6 Beaded hair is pathognomonic of monilethrix.

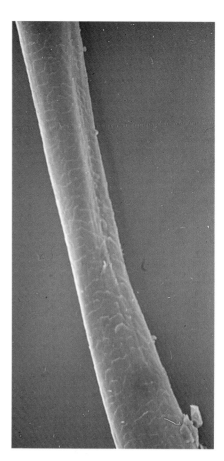

Fig. 10.7 Electron microscopy shows weathering and fluting at the internode. Fractures tend to occur at the internodes.

improve less severely affected cases. Retinoids and minoxidil have been used with variable success.

Key points

Monilethrix is a hereditary hair shaft disorder characterized by a short stubble of broken hairs and keratosis pilaris. Diagnostic beading of the hair can be seen on light microscopy. Monilethrix hairs do not twist, but are fragile.

10.4 Pseudomonilethrix

Introduction

Some patients with features suggestive of a hair shaft disorder have been found on light microscopy to have an irregular beading of hair that superficially resembles the nodes seen in monilethrix and are thus called pseudomonilethrix (Fig. 10.8). The beading is produced as an artefact of mounting hairs on glass slides and is of no significance. On scanning electron microscopy, the widened beads can be seen to be an optical illusion. They merely represent artefactual indentations of the shaft viewed in cross-section.

Key points

Pseudomonilethrix does not exist as a specific disease entity. Artefactual nodes on light microscopy due to hair shaft soft-

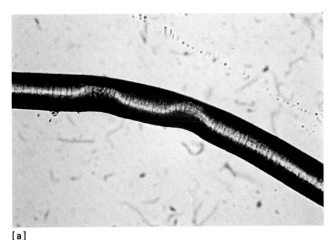

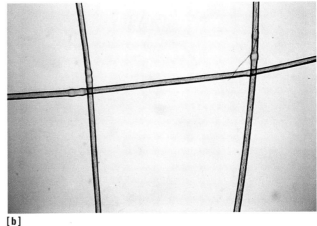

[a] [b]

Fig. 10.8 Pseudomonilethrix. The soft hair is compressed between the slide and the cover slip, producing indentations in the hair, which resemble nodes when viewed from the side. (Courtesy of Dr M. Rogers, Sydney.)

ness may be seen in some patients but are not specific to any particular disorder and can occur in normal hair.

10.5 Pili torti

Definition

Flattened and twisting hairs may occur in a number of hair dystrophies. One type of twisting hair dystrophy, where the flattened hairs rotate completely through 180° at irregular intervals, is called pili torti.

Occasional twists of less than 180° do not qualify as true pili torti. These incomplete twists may occasionally occur in normal hair as well as in a number of poorly characterized hair shaft disorders. Until a better classification exists they are best called twisting hair dystrophy.

Epidemiology

Uncommon.

Aetiology

Pili torti may occur as an isolated autosomal dominant abnormality, or it may occur as part of a syndrome (Table 10.3).

Pathogenesis

Unknown.

Clinical features and investigation

In pili torti hair is normal at birth, but the lanugo hairs are gradually replaced by abnormal twisted hairs that may be detected as early as the third month. Affected hairs are brittle, fracture easily and do not grow to any considerable length (Fig. 10.9). Generally the hairs snap at about 5 cm, however, they may break earlier if they are subjected to trauma. The patient presents with a short coarse stubble over the entire scalp and a few circumscribed bald patches. Scattered hairs

Table 10.3 Syndromes associated with pili torti.

Menkes' kinky hair syndrome	Pale skin and progressive psychomotor retardation due to an X-linked inborn error of copper transportation
Bjornstad's syndrome	Autosomal dominant condition with sensorineural deafness
Basex syndrome	Basal cell carcinoma and follicular atrophoderma
Conradi–Hünnermann syndrome	Chondrodysplasia punctata, limb asymmetry, characteristic facies, spontaneously resolving congenital ichthyosiform erythroderma, hypotrichosis, cicatricial alopecia, follicular atrophoderma, limb asymmetry, abnormal nails and cataracts
Crandall's syndrome	Sex-linked with deafness and hypogonadism
Citrullinaemia	Hereditary arginosuccinic acid synthetase deficiency
Trichothiodystrophy	Ichthyosis, photosensitivity, brittle sulphur deficient hair, mental and growth retardation, neutropenia and decreased fertility
Salti-Salem syndrome	Hypogonadotrophic hypogonadism
Some ectodermal dysplasias (see Table 10.4)	Characteristic facies; nail, sweating and dental defects.

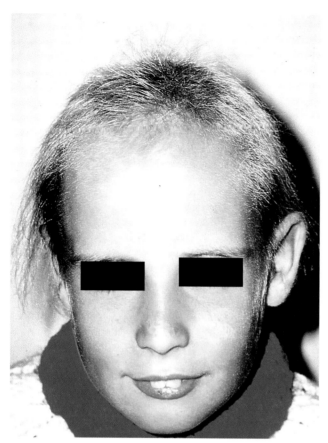

Fig. 10.9 Pili torti.

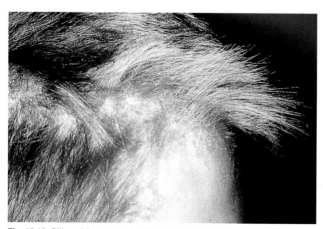

Fig. 10.10 Pili torti demonstrating the spangled effect due to reflection of light from the twisted hairs.

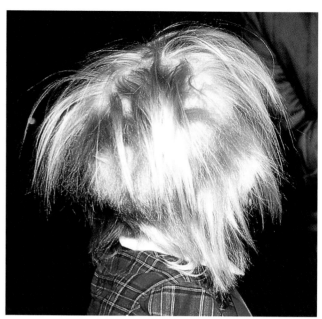

Fig. 10.11 Pili torti showing unruly hair that resembles uncombable hair syndrome or loose anagen syndrome.

have a spangled appearance due to light reflecting off the twists (Fig. 10.10). Occasionally the hairs are unruly, resembling uncombable hair syndrome (Fig. 10.11).

As adolescence approaches, the hair improves and normal (untwisted) hairs repopulate the scalp (Fig. 10.12). In some cases, spangled, twisted hairs may have to be carefully sought and a hand-held epiluminescence microscope is useful for this. However, not everyone improves, and some less fortunate patients remain severely affected

throughout life. A late-onset variant of isolated pili torti that first presents after puberty with patchy alopecia has also been described.

Involvement of body hair is variable, but occurs most commonly on the eyebrows.

Menkes' kinky hair syndrome (Figs 10.13 & 10.14) is an X-linked recessive syndrome. Affected males have pili torti, growth retardation and progressive psychomotor retardation. There is an abnormality in copper metabolism, but why this makes the hair twist is not known. Defects in copper metabolism have not been demonstrated in other forms of pili torti. As copper is a cofactor for tyrosinase, affected hairs are lighter in colour. Female carriers may manifest limited features due to random X inactivation. Affected females demonstrate patchy areas of short, broken and twisted hairs, along Blaschko's lines, on their scalp.

Associated features

Other ectodermal abnormalities that may occur in association with pili torti include keratosis pilaris, nail dystrophy, dental defects, corneal opacities and mental retardation. Specific syndromes of which pili torti is a component are listed in Tables 10.3 and 10.4.

Investigation

Hairs should be plucked and mounted for examination by light microscopy. Electron microscopy is not required to establish the diagnosis, however, it may better delineate the degree of hair weathering.

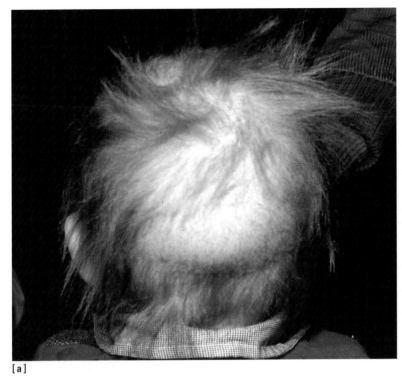

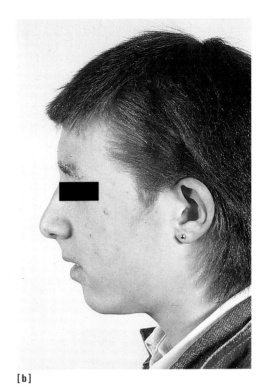

[a]

[b]

Fig. 10.12 Pili torti tends to improve with age.

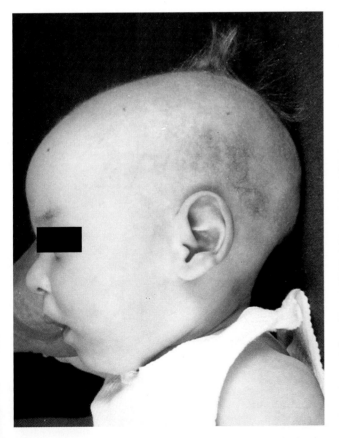

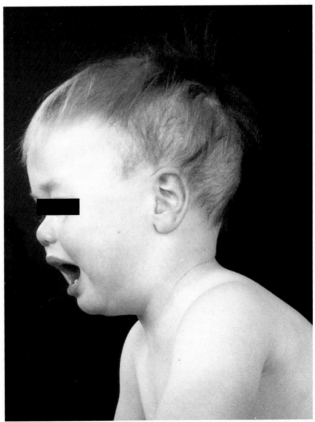

[a]

[b]

Fig. 10.13 (a) An infant with Menkes' kinky hair syndrome, and (b) shown again at the age of 12 months. (Courtesy of POSSUM.)

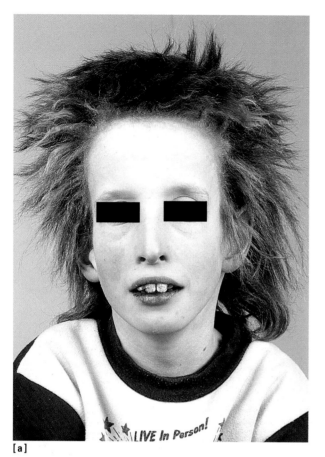
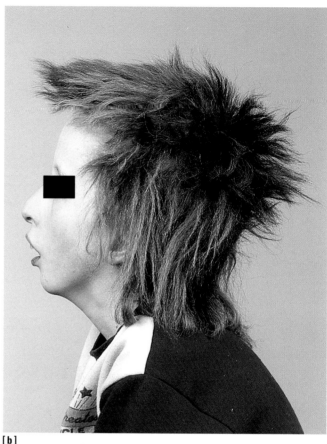

[a]   [b]

Fig. 10.14 The same child aged 12 years with Menkes' kinky hair syndrome following treatment from birth with systemic copper histidine. (Courtesy of POSSUM.)

Pathology

The diagnosis is confirmed by demonstrating the perfect 180° twists on light microscopy (Fig. 10.15). To the inexperienced observer the twists may look like beads on light microscopy and this is a source of confusion in the literature. With scanning electron microscopy extensive proximal weathering can be seen and trichorrhexis nodes and fractures are seen at the twists (Fig. 10.16).

Differential diagnosis

It is common to see patients with clinical features suggestive of a hair shaft defect, who are not easily classified. A proportion of these people have some incomplete twists in their hair and are accordingly diagnosed as having a twisting hair dystrophy. These patients are heterogeneous and more work is required to determine the significance of this finding, which may also be seen occasionally in normal hair. Twisted hairs may also occur at the edge of an area of cicatricial alopecia, due to deformity of the hair infundibulum by the scarring process. It is of no diagnostic significance.

Prognosis

Patients with true pili torti can be reassured that most will improve at puberty. Without treatment Menkes' patients slowly deteriorate, and die within a few years of life. Partially treated males may develop long unruly hair that resembles uncombable hair (Fig. 10.14) The twisting hair dystrophies are a diverse group and the prognosis is very variable.

Table 10.4 Ectodermal dysplasias associated with pili torti.

Salamon syndrome
Arthrogryphosis and ectodermal dysplasia
Ectodermal dysplasia with syndactyly
Tricho-odonto-onycho-dysplasia with syndactyly
Pili torti and enamel hypoplasia
Pili torti and onychodysplasia
Rapp–Hodgkin's syndrome
Ankyloblepharon–ectodermal dysplasia–cleft lip and palate (AEC) syndrome

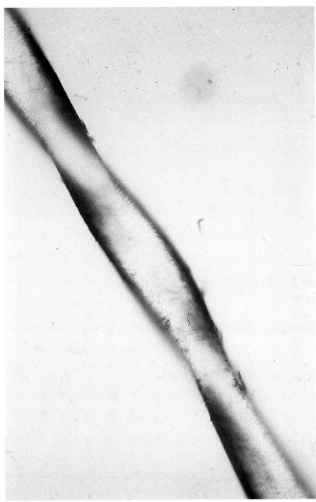

Fig. 10.15 Light microscopy showing neat 180° twists.

10.6 Netherton's syndrome (trichorrhexis invaginata)

Definition

Netherton's syndrome is characterized by a specific ichthyosiform erythroderma; ichthyosis linearis circumflexa (ILC) combined with a specific hair shaft defect known as trichorrhexis invaginata.

Epidemiology

Netherton's syndrome is very rare. Females tend to have more severely affected hair, while males have more severe skin disease.

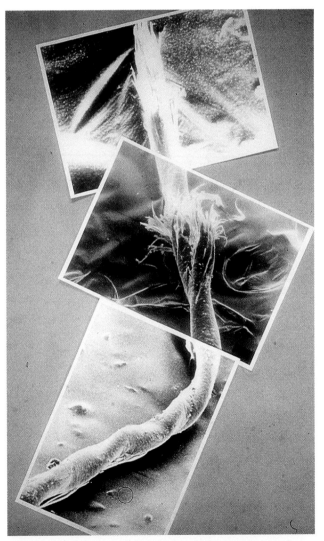

Fig. 10.16 Electron microscopy of a twisted hair showing the weathering that occurs at the twist and ultimately leads to tapered fractures.

Treatment

While awaiting possible spontaneous improvement, minimizing hair trauma is desirable. If the diagnosis of Menkes' is made prenatally then labour should be induced at 32 weeks gestation to commence early intramuscular copper histidine replacement therapy.

Key points

Pili torti is an autosomal dominant, self-limiting hair shaft disorder of childhood characterized by spangled hair, that is fragile and breaks easily to produce a sparse stubble. Pili torti most commonly occurs as an isolated finding, but in some cases pili torti is part of a syndrome. Hair microscopy is diagnostic when the hairs are twisted completely through 180° at irregular intervals. Incomplete twists are nonspecific and occur in a variety of poorly characterized hair shaft disorders collectively known as twisting hair dystrophies.

Aetiology

The disorder is inherited in an autosomal recessive fashion with intrafamily variation in expression.

Pathogenesis

Trichorrhexis invaginata occurs due to intussusception of the distal portion of the hair shaft into the proximal portion.

Clinical features and investigation

The patient may present primarily with either the cutaneous changes or with sparse and fragile hair (Figs 10.17 & 10.18). Generalized erythema and scaling is usually present at birth (without a collodion membrane), but the degree, extent and persistence are variable. In general the ichthyosiform

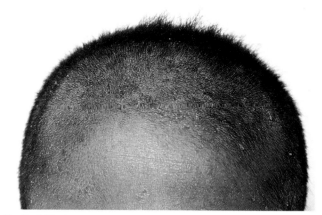

Fig. 10.18 The hair in Netherton's syndrome.

erythroderma tends to improve in late childhood. Pruritus aggravated by heat is a prominent symptom. Failure to thrive is a prominent feature in infancy and intensive nutritional support and prolonged hospitalization may be required.

The characteristic skin lesion, ILC has been present in three-quarters of reported cases. It is a polycyclic and serpiginous eruption with a keratotic margin, characterized by a double-edged scale, which slowly migrates and changes pattern (Figs 10.17 & 10.19). Rarely a subcorneal blister can be seen in the margin. Ichthyosis linearis circumflexa tends not to develop until after the age of 2 years and is episodic. Attacks last 2–3 weeks and then clear for weeks or months at a time.

Pathology

Histology of the active margin is diagnostic. Eosinophilic degeneration of the cells in the upper malpighian layers with overlying parakeratosis is seen. Infections of any kind may aggravate the erythroderma. Other types of ichthyosis such as ichthyosis vulgaris and X-linked ichthyosis may also occur

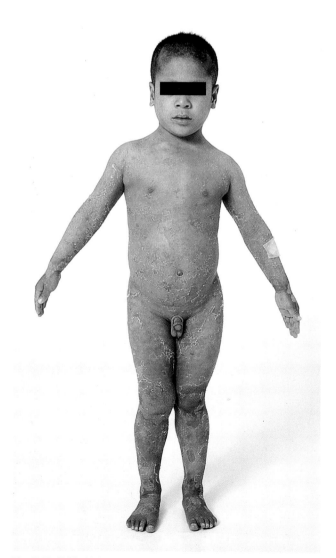

Fig. 10.17 Child with Netherton's syndrome. (Courtesy of Dr J. Wishart, New Zealand.)

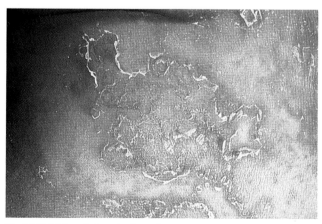

Fig. 10.19 Ichthyosis linearis circumflexa.

with Netherton's syndrome. Rarely epilepsy or growth retardation may be associated.

The hair changes appear in infancy. All cases of ILC can be shown to have bamboo hairs if sought carefully. In some cases only the proximal fragment of a fractured invaginate node remains and resembles a golf tee. In most cases abnormal hairs are readily found and consist of torsion nodules, invaginate nodules and trichorrhexis nodosa, giving individual hairs a bamboo-like appearance (Figs 10.20–10.22). The patient presents with short, dry and brittle hair on the scalp, and sparse or absent eyebrows and eyelashes.

Investigation

Skin biopsy and hair shaft microscopy may show diagnostic features, but frequently the findings are nonspecific. Multiple hair shaft examinations and skin biopsies repeated at regular intervals may be required.

Differential diagnosis

In the absence of a family history the diagnosis is often missed in infancy. Common misdiagnoses include congenital nonbullous ichthyosiform erythroderma, Leiner's disease, acrodermatitis enteropathica and the peeling skin syndrome.

Associated features

Up to 75% of patients also have an atopic diathesis. Failure to thrive in infancy is common and potentially life threatening.

Other associated features are:
• a characteristic facies due to prominent perioral erythema and maceration;
• flexural lichenification;
• nail dystrophy (including pterygium);
• a persistent tender, verrucous hypertrophy of the axillae, inguinal folds and lower legs that develops in early adult life.

Sixteen per cent of patients are said to be intellectually subnormal, but normal intelligence is the rule if perinatal complications are minimized.

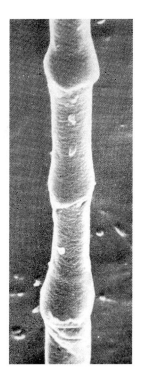

Fig. 10.21 Electron microscopy of Bamboo hair.

Prognosis

Spontaneous improvement may occur as the patient gets older (Fig. 10.23), but is not seen in every case.

Treatment

There is no specific treatment for the hair. Retinoids may improve the skin but their effect is variable and in many cases they make the rash worse; reminiscent of the effect of retinoids on atopic eczema. Worsening of the skin with retinoids helps to distinguish Netherton's syndrome from other ichthyosiform erythrodermas. Retinoids have minimal impact on the hair.

Emollients, keratolytics and antibiotics help the skin and photochemotherapy is useful for difficult cases. Calcipotriol has recently been used successfully in one child and warrants further investigation. It is important to control any itchy eczema on the scalp to minimize hair trauma. However, the ichthyosis does not respond to topical steroids and over treatment of the skin may produce Cushingoid features.

Key points

Netherton's syndrome is an autosomal recessive hair shaft disorder characterized by increased hair fragility and alopecia, associated with a nondistinct ichthyosiform erythroderma at birth, which later evolves into the hallmark ichthyosis: ILC. Atopy occurs in 75% of cases, and many infants fail to thrive. Trichorrhexis invaginata, when seen on hair microscopy is diagnostic. Skin biopsy of the active

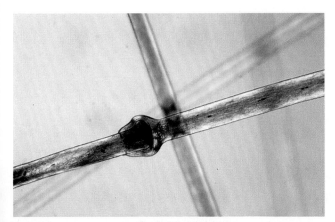

Fig. 10.20 Light microscopy of trichorehexis invaginata.

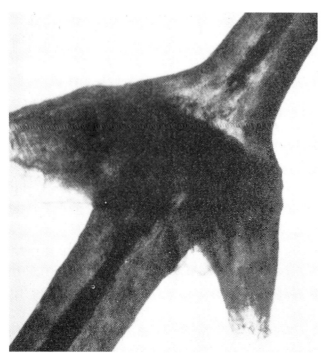

Fig. 10.22 Electron microscopy of an invaginate node.

margin of ILC is diagnostic and shows eosinophilic degeneration in the stratum malphighii.

10.7 Trichothiodystrophy

Definition

Trichothiodystrophy (TTD) is characterized by brittle sulphur deficient hairs. The syndrome may also involve other organs of neuroectodermal origin. The characteristic finding is alternating light and dark bands on polarized light microscopy of hair shafts, and this serves as an important marker for this condition.

Epidemiology

Rare.

Aetiology

Trichothiodystrophy is an autosomal recessive genodermatosis. Some patients with TTD also have a fault with repair of DNA damaged by UV light, identical to that seen in xeroderma pigmentosum group D. However, these patients are not necessarily photosensitive and do not have an increased susceptibility to skin cancer.

Pathogenesis

The hair cysteine content is less than 50% of normal and the fragility is due to failure of high-sulphur protein to migrate to the exocuticular part of the hair cuticle cells (Fig. 10.24). The normally homogeneous band of high sulphur proteins in the A-layer becomes fragmented in TTD.

Clinical features

Patients have persistent alopecia of the scalp, eyebrows and eyelashes due to breakage of the hairs close to the scalp (Figs 10.25–10.27). After puberty, other hairs on the body may also be affected, and diffuse follicular keratosis with or without an ichthyosiform erythroderma sometimes develops. The nails are brittle and dystrophic.

Pathology

Hair microscopy shows brittle and badly weathered hair. One relatively characteristic abnormality is trichoschisis, which is a clean, transverse fracture across the hair shaft at a site that has lost its cuticle. Trichoschisis can occur sporadically in normal hairs as a manifestation of excessive weathering,

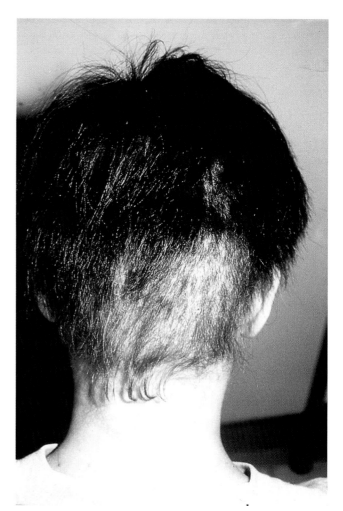

Fig. 10.23 An older child with Netherton's syndrome in whom the hair has grown longer and only breaks at sites of maximal trauma, such as the occiput.

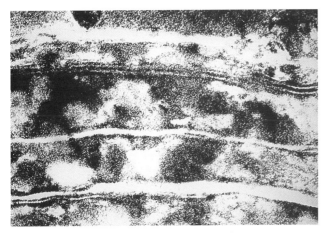

Fig. 10.24 Electron microscopy showing the absent A-layer.

however it is more usual for normal hairs to fracture at trichorrhexis nodes (trichoclasis). Light microscopy also shows flattened and twisted ribbon-like hairs. On scanning electron microscopy the shaft can be seen to be irregular with ridging and fluting and the cuticular scales are completely deficient in places (Fig. 10.28).

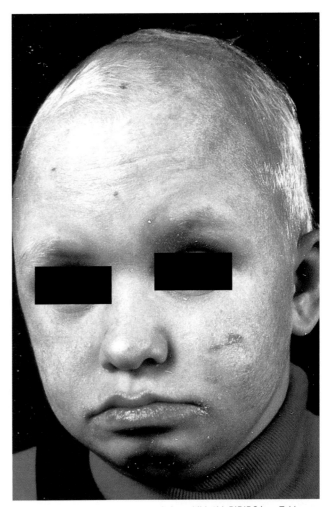

Fig. 10.26 Moderately severe alopecia in a child with PIBIDS (see Table 10.5).

Polarized light microscopy shows the characteristic 'tiger tail' pattern of alternating dark and light diagonal bands (Fig. 10.29).

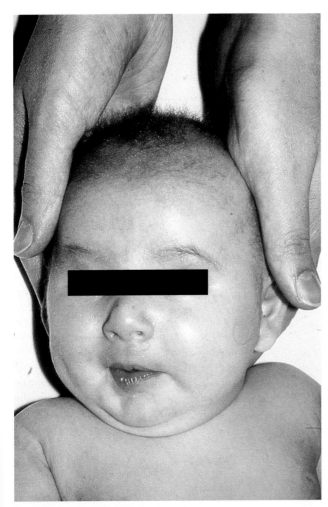

Fig. 10.25 An infant with trichothiodystrophy.

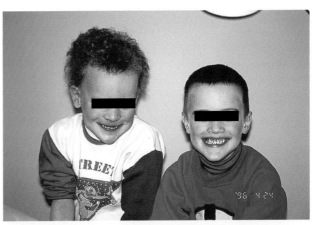

Fig. 10.27 The twin on the left has IBIDS (see Table 10.5). While her brother has his hair cut every 6 weeks, her hair rarely if ever requires cutting.

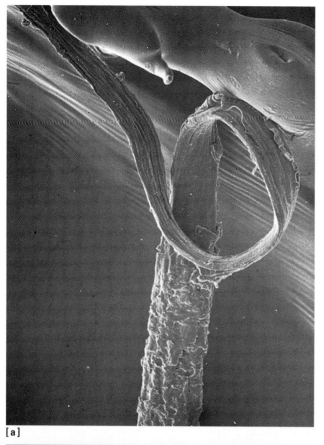

[a]

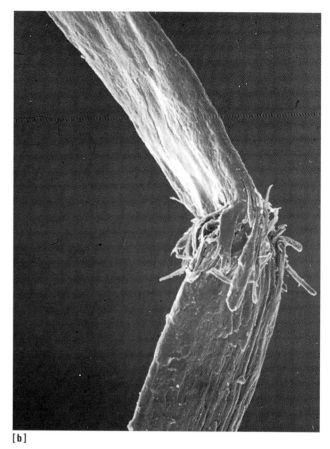

[b]

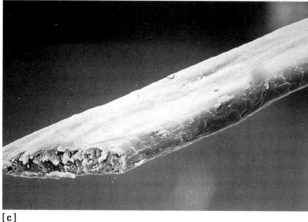

[c]

Fig. 10.28 (a) The hair is weathered and flattened and resembles a ribbon. (b) Trichorrhexis nodes are the most common finding in trichothiodystrophy, while (c) trichoschisis is more specific.

Investigation

Hair should be examined by light microscopy and polarized light microscopy. Confirmation of the diagnosis requires measurement of the sulphur content by hydrolysis and 2D electrophoresis and spectrophotometry. However, this is not readily obtained outside of specialized centres.

Differential diagnosis

The changes seen on light microscopy are frequently non-specific and could simply represent hair weathering. The occurrence of these changes near to the root is suggestive of an intrinsic hair shaft defect. If the tiger tail is seen on polarized light microscopy, that is very helpful, however, this is not present in all cases. It is also important to realize that this pattern is not exclusive to TTD. It is also seen in arginosuccidase deficiency. For a definite diagnosis the hair cysteine content should be measured and this is pathognomonic.

Associated features

In addition to the nail changes, patients may have an as-

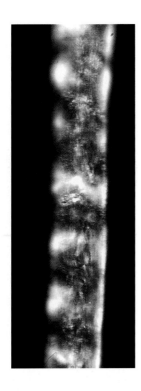

Fig. 10.29 Tiger tail pattern seen with polarized light microscopy in trichothiodystrophy. (Courtesy of Dr D. de Berker, Bristol.)

sociated ichthyosis, photosensitivity, short stature, intellectual impairment, decreased fertility and low fertility. A number of syndrome complexes are described by acronyms (Table 10.5).

Prognosis

The disorders seen in TTD tend to be fixed with no tendency to spontaneous improvement.

Treatment

No specific therapy for the hair is available. It is generally not possible to decrease weathering sufficiently to allow the hair

to grow to any significant length. The associated abnormalities often dominate the picture and require specific supportive treatment, particularly minimizing sun-induced skin damage. Genetic counselling is important, but is made difficult by genetic heterogeneity. Second trimester prenatal diagnosis of those cases associated with a DNA repair defect has already been accomplished.

Recently hairs collected from the scalp of TTD patients have been grafted onto nude mice. The hairs produced by the graft-bearing mouse display the same biochemical profile as the original hairs from the donor. This animal model will allow *in vivo* investigations modulating gene expression and may ultimately lead to treatment for this condition.

Key points

Trichothiodystrophy is an autosomal recessive disorder. Impaired incorporation of sulphur-rich protein into the hair cuticle leads to the production of structurally unsound hair. There may be a number of associated neuroectodermal disorders. Hair microscopy shows trichoschisis, polarized light microscopy shows a tiger-tail pattern and chemical analysis of the hair demonstrates a profound sulphur (cysteine) deficiency.

10.8 Pili annulati

Definition

Pili annulati or ringed hair is a distinctive hair shaft abnormality that produces alternating light and dark bands that can give a spangled appearence to the hair.

Epidemiology

Uncommonly diagnosed, as most patients are asymptomatic and do not present to dermatologists.

Table 10.5 Syndromes associated with trichothiodystrophy.

	P	I	B	Ich	D	S	n	Other abnormalities
Trichoschisis			+					
Sabinas syndrome			+	+	+			Ocular
BIDS syndrome			+	+	+	+		Quadriplegia, fits
IBIDS or Tay's syndrome		+	+	+	+	+		Dental, ocular and cardiac
PIBIDS syndrome	+	+	+	+	+	+	+	XP
SIBIDS		+	+	+	+	+	+	Osteosclerosis and cataracts
ONMR syndrome			+	+		+	+	Recurrent infections
Marinesco–Sjogren's syndrome			+	+		+		Neurological and dental

B, brittle, sulphur deficient hair often associated with brittle nails; I, intellectual impairment; D, decreased fertility; S, short stature; Ich, ichthyosis; P, photosensitivity; n, neutropenia; ONMR, onychotrichodysplasia, neutropenia, mental retardation; XP, xeroderma pigmentosa.

Aetiology

Pili annulati is an autosomal dominant condition with variable expressivity.

Pathogenesis

A defect of hair shafts causes randomly distributed clusters of air-filled cavities to appear within the cortex that are between 0.1 and 2 mm wide. These are seen on light microscopy as alternating light and dark bands Increased hair fragility is not generally a feature of pili annulati, and the hairs are in all other respects normal.

Clinical features

Pili annulati is frequently an incidental finding during patient examination. Fair haired patients may present having detected a spangled appearance in their hair (Fig. 10.30). In dark haired people the banding is obscured by the pigment.

Rarely patients present with slow hair growth, or with hair breakage, which may occur in the abnormal bands if the hairs are subjected to unusual trauma. Nevertheless, hair tension studies do not demonstrate increased hair fragility. Axillary hairs may also be affected.

Pathology

With the naked eye or the epiluminescent microscope one sees the abnormal pale bands alternating with normal darker bands. When viewed by light microscopy the pattern is reversed, with the normal bands appearing pale (Figs 10.31 & 10.32). Electron microscopy shows cobblestoning of the cuticle, and examination of the hair in cross-section shows air filled cavities lying partly within cortical cells and between macro fibrils (Fig. 10.33).

Investigation

Light microscopy is sufficient for diagnosis.

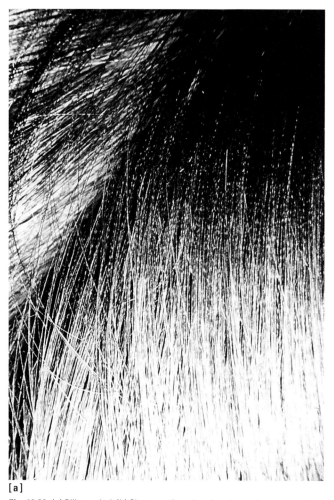
[a]

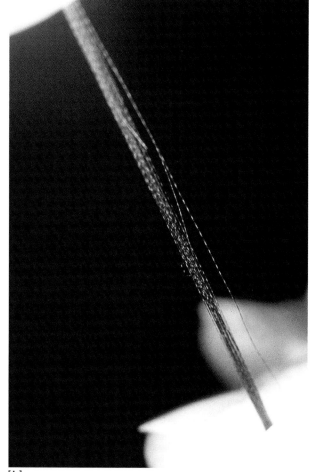
[b]

Fig. 10.30 (a) Pili annulati. (b) Close-up view showing alternating dark and light bands.

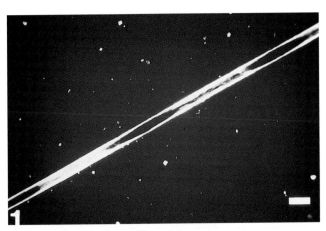

Fig. 10.31 Light microscopy of pili annulati.

Differential diagnosis

Pseudo pili annulati is sometimes seen in normal hair. An apparent banding that resembles pili annulati is seen when the hair is examined by light microscopy and is due to an optical effect. The illusion is created by regular partial twisting back and forth of elliptical hair. Clinically the hair is normal and electron microscopy of the hair is also normal.

Associated features

Usually none, however blue naevi have been reported.

Prognosis

The patient can be reassured that the abnormality does not worsen with age.

Treatment

No treatment is usually required. In those cases where hair fragility is a problem, hairdressing procedures that excessively traumatize the hair should be avoided.

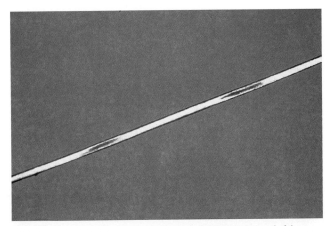

Fig. 10.32 Polarized microscopy of pili annulati showing reversal of the banding.

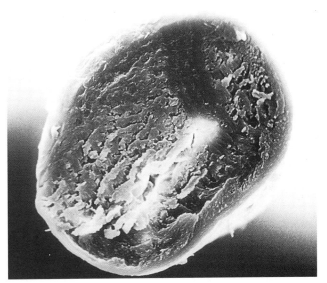

Fig. 10.33 Cross-section of the hair in pili annulati shows air-filled cavities lying within the cortical cells.

Key points

A hereditary hair shaft disorder without increased fragility characterized by alternating dark and light bands that may sometimes be seen with the naked eye. Hair growth tends to be slow, and patients may present having detected a spangled appearance in their hair.

10.9 Woolly hair

Definition

Woolly hair is the occurrence of tightly coiled scalp hair in a non-black individual. The name derives from a resemblance to sheep's wool. The condition may be localized or generalized and congenital or acquired.

Epidemiology

Uncommon.

Aetiology

The congenital diffuse form is usually inherited as an autosomal dominant trait, although recessive inheritance has been described. Congenital localized woolly hair naevus occurs sporadically. Acquired woolly hair or acquired progressive kinking may occur either as a prodrome to androgenetic alopecia or as a side-effect of etretinate drug treatment.

Pathogenesis

The basis for the woolly appearence of the hair is unknown, but may relate to its cross-sectional morphology.

Clinical features

In diffuse woolly hair, excessively curly hair is present at birth (Figs 10.34 & 10.35). Though tightly coiled, the hair is brittle and may develop proximal trichorrhexis nodes and fractures. Frequently, the hair never grows to more than 2 or 3 cm. Hair diameter is reduced and the colour may be lighter than that of unaffected family members.

Woolly hair naevus occurs as one or more circumscribed patches of tightly curled hair (Fig. 10.36), which are often slightly lighter in colour than the rest of the hair. It is present at birth or appears during the first 2 years of life.

Acquired woolly hair has been variously described under the names of acquired progressive kinking, whisker hair or symmetrical circumscribed allotrichia. All three appear to be variants of the same condition. It first presents at adolescence with an irregular band around the edge of the scalp, that runs from above the ears to the occipital region. This hair becomes coarse, unruly, kinky, dry and lustreless (Fig. 10.37). Patients may also notice that the area rarely requires cutting.

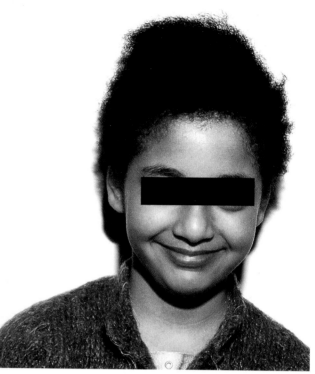

Fig. 10.35 Generalized woolly hair in a child of Indian descent.

Pathology

Hair microscopy shows a general waviness and half-twists. Scalp biopsy is normal (Fig. 10.38).

Investigation

Hair microscopy is sufficient.

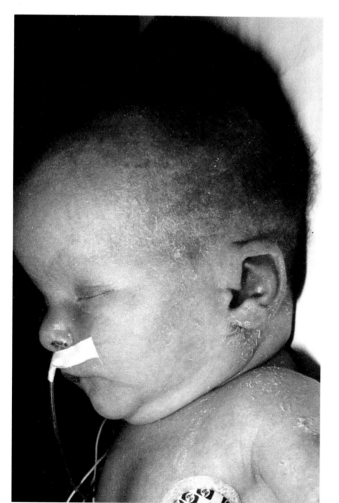

Fig. 10.34 Generalized woolly hair in an infant. (Courtesy of POSSUM.)

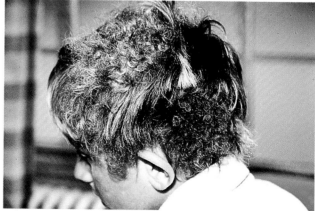

Fig. 10.36 Woolly hair naevus.

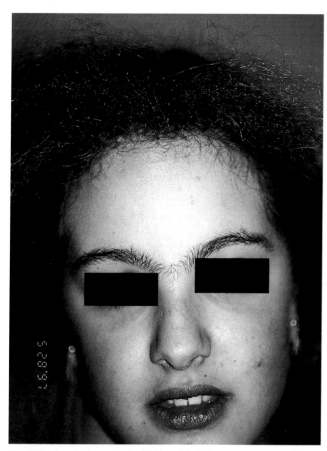

Fig. 10.37 Acquired progressive kinking of the hair.

Differential diagnosis

The unruly hair may be confused with pili torti, the uncombable hair syndrome and the loose anagen syndrome.

Associated features

Usually none, although there is an association with verrucous or linear epidermal naevus, usually on the neck or arm, in a

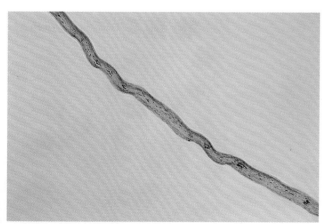

Fig. 10.38 Light micrograph of a woolly hair.

proportion of cases. An epidermal naevus directly beneath the woolly hair naevus has also been reported and has been associated with a variety of ectodermal defects and called the woolly hair naevus syndrome. Other occasional associations include keratosis pilaris atrophicans, pili torti, pili annulati and a variety of ocular, skeletal and developmental defects. An eye examination is recommended for woolly-haired patients.

Prognosis

The diffuse type of congenital woolly hair tends to improve with age. Usually, but not invariably, acquired progressive kinking heralds the onset of androgenetic alopecia.

Treatment

No therapy is available.

Key points

Woolly hair is the occurrence of curly and wiry hair on the scalp of a non-Negroid person, that resembles pubic hair. It may appear either at birth diffusely as an autosomal dominant trait, at birth as a circumscribed developmental defect, in adolescence as a possible precursor of androgenetic alopecia (acquired progressive kinking) or in a person receiving etretinate.

10.10 Uncombable hair syndrome

Definition

Unruly hair due to a distinctive hair shaft defect that leads to the production of hair with a triangular or kidney shaped cross-section. Also known as pili trianguli et canaliculi.

Epidemiology

Uncommon.

Aetiology

Uncombable hair is most likely to be an autosomal dominant genodermatosis. However, many patients do not have a positive family history.

Pathogenesis

A disturbance of hair shaft shape, with hairs that are kidney shaped and almost triangular in cross-section rather than round or oval, and which have a well-defined longitudinal depression, produces the unruly hair. The hairs may twist, but tend to be resistant to weathering. It has been suggested that the cross-sectional shape of the hair renders it more rigid, and this, combined with the minimal cuticular weathering, encourages the hair to stand on end.

Clinical features

The hair is difficult to manage and unruly. The unruly hair usually first becomes manifest at the age of 3 or 4 years, however it may not be noticed until the child is 12 years old. The hair is normal in quantity and often also in length. The hair is difficult to brush, comb or style and sometimes these efforts may lead to hair breakage. The hair is often a distinctive silvery-blond due to reflection of light from the flat surface of differently angulated hair shafts, although the hair may occasionally be red (Figs 10.39 & 10.40). An alternate name for this condition is spun glass hair. The eyebrows and eyelashes are normal.

Pathology

Hair microscopy may appear normal or show twists and homogenous longitudinal shadowing to one side suggestive of a groove (Fig. 10.41). Electron microscopy shows the longitudinal depression and triangular or kidney-shaped cross-section (Fig. 10.42). Not all the hairs are affected, but in most cases over half will show the abnormal cross-section.

Horizontal scalp histology shows the irregular shape of some of the hair follicles and can be used to confirm the diagnosis in difficult cases or if an electron microscope is not handy.

Investigation

While the diagnosis can be suspected on light microscopy, electron microscopy is very helpful.

Differential diagnosis

Occasional triangular hairs may occur in the normal population as well as in a variety of ectodermal dysplasias and the

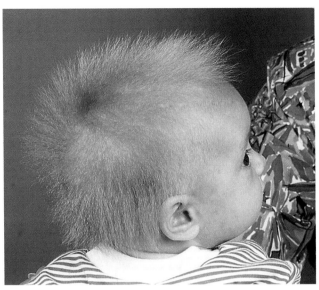

Fig. 10.40 Uncombable hair syndrome in a redhead.

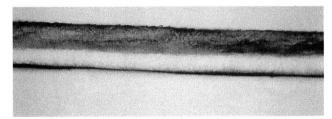

Fig. 10.41 Light microscopy demonstrating the eccentric medulla indicating the hair is triangular rather than round.

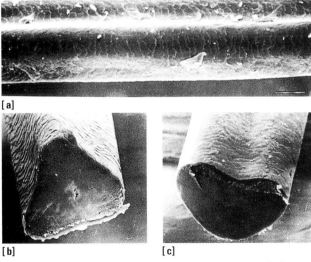

[a]

[b]   [c]

Fig. 10.42 Scanning electron micrograph of a hair showing canalicular gutter along the hair shaft (a). In cross-section the hair can be seen to be triangular (b) or kidney shaped (c).

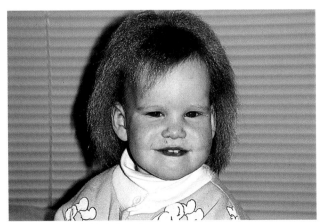

Fig. 10.39 Uncombable hair syndrome.

Marie Unna syndrome also has grooved hairs. Thus the microscopy is only pathognomonic, if the groove is seen in more than 50% of the plucked hairs and the diagnosis often requires clinicopathological correlation.

Associated features

While uncombable hair has been reported in asssociation with ectodermal dysplasia, it is unlikely that these were true cases of uncombable hair syndrome.

Prognosis

The condition usually improves with age.

Treatment

None is required other than reassurance and advice to keep the hair short so it is more easily managed. Biotin has been reported to be helpful although in our experience it has not been effective.

Key points

Uncombable hair syndrome is a hereditary syndrome characterized by silvery unruly hair that is first noticed when the child is between 3 and 12 years old. There is a distinctive triangular hair shaft abnormality that is best seen with scanning electron microscopy.

10.11 Straight hair naevus

Definition

A straight hair naevus is the opposite of a woolly hair naevus. The hairs in a localized area of a Negroid scalp are straight.

Epidemiology

Uncommon.

Aetiology

Unknown.

Pathogenesis

The straight hairs are round in cross-section. The cross-sectional shape is thought to determine whether the hair is straight or curly.

Clinical features

A straight hair naevus is usually present at birth (Fig. 10.43), but in one case it developed from a patch of apparently normal hair at the age of 6 months.

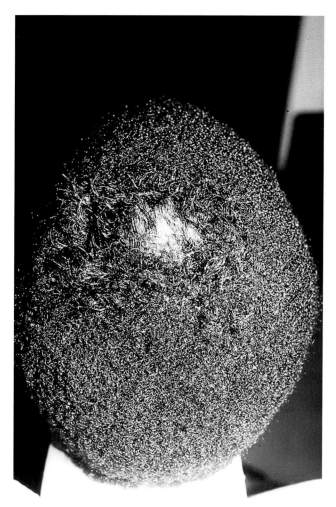

Fig. 10.43 Straight hair naevus in a black child.

Pathology

As well as having a circular cross-sectional shape, the hairs are about one-half the normal diameter. The cuticular scales are small and their pattern disorganized.

Investigation

Light microscopy is recommended.

Differential diagnosis

It was suggested that straight hair naevus represented a localized form of uncombable hair syndrome, however, this has been discounted as the hairs do not show a longitudinal groove or triangular cross-section on electron microscopy.

Recently local or diffuse straight hair has been described in patients with the acquired immune deficiency syndrome (AIDS) and scalp biopsy in these patients has shown a lymphohistiocytic infiltrate and fibrosis around the upper and mid-follicle.

Associated features

The abnormal hair may be associated with an underlying epidermal naevus, but more commonly the scalp is normal.

Prognosis

Uncertain.

Treatment

None has been shown to be effective.

Key points

A naevus consisting of a localized patch of straight hair on a Negroid scalp.

10.12 Loose anagen syndrome

Definition

Loose anagen syndrome is a disorder of anagen hair anchorage to the hair follicle, characterized by ability to easily and painlessly pull out large numbers of anagen hairs from the scalp.

Epidemiology

Loose anagen syndrome was first described in 1986 but despite the paucity of reported cases, it is by no means rare.

Aetiology

The condition is frequently familial and anagen hairs can often be plucked without force from one or other of the apparently normal parents, suggesting an autosomal dominant mode of inheritance (Fig. 10.44).

Pathogenesis

There is a generalized disturbance of cellular adhesion, that is most pronounced between the inner root sheath and the hair cuticle. Traction on the hair causes separation of the hair from the inner root sheath which remains attached to the rest of the follicle.

Clinical features

Females are more often affected than males, and usually have fair hair which is dry and lustreless (Fig. 10.45). The condition does not present until the ages of 2–9 years. Parents complain that the child has easily pluckable hair that infrequently requires cutting. Some children have diffuse thinning of their hair and hair of uneven lengths while others have focal areas of alopecia.

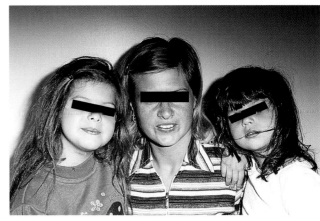

Fig. 10.44 The mother and two daughters all have loose anagen syndrome.

In addition the hair is frequently unruly and may have a tacky feel about it.

Pathology

The trichogram of the plucked hairs is striking in showing 98–100% anagen hairs. This relates to the fact that plucking normal hairs precipitates the onset of the next anagen (p. 7). Microscopy of the hair shows distinctive misshapen hairs with a distorted bulb, pronounced cuticular ruffling distal to the bulb and a short segment of twisted hair shaft between the bulb and the roughened and frayed cuticle. Additionally, the external root sheath is absent from the plucked anagen hair, while the internal root sheath and the cuticle are absent distal to the bulb (Fig. 10.46).

Examination of the distal hair shafts may show kinking similar to that seen in woolly hair (Fig. 10.47). In addition trichorrhexis nodes and longitudinal grooves are occasionally seen.

Electron microscopy shows that the hairs have abnormal shapes, being triangular, quadrangular, trapezoid, kidney

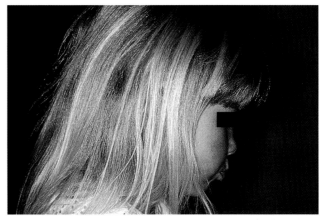

Fig. 10.45 Child with loose anagen syndrome showing the characteristic blond wavy hair.

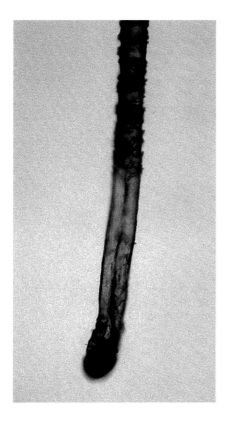

Fig. 10.46 Light micrograph showing the ruffling of the cuticle in loose anagen syndrome.

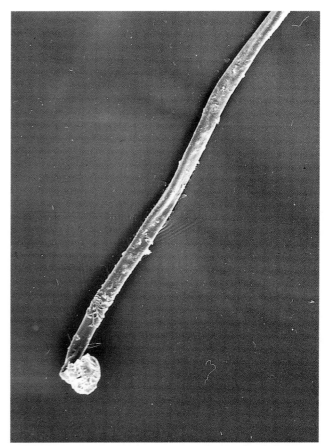

Fig. 10.48 Electron micrograph of a loose anagen hair showing cuticular ruffling.

shaped or heart shaped. The hairs may have longitudinal grooves with slight twisting about their axis resembling uncombable hair syndrome or woolly hair. Distal to the bulb the cuticular scales are rolled backward creating a rippled appearance (Fig. 10.48).

Scalp histology shows a cleft between the inner and outer root sheaths, and the inner root sheath appears homogenized due to premature keratinization of the layers of Huxley and Henle. There is no perifollicular inflammation, and some hairs are not involved in the process.

Investigation

Light microscopy of the hair bulb is usually sufficient to make the diagnosis.

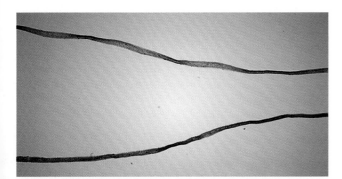

Fig. 10.47 The distal hair shaft shows changes similar to those seen in woolly hair, which may explain the unruly nature of the hair.

Differential diagnosis

It is important to distinguish this syndrome from AA, in which exclamation mark hairs may be found, and from telogen effluvium in which the plucked hairs are club hairs. The unruly hair may lead to confusion with pili torti, uncombable hair syndrome or woolly hair.

Associated features

The child is otherwise well and there are no associated abnormalities of nails or dentition.

Prognosis

While cases of loose anagen syndrome have been described in adults, on the whole the condition improves spontaneously in the mid to late teens.

Treatment

None is required other than to reassure the patient while awaiting spontaneous improvement.

Key points

Loose anagen syndrome is most commonly seen in young blond girls and is characterized by loose, anagen hairs, that are easily and painlessly removed in clumps, to leave patches of alopecia, which always regrow. Hairs show a distinctive cuticular ruffling just distal to the bulb on microscopy. The condition improves with age and is associated with unruly hair with a tacky texture.

10.13 Pohl–Pinkus lines

Definition

Pohl–Pinkus lines are a zone of decreased hair shaft diameter.

Epidemiology

Relatively common, but frequently unrecognized.

Aetiology

Pohl–Pinkus lines may follow serious illness, major surgery or antimitotic chemotherapy.

Pathogenesis

Early anagen hairs are susceptible to events which may produce a temporary disturbance of protein synthesis in the hair matrix. This is manifest by a zone of decreased hair shaft diameter.

Clinical features

Some months after the insult, a band becomes obvious along the growing hair that can be seen with the naked eye to represent a focal area of hair constriction. Longer narrowings or anagen effluvium may occur with ongoing injury or larger doses of chemotherapy.

Pathology

Hair microscopy and electron microscopy show the transition in hair calibre (Fig. 10.49).

Investigation

Light microscopy is sufficient.

Associated features

Pohl–Pinkus lines are to hair what Beaus lines are to nails. Frequently, Beaus lines accompany Pohl–Pinkus constrictions.

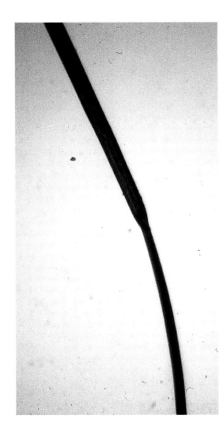

Fig. 10.49 Light micrograph of a Pohl–Pinkus hair showing the alteration in calibre.

Prognosis

Cessation of the insult allows the hair to return to its normal diameter.

Treatment

Appreciation that the constriction relates to a recent illness or medication is all that is required.

Key points

Pohl–Pinkus lines are the hair equivalent of Beaus lines in the nail. They are a zone of hair narrowing.

10.14 Peripilar casts

Definition

Hair casts are sleeve like tubular structures that encircle the hair shaft.

Epidemiology

Relatively common.

Aetiology

Disorders of keratinization and inflammation of the follicular ostium produce the casts, that are predominantly composed of retained internal root sheath adhering to the emerging hair shaft.

Pathogenesis

Peripilar casts are variably sized, tubular masses composed of amorphous keratinous material that encircle hair shafts. They are produced within the follicular infundibulum and remain attached to the hair.

Clinical features

Peripilar casts are also called pseudo-nits. They are often found in the hair of normal children and adults as whitish-yellow scales that can be easily moved up and down the hair shaft (Fig. 10.50).

Pathology

Light microscopy demonstrates the amorphous cast around the hair shaft.

Investigation

Light microscopy of an affected hair shaft quickly confirms the diagnosis (Fig. 10.51). Electron microscopy is not generally performed (Fig. 10.52).

Differential diagnosis

The ability to slide peripilar casts along the hair, distinguishes them from true nits, due to pediculosis capitis, which are eccentric and fixed tightly to the hair shaft, as well as from trichorrhexis nodes and trichonodosis. When the casts bulge out of the follicular opening they can look like comedones.

Associated features

Peripilar casts are more common in scaly scalp disorders such

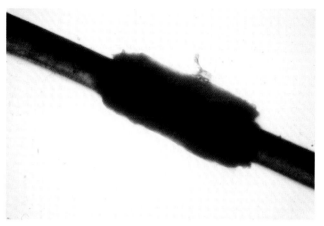
Fig. 10.51 Light photomicrograph showing the circumferential cast.

as psoriasis and seborrhoeic dermatitis, and may also accompany lichen planopilaris and traction alopecia.

Prognosis

The condition is intermittent, and casts often disappear spontaneously only to recur at some later stage.

Treatment

The casts can be removed manually with a fine toothed comb. Vitamin A lotion may reduce the number of casts formed.

Key points

Hair casts are sleeve-like tubular structures, encircling the hair shaft, consisting of retained internal root sheath. They can be diagnosed by sliding the casts up and down along the hair, and by light microscopy of the hair shaft.

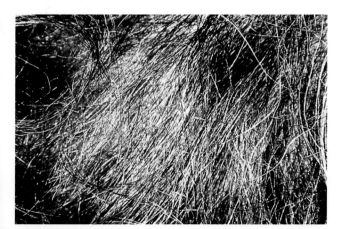
Fig. 10.50 Hair casts.

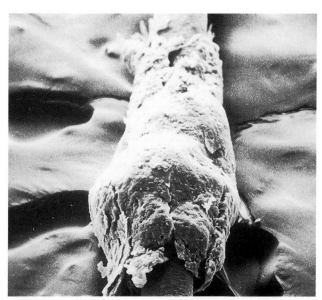
Fig. 10.52 Electron micrograph showing the circumferential cast.

10.15 Pili multigemini

Definition

Pili multigemini is a disorder characterized by bundles of hairs emerging from a single pore.

Epidemiology

Uncommon.

Aetiology

Unknown.

Pathogenesis

It has been postulated that the dermal papilla of a follicle splits into a number of parts, each giving rise to a separate hair shaft within the infundibulum.

Clinical features

Multigeminate follicles mainly occur in the beard area in adults, and on the scalp of children. Tufts of large thick terminal hairs emerge from dilated pores. Numerous pores are sometimes involved.

Pathology

Histologically the follicle can be seen to be distorted. Multiple matrices and hair papillae (2–8) give birth to numerous terminal hairs that all converge on a single infundibulum. The abnormal follicle is lined by a common outer root sheath, but each hair has its own inner root sheath. The individual hairs are distorted, being either flattened, ovoid or triangular in configuration. Neighbouring hairs may adhere to one another; some then bifurcate and later readhere. When this happens it is called pili bifurcati. It also occurs as an isolated defect in otherwise normal follicles.

Investigation

A skin biopsy will demonstrate the nature of the follicular disturbance.

Differential diagnosis

Open comedones and trichostasis spinulosa frequently contain multiple trapped vellus hair, and their distinction from multigeminate follicles is based on the size of the hairs that emerge from the follicle.

Within a patch of cicatricial alopecia it is common to see two or three hairs emerging from a single follicle. When multiple hairs emerge in clumps, this is called tufted folliculitis (p. 108), and this is most frequently seen in folliculitis decalvans.

Associated features

Pili multigemini has been reported in association with cleidocranial dysostosis, but this is exceptional. Isotretinoin has been known to cause this condition.

Prognosis

The lesions tend to persist.

Treatment

None is satisfactory. Plucking the hairs is followed by recurrence. If only one follicle is involved, punch excision including the dermal papillae is curative. If only a few follicles are involved cryosurgery could be used in an attempt to ablate the follicle, but the doses required (30 seconds, two freeze–thaw cycles) produce significant short-term morbidity and permanent hypopigmentation.

Key points

Pili multigemini is the name given to multiple terminal hairs emerging as a tuft from a single follicular opening on the face or scalp. It may be a primary isolated abnormality or secondary to follicular distortion within a patch of scarring alopecia.

10.16 Trichonodosis

Definition

When a single or double knot occurs in the hair shaft, either spontaneously or in response to rubbing or scratching it is called trichonodosis.

Epidemiology

Trichonodosis is relatively common, especially in people with short, curly hair.

Aetiology

Mechanical knotting of the hair may occur with rubbing or scratching the skin.

Pathogenesis

Short and curly hairs are prone to developing knots when rubbed in a circular motion.

Clinical features

Trichonodosis is usually an incidental finding of little significance. Some patients may present thinking they have nits, especially when the knots occur on pubic or axillary hair.

The knots can be seen on close inspection with the naked eye, and are easily demonstrated with a hand-held epiluminescence microscope.

Pathology

Light microscopy of a plucked hair (Fig. 10.53) can be used to demonstrate the knot. Electron microscopy shows damage to the cuticle where it has been extended (Fig. 10.54). Brushing or combing may cause the hair shaft to fracture at the site of the knot.

Investigation

Usually none required.

Associated features

Any abnormalities of the hair shaft are secondary to the knot. An associated dermatitis or louse which precipitated the itch and subsequent scratching may be seen.

Differential diagnosis

The knots on superficial inspection may resemble lice.

Prognosis

The condition is temporary but may be recurrent.

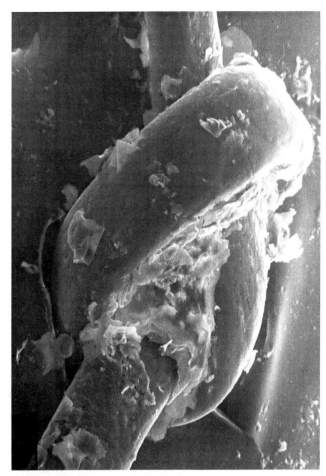

Fig. 10.54 Electron micrograph of trichonodosis.

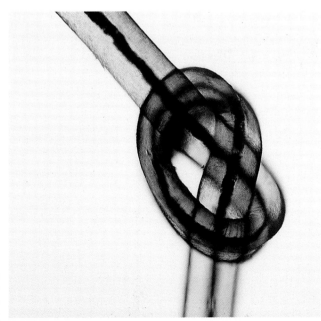

Fig. 10.53 Light micrograph of trichonodosis.

Treatment

If excessive scratching is producing the knots, treatment of the itch should lead to resolution. Combing often tightens the knots, pulls the hair out at the root or fractures the hair at the site of the knot.

Key points

Trichonodosis is an acquired knotting of the hair caused by rubbing. It may be mistaken for pediculosis. No treatment is required.

10.17 Bubble hair

Definition

Bubble hair is an acquired, localized hair shaft defect characterized by air bubbles within the hairs.

Epidemiology

Relatively common among women who use heated tongs and curling devices in their hair.

Aetiology

Overheating moist hairs produces air bubbles within the cortex.

Pathogenesis

It is thought that water seeps into the hair cortex and boils when heated with the curling tongs. Curling tongs may generate temperatures in excess of 180°C. The steam thus generated produces the bubbles. The bubbles in the hair can be focal or diffuse. The hair is weakened at the sites of the bubbles and may break.

Clinical features

Patients present with a focal area of brittle hair on the scalp. There is also a change in the texture of the involved hairs which have become straight and stiff. In affected areas the hair may fracture and come off in clumps.

Pathology

The air bubbles within the cortex that distort the entire appearence of the fibre are well seen on light microscopy (Fig. 10.55 & 10.56).

Investigation

Light microscopy.

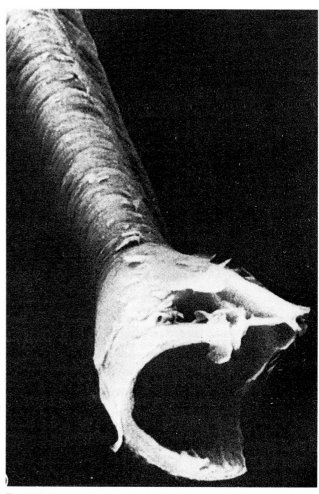

Fig. 10.56 Fracture at the site of a bubble. (Courtesy of Dr C. Gummer, London.)

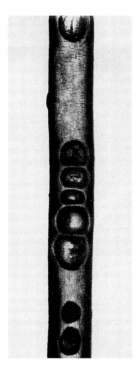

Fig. 10.55 Numerous bubbles within the hair. (Courtesy of Dr C. Gummer, London.)

Differential diagnosis

Bubble hair may clinically resemble acquired trichorrhexis nodosa; however, the two conditions are easily distinguished by light microscopy.

Associated features

Other coincidental features of weathering may be evident.

Prognosis

The condition is self-limiting if patients avoid the precipitating factors.

Treatment

Avoiding the use of curling tongs, especially on wet hair, may be sufficient. Hair dryers should not be used on the hottest setting in predisposed individuals.

Key points

An acquired hair shaft defect in which air bubbles form inside the hair. The bubbles are produced by heating wet hair sufficiently to cause any water that has seeped into the cortex to boil and produce steam.

10.18 Trichostasis spinulosa

Definition

Trichostasis spinulosa is a variant of a comedo that contains numerous vellus hairs.

Epidemiology

Common.

Aetiology

It is a normal age-related process.

Pathogenesis

It is due to follicular hyperkeratosis retarding expulsion of telogen hairs.

Clinical features

Trichostasis spinulosa is seen most commonly in the large pilosebaceous follicles on the nose and face, but has also been seen on the trunk and limbs (Fig. 10.57). Often hairs are visible in the follicular papule.

Pathology

From 5 to 50 hairs may be present in a single follicle (Fig. 10.58), which looks like a horny plug. There may be a mild perifolliculitis. Numerous follicles may be involved.

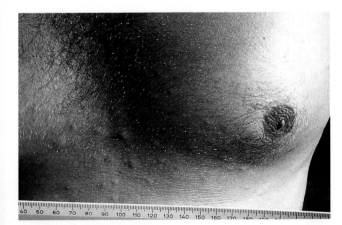

Fig. 10.57 Trichostasis spinulosa.

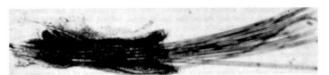

Fig. 10.58 Trichostasis spinulosa. Microscopy of a hair tuft showing numerous hairs embedded in a horny plug.

Investigation

A small skin biopsy will demonstrate the condition.

Differential diagnosis

Distinction from a comedo may be academic.

Associated features

None.

Prognosis

More tend to appear with time.

Treatment

The lesions can often be extruded without recurrence. Topical retinoic acid has been shown to be helpful as has depilatory wax. However, patients may consider the waxing a greater inconvenience than the disorder.

Key points

The presence of large comedo-like lesions that contain numerous telogen vellus hairs is called trichostasis spinulosa. The hairs have been retained in the dilated follicle as a result of follicular hyperkeratosis.

10.19 Bird's nest hair and dreadlocks

Definition

Matting of the scalp hair, or bird's nest hair is a sudden, usually irreversible tangling that occurs when shampooing.

Epidemiology

Uncommon, but most cases are localized and dealt with by hairdressers.

Aetiology

The tangling is due to an interaction between the electrostatic forces generated by the rotary action of washing on weathered, high-friction hairs.

Pathogenesis

Long hair that has not been cut for a number of years is a predisposing factor, as is badly weathered hair. The process is akin to felting, as utilized in the textile industry and recognized in the home when woollen clothing shrinks after incautious washing. The individual fibres become fused together and can only be teased apart with considerable force.

Electrostatic forces are normally present between hairs. They are increased by wetting the hair. The rotatory motion with which the shampoo is massaged into the scalp, together with the above factors, combine to produce this event.

Clinical features

Usually the hair is long and has not been cut for a number of years, often on religious grounds. Bird's nest hair is a sudden and dramatic event that fortunately is uncommon (Fig. 10.59 & 10.60). Such hair is presumably severely weathered and cuticular damage increases the friction between hairs.

Focal matting of the hair is probably a common occurrence, easily remedied by cutting or untangling the hair. Dreadlocks, as worn by Rastafarians, represent controlled matting of hair. The hair is deliberately styled in this fashion. After 2–3 years without washing or combing the hair, tightly bound locks form (Fig. 10.61). Scanning electron microscopy of a lock does not always show fusion of adjacent shafts, but does show extensive hair weathering (Fig. 10.62) and some intertwining loops.

Pathology

With the electron microscope, deposits of shampoo can be seen bound to the hairs and matting individual fibres

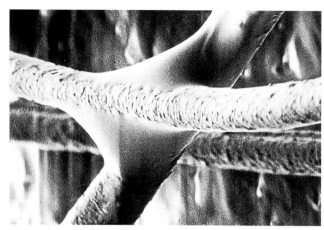

Fig. 10.60 Electron micrograph showing fusion of the individual hair fibres. In this case it is most likely to be due to hair spray.

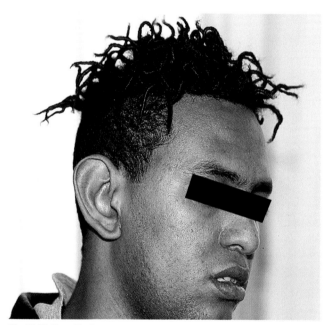

Fig. 10.61 Dreadlocks.

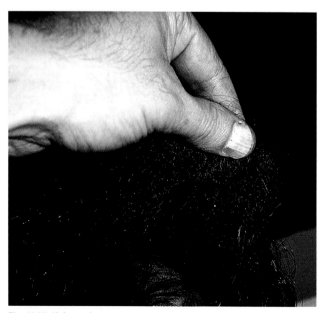

Fig. 10.59 Hair matting.

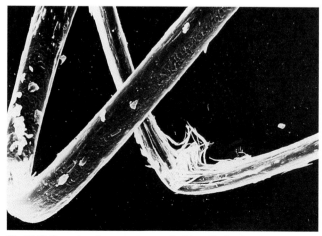

Fig. 10.62 Scanning electron micrograph of dreadlocks showing extensive weathering.

together (Fig. 10.60). The hairs are not knotted, but actually fused together and thrown into intertwining loops.

Investigation

Light and electron miscroscopy demonstrate the fusion of individual hairs.

Differential diagnosis

The clinical presentation is distinctive.

Associated features

Other evidence of weathering is usually seen.

Prognosis

If the matted hair is shaved off recurrence is exceptional. If the hair is manually unmatted, the condition is likely to recur.

Treatment

One case was successfully disentangled after 3 months of diligent lubrication of the mass with olive oil and separation of the hair with a knitting needle, however, in all other cases the affected hair had to be cut off.

Key points

Matting is a sudden, widespread, often irreversible fusion of individual hair fibres during shampooing. It produce a mass of hair that resembles a bird's nest.

Section F
Infectious, inflammatory and neoplastic disorders

Chapter 11

Infections and infestations of the hair

11.1 Tinea capitis

Definition

Tinea capitis is the invasion of scalp hair by dermatophyte fungi.

Epidemiology

The predominant organism causing tinea capitis varies from country to country (Table 11.1). *Microsporum canis* is the dominant organism in Europe, while *Trichophyton tonsurans* accounts for over 90% of tinea capitis in the USA.

Aetiology

Nearly all dermatophytes are able to parasitize hair (Table 11.2). Anthropophilic infections are acquired from close person to person contact as well as from material left on hairbrushes, combs and hats. Trauma assists inoculation. Zoophilic infections are acquired exclusively from animals, with the exception of *M. canis*, which can be secondarily spread from person to person in a limited fashion. Geophilic infections arise in children playing on infected soil. Some infections can be both zoophilic and geophilic.

Pathogenesis

Scalp ringworm is classified according to the pattern of hair invasion (Fig. 11.1). The two main forms of invasion are ectothrix (Gk *ectos* from outside) and endothrix (Gk *endon* from within). Ectothrix infections may be further classified as small spored (2–3 μm) or large spored (5–10 μm). Small spored ectothrix are only caused by *Microsporum* species.

Large spored ectothrix may be due to either *Microsporum* or *Trichophyton* species. Endothrix infections are only due to *Trichophyton* species.

Clinical features

Generally anthropophilic fungi produce noninflammatory lesions while zoophilic and geophilic fungi produce lesions with marked inflammation such as kerion and favus. Inflammatory tinea capitis tends to be self limiting over 6–10 weeks, but generally heals with scarring. Children are far more susceptible to infection than adults.

Small spore ectothrix infections classically produce annular lesions or grey patch ringworm. Brittle hairs break off close to the scalp surface to create circular patches of partial alopecia (Fig. 11.2). The broken hairs have a dull grey appearance due to their coating of arthrospores. Inflammation of the scalp is minimal, but fine scaling is characteristic. There is usually a fairly sharp margin. There may be several such patches arranged more or less randomly throughout the scalp. Each fluoresces green with a Wood's light (Fig. 11.2). Occasional nonfluorescent *Microsporum* species may occur particularly with *M. ferrugineum.* The responsible fluorescent substance (possibly pteridines) is formed only when hair keratin is invaded and fluorescence can be masked by scalp lotions or creams. These should be washed off prior to Wood's light examination. Plucked hairs do not fluoresce. With some infections due to *M. audouinii* there may be minimal hair loss and the mild scaling may mimic seborrhoeic dermatitis. The Wood's light is invaluable for these cases.

Large spored ectothrix infections may produce scalp ringworm that resemble small spored ectothrix. Alternatively, there may be more marked inflammation of the scalp. Occa-

Table 11.1 Most common causes of tinea capitis by continent.

Europe	Australia	N. America	S. America	Africa	Asia
M. canis	M. canis T. tonsurans (aborigines)	T. tonsurans M. canis M. audouinii	T. violaceum M. canis	T. violaceum T. soudanense M. audouinii M. canis T. yaoundi	T. violaceum

sionally a folliculitis or a kerion occurs, especially with zoophilic and geophilic fungi. Agminate folliculitis is a moderately severe inflammatory response and consists of well-defined dull-red plaques studded with follicular pustules (Fig. 11.3). A kerion is a painful, boggy, elevated, purulent inflammatory mass. Hairs fall out rather than break off and any remaining hairs can be easily and painlessly pulled out. Thick crusting with matting of adjacent hairs is common. The usual organisms responsible are *T. verrucosum* and *T. menta-*

grophytes. Occasionally an anthropophilic infection smouldering on for many months will suddenly develop into a kerion. Histology of a kerion shows intense folliculitis and hyphae can be readily seen with a PAS stain.

In endothrix infections the arthrospores remain confined within the cuticle. Affected hairs are severely damaged and break off at the scalp surface. Patients present with black dot ringworm, where broken hairs within an angular patch of alopecia appear as black dots. With the anthropophilic fungi,

Table 11.2 Fungi that cause tinea capitis.

		Anthropophilic	Zoophilic	Geophilic
Small spored ectothrix infections: green fluorescence with Wood's lamp	Microsporum species	M. audouinii (worldwide) M. ferrugineum (Europe, Asia, Africa)	M. canis (cats and dogs, worldwide) M. equinum (horses, widespread) M. distortum (cats, dogs, New Zealand, Australia, USA)	
Large spored ectothrix infections: no fluorescence with Wood's lamp (except rarely with M. nanum and M. gypseum)	Microsporum species		M. persicolor (field vole, West Europe) M. nanum (pigs, worldwide)	M. gypseum (worldwide) M. nanum (worldwide)
	Trichophyton species	T. megninii (Africa, Southern Europe) T. rubrum (worldwide)	T. verrucosum (cattle, widespread) T. mentag var. mentag (various animals, worldwide) T. mentag var. erinacei (hedgehogs, Europe, New Zealand) T. mentag var. quickeaneum (mice, widespread)	
Endothrix infections: no fluorescence with Wood's lamp (except pale greenish-grey with T. schoenleinii favic type)	Trichophyton species	T. tonsurans (widespread especially USA) T. schoenleinii (Middle East, North Africa) T. soudanense (Central Africa) T. violaceum (Middle East, Europe, Africa) T. gourvilii (West Africa) T. yaoundi (Africa especially Cameroon)	T. simii (monkeys, India) T. equinum (horses, widespread) T. gallinae (chickens, worldwide)	

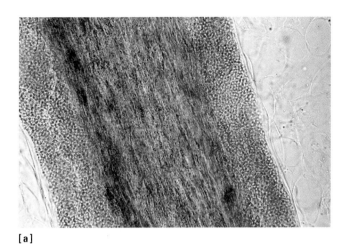

[a]

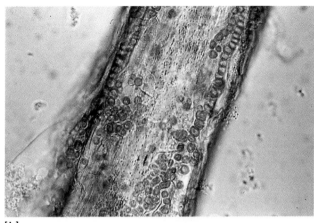

[b]

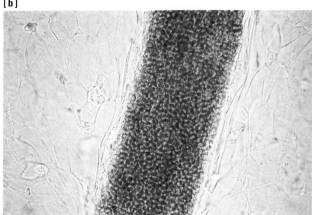

[c]

Fig. 11.1 (a) Endothrix infection of the hair. (b) Small spored ectothrix infection of the hair. (c) Large spored ectothrix infection of the hair. (Courtesy of Dr D. Ellis, Adelaide.)

there is usually minimal scaling or inflammation of the scalp. Sometimes hair loss is minimal and all that can be seen is a mild folliculitis or seborrhoeic dermatitis-like scaling. This is particularly common in black Americans infected with *T. tonsurans* and *T. violaceum*. Fluorescence is negative and the diagnosis depends on first considering the possibility and subsequent confirmation by microscopy and fungal culture.

Trichophyton schoenleinii tends to produce a distinctive type of tinea capitis known as favus. This is characterized by cutaneous atrophy, scar formation and cicatricial alopecia with yellowish cup-shaped crusts known as scutula (Fig. 11.4). Each scutulum develops around a hair that pierces it centrally. Adjacent crusts adhere and form a confluent mass of yellow crusting. The initial infection is usually in childhood, but unlike other forms of tinea capitis there is no tendency to spontaneous clearing at puberty. The lesions fluoresce a characteristic greyish green. Hair microscopy shows characteristic air spaces as hair invasion occurs without spore formation. Tinea corporis and onychomycosis sometimes occur simultaneously. Favus, like kerion generally heals with scarring to produce a cicatricial alopecia.

Tinea imbricata due to *T. concentricum* may occur on the bald scalp, but it is not known to invade hair.

Majocchi's granuloma and tinea incognito can result from treatment of tinea capitis with potent topical steroids. Typically with tinea incognito the raised margin is lost, scaling and itch are absent and the inflammation is reduced to a few nondescript nodules. Majocchi's granuloma on the scalp is rare and presents as a granulomatous folliculitis with inflammatory nodules bordering flat, scaly patches

A mycetoma is a very rare indolent infection of soft tissue, characterized by tumefaction, with or without draining sinus tracts to the skin with dark or pale granules. They occur when there is traumatic inoculation of the dermatophyte into the skin, soft tissues or bone and appear almost exclusively in Africans. The cutaneous nodules are painless, smooth, firm and mobile. They may grow very slowly for years and involvement of underlying bone produces hideous deformities.

Yeast infection of the scalp with candida is uncommon and generally only occurs in the context of immunodeficiency.

Investigation

The scalp should be examined with a Wood's light and hairs plucked for fungal microscopy and culture. A scalp biopsy

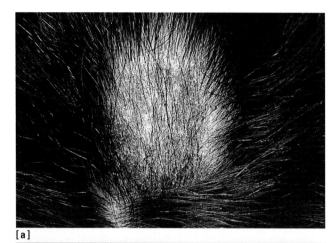

[a]

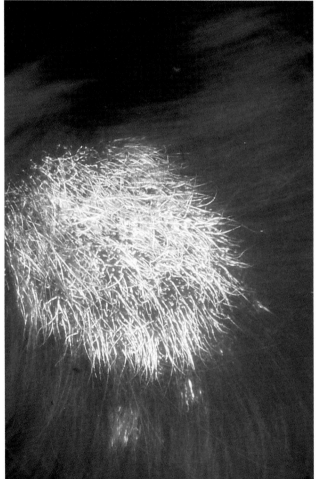

[b]

Fig. 11.2 (a) Tinea capitis. (b) Positive fluorescence of tinea capitis.

will rarely be required, but is useful in difficult or part-treated cases.

Treatment

The fungus should be cultured to confirm the diagnosis and to identify the species involved. While the management is not

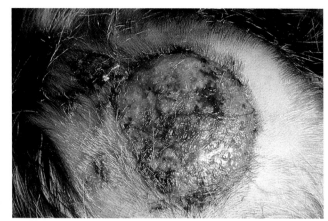

Fig. 11.3 Kerion in a young child.

influenced by the species, determination allows an animal or human reservoir to be traced and treated.

The treatment of choice in all ringworm of the scalp is still griseofulvin. Given late in inflammatory infections (which have a tendency to spontaneously heal), it may not alter the course of existing lesions, but it will prevent the development of new ones. Grey patch ringworm requires the full dose, which is 15 mg/kg daily of microsize griseofulvin for adults (or 10 mg/kg/day of ultramicrosize griseofulvin) and 10 mg/kg for children for at least 6 weeks. Cultures should be repeated after 4 weeks and every 2 weeks thereafter until mycological cure. Black dot ringworm may require slightly longer treatment and treatment should be continued for 2 weeks beyond clinical and mycological cure. Kerion generally requires 6 weeks of therapy.

Headache from the drug may be overcome by reducing the dose and slowly increasing it again. Griseofulvin interacts with a number of drugs, such as warfarin and phenobarbitone and dose adjustments may be required. An id eruption consisting of multiple small papules on the side of the face and the trunk may occur after commencing therapy with griseofulvin for tinea capitis; however, a true drug hypersensitivity to griseofulvin is rare.

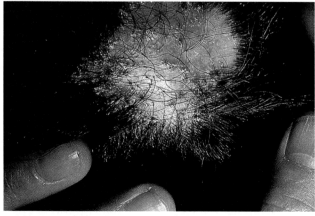

Fig. 11.4 Scutula seen in favus. (Courtesy of Dr D. Ellis, Adelaide.)

Secondary bacterial infection occasionally occurs and if suspected swabs should be taken and a broad spectrum oral antibiotic such as erythromycin given.

Alternatives to griseofulvin are ketaconazole, itraconazole, fluconazole and terbinafine. Cure rates are similar, shorter treatments are required and there are fewer drug interactions. The drawbacks are that ketaconazole has problems with hepatotoxicity (approximately 1 in 50 000) and many of these newer drugs are not licensed for use in children. Few comparative studies for these newer agents in tinea capitis are available, but those to hand suggest griseofulvin is still the drug of first choice, if only on cost.

The source of infection should be traced. It is usual to advocate in cases of *M. canis* that cats and dogs should be examined with a Wood's light by a veterinary surgeon and infected animals treated with griseofulvin. However, infection among kittens is ubiquitous and despite treatment the kittens frequently become reinfected, and so the value of treating the animal reservoir is uncertain.

Griseofulvin treatment of kerion does not tend to prevent the development of scarring alopecia and so it is prudent to combine the griseofulvin with prednisolone 25 mg daily for the first week or two, and this may also hasten resolution of the symptoms. Oral antibiotics are generally not required unless secondary bacterial infection is proven. Selenium sulphide or ketaconazole shampoo may also decrease the period of fungal shedding.

In very young children, unable to swallow tablets, a griseofulvin suspension can be used, or if unavailable, the tablets can be crushed and mixed into ice cream. Ketaconazole shampoo alone is unlikely to be helpful but is a useful adjunctive treatment to reduce fungal shedding and infectivity.

Children with infection due to anthropophilic fungi and *M. canis* should be kept home from school until the infection has cleared. In school epidemics classmates should be examined with a Wood's light; however, in recent infections the fluorescent part of the hair may not yet have emerged from the follicle and fluorescence will only be detected if the hair is plucked and the root examined.

Key points

Tinea capitis is a dermatophytic trichomycosis of the scalp that may be caused by a number of *Trichophyton* and *Microsporum* species. Acute infection (kerion) is characterized by follicular inflammation with painful, boggy nodules that drain pus and produce scarring; or by a scutula (favus). Chronic infection manifests as grey scaling patches with broken hairs that may (small spore ectothrix) or may not (large spore ectothrix and endothrix) fluoresce with a Wood's light.

11.2 Tinea barbae

Introduction

Tinea barbae is ringworm of the beard and moustache areas of adult males. Tinea of the chin and upper lip of females is considered a ringworm of the glabrous skin of the face and is called tinea faciei.

Clinical features and investigation

Trichophyton verrucosum and *T. mentag* var. *mentag* are common in farmers who present with a kerion. *M. canis* and *T. rubrum* tend to be less inflammatory (Fig. 11.5). Other patterns seen in tinea capitis such as agminate folliculitis and diffuse erythema and scaling are also seen in tinea barbae.

Management

Hairs from follicular pustules should be extracted for microscopy and culture. With very inflammatory tinea the culture is often negative. Ultramicrofine griseofulvin in a dose of 330 mg daily for 4–6 weeks is usually sufficient for noninflammatory lesions and early inflammatory kerions. Late inflammatory lesions usually resolve spontaneously, but griseofulvin may shorten the course of events and is generally given. Secondary bacterial infection may occur and requires oral antibiotics.

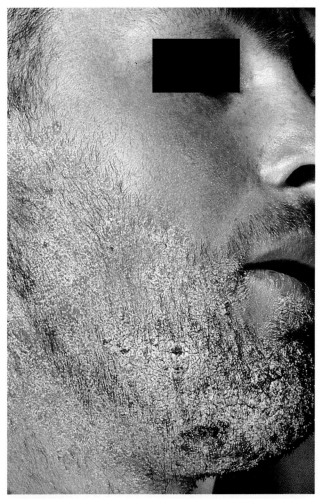

Fig. 11.5 Tinea barbae.

Key points

Tinea invading the terminal hairs of the beard of an adult male is called tinea barbae, while tinea involving the glabrous skin of the face of a child or adult female is called tinea faciei. Kerion may occur with tinea barbae due to zoophilic fungi. Griseofulvin for 4–6 weeks is the treatment of choice.

11.3 Pediculosis and scabies

Aetiology

Lice feed on the skin and deposit their eggs (nits) on the hair. Two species of louse infest man, *Pediculus humanus* and *Phthirus pubis*. There are two subspecies of *P. humanus*: *P. humanus capitis*, the head louse, and *P. humanus corporis*, the body or clothing louse. Head lice and body lice look almost identical, and are capable of interbreeding, but on the host they tend to maintain their territorial preferences. Although the head louse occasionally wanders onto the body, the body louse rarely ventures onto the scalp.

Pathogenesis

The female head louse is 3–4 mm long. The male is slightly smaller and banded across the back (Fig. 11.6). During her 40 day life span, the female lays approximately 300 eggs at a rate of 8 a day. The eggs are oval, white capsules with a lid (operculum) and are firmly cemented to the side of the hair shaft adjacent to the scalp (Fig. 11.7). After about a week the larvae hatch close to the scalp. Larvae resemble small adults and begin feeding on the blood of the host soon after hatching. Digestion of the blood is dependent on Gram-negative bacteria which colonize the intestine of the larvae. After undergoing three moults in 10 days, the louse reaches maturity and commences mating.

The life cycle of the body louse is similar to that of the head louse. Its natural habitat is clothing and it only visits its host to feed. Nits are cemented to clothing fibres, especially in the seams closest to the body. Washing in hot water and ironing kill lice, so this tends to be a disease of vagrants and refugees.

Phthirus pubis, the pubic louse is structurally and morphologically different to *P. humanus*. The term crab louse is appropriate as its body is squat and the second and third pairs of legs carry heavy, pincer-like claws. In addition to pubic hair the pubic lice can colonize the axillae, eyebrows, eyelashes, beard and trunk (of hairy men) and also the scalp margin.

Pubic lice are vessel feeders and have specially adapted mouthparts to probe the skin and pierce blood vessels. Eggs only attach to coarse terminal hairs and so this infestation is rare prior to puberty, and can be extensive in the hirsute male. Eggs hatch in 6–8 days and the nymphs reach maturity in 15–17 days.

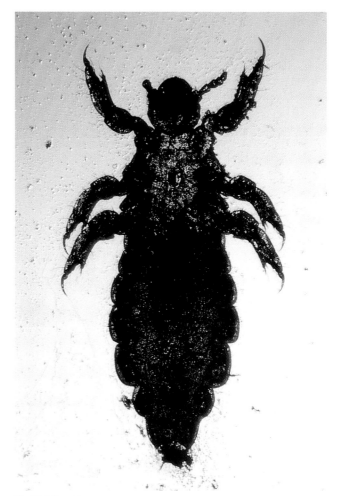

Fig. 11.6 Head louse.

Clinical features

In most established infestations of head lice there are fewer than 10 adult lice and counts of more than 100 are uncommon. Most infections are acquired by direct head to head contact, but combs, brushes and hats are important in some cases. Pruritus is variable. It is often intense and only rarely absent. It is usually worst in the occipital region where the infestation is heaviest. Scratching leads to impetiginization and the hair may become matted down by exudate to produce plica polonica. Nits can be seen with the naked eye (Fig. 11.8) and are very easily seen with a Wood's light. This is useful for screening in schools during epidemics. Head lice are rare in Negroids as the lice appear not to grab tightly curled hair as well.

Transmission of body lice is by close contact or by shared clothing. Usually only a few lice infest an individual although in some there may be thousands. Body lice infestation requires the individual to be in constant contact with a particular outfit of infested clothing, hence this louse flourishes in the homeless. The patient presents with generalized itch, often with no rash or only scattered excoriations. Secondary bacterial infection is common and papular urticaria occurs in

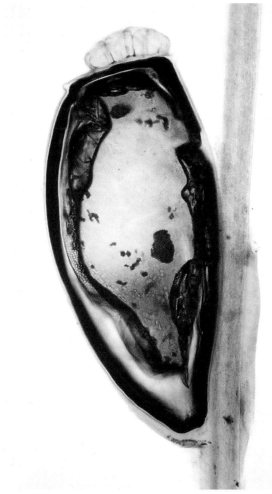

Fig. 11.7 Nit attached laterally to a hair shaft.

some cases. Prolonged infestations result in patchy post-inflammatory hyperpigmentation, which is known as vagabond's disease. Infected lice may transmit epidemic typhus, trench fever and louse-borne relapsing fever.

Pubic lice are spread by sexual contact and other sexually transmitted diseases frequently coexist. Occasionally they

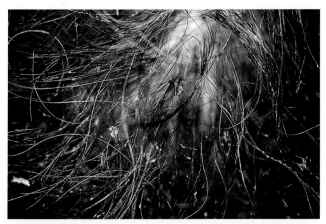

Fig. 11.8 Pediculosis capitis.

may be transmitted by shed hairs in clothing, towels or sleeping bags. The host immunological reaction to louse salivary antigens is variable and some subjects have intense irritation with a small louse population, while others with numerous lice are symptom free. The mites tend to feed at night and itching in the evening and night is the principal symptom.

Blue-grey macules known as maculae ceruleae or *taches bleues* on the abdominal wall and thighs are characteristic, but rare. They are due to altered blood at the sites of bites. Lice and nits are visible with the naked eye on close inspection and louse faeces can be seen on the skin as rust coloured speckles.

Scabies is an infestation caused by the mite *Sarcoptes scabiei* var. *hominis*. Involvement of the scalp is rare except in infancy and in the immunocompromised. Thus when scabies is present on the scalp, immunosuppression should be suspected. Such cases tend not to be itchy and the resulting high density of mites makes this condition highly infective. Scalp lesions may occur without evidence of infestation elsewhere and simulate seborrhoeic dermatitis, or may be associated with crusted lesions on the trunk and limbs in the Norwegian scabies variant. The diagnosis requires identification of the mite.

Investigation

Parasitophobia is not uncommon and the diagnosis of infestation should not be accepted unless the insect or its eggs have been positively identified Peripilar hair casts or pseudonits (p. 180) are a source of confusion but these can be readily slid up and down the hair shaft and are circumferential rather than eccentric. This can be visualized by light microscopy.

Treatment

In the presence of severe itch, scratching may cause secondary bacterial infection, for which systemic antibiotics are usually required. Malathion and carbaryl became the mainstays of therapy for head louse infection following emergence of resistance to the organochloride antiseptics. They should be left on the scalp for 12 hours before being washed off. Blow drying should be avoided as heat degrades these insecticides. Both agents effectively kill lice, although they do not kill all the eggs and a second application after 7–10 days is usually recommended. Malathion coats the hair making it resistant to reinfection for 6 weeks. Permethrins are another treatment alternative that generally only requires a 10 minute scalp application after shampooing. While a single treatment may suffice it is usually reapplied after 7–10 days. Again hair dryers should be avoided.

Multiresistant head lice have emerged in a number of areas around the world. In such cases oral treatment with cotrimoxazole can be used. The circulating cotrimoxazole, ingested by the mite works by eradicating the Gram-negative bacteria in the intestines of the mite. Alternatively the mites can be suffocated by topical applications of oils such as petrolatum or conditioner. Another emerging treatment for multiresistant lice is ivermectin, which may be used orally or formulated into a 1% shampoo. The safety and efficacy of oral ivermectin in children has not yet been established.

None of these treatments remove the dead nits. Combing with a fine toothed comb is tedious and can be painful unless the hair is pretreated with conditioner. Nits will eventually wear away after repeated washing but 8% formic acid in a cream rinse can be used as a nit-remover.

Head lice epidemics are common and in general malathion, carbaryl and permethrin are rotated every 3 years to prevent resistance. Infected children should be kept home from school until the first treatment is completed.

With body lice infestations, it is the clothing and not the patient that requires treatment. A hot wash, a tumble dry and ironing will kill both the lice and the eggs. The opportunity created by separating the client from his or her clothes can also be utilized to give him or her a bath!

As pubic lice may wander it is preferable to treat the whole trunk and limbs. Preparations containing γ-benzene hexachloride, malathion, carbaryl and permethrins are all effective. Eyelash infection can be treated with vaseline, 20% fluorescein drops or malathion liquid which does not tend to irritate the eye.

Key points

Itch without a rash, or with only excoriations, requires careful inspection of hairy regions for lice and nits. In addition the clothing in contact with the skin should be inspected paying particular attention to the seams. Impetigo of the scalp should never be accepted as the primary diagnosis until lice have been excluded. Lice should be captured and viewed under a microscope to confirm the diagnosis.

11.4 Piedra (trichomycosis nodularis)

Definition

Piedra is Spanish for stone. Piedra is a fungal infection of the hair shafts that produces gritty, adherent nodules attached to the hair cortex that are difficult to scrape off.

Epidemiology

Black piedra is endemic to tropical regions of South and Central America and South-East Asia. Rare cases have been reported in the USA and South Africa. Infection is acquired either from the soil or spread from person to person. Young girls are most commonly affected. Familial outbreaks are common and epidemics have occurred in schools.

White piedra occurs in tropical climates and infection is acquired either from prolonged intimate human contact or from the soil.

Aetiology

There are two varieties of piedra, black and white caused by *Piedraia hortae* and *Trichosporon beigelii*, respectively.

Clinical features

Black piedra is characterized by 1.5 mm long, discrete, hard, stony, black nodules that cling firmly to the scalp hairs (Fig. 11.9). The fungus is confined to the hair cuticle where it proliferates, but it does not penetrate the hair cortex and so there is no loss or breakage of the hair. Combing the hair with a metal comb produces a characteristic rattling sound or a metallic click. Nodules may be present along the entire length of the hair. The hair is normal between nodules. Many patients do not seek treatment for this condition, despite being aware of its presence. In Malaysia the condition is well known to the indigenous population of the peninsula as 'rambut berbuah' (fruit bearing hair).

White piedra may involve the hair of the scalp, beard, eyelashes, eyebrows, axillary and especially the pubic regions. Homosexual males are commonly infected in the

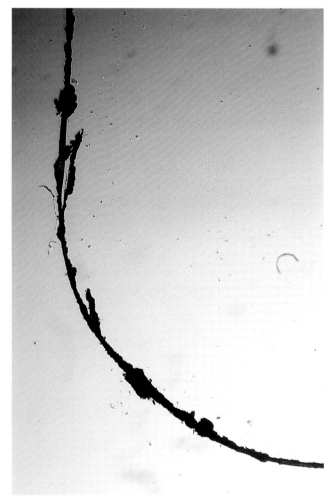

Fig. 11.9 Black piedra.

pubic region. The nodules are composed of closely packed septate hyphae and blastoconidia in a dense geometric array. Characteristic soft, spongy, white or light-brown concretions cling to hairs either as discrete nodules or a coalesced sheath (Fig. 11.10). Unlike black piedra, the concretions can be scraped off. Itch often accompanies white piedra and intertrigo can occur in the groin. Wood's light examination is negative.

Investigation

In black piedra, Wood's light examination is negative, but light microscopy shows hyphae within the nodules. Fungal culture produces a slow growing black colony that develops green aerial hyphae.

Treatment

Treatment is not required in all cases. In parts of Malaysia, the nodules of black piedra are considered attractive and young girls encourage its growth by sleeping with their hair in the soil. If treatment is desired, affected hairs can be cut short and

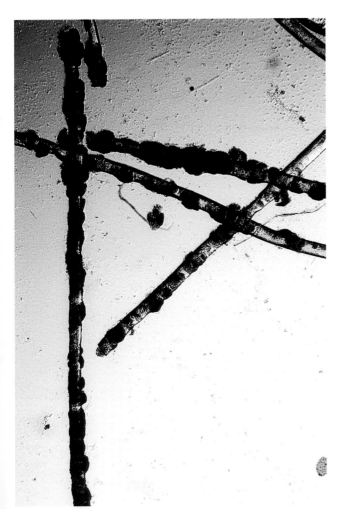

Fig. 11.10 White piedra.

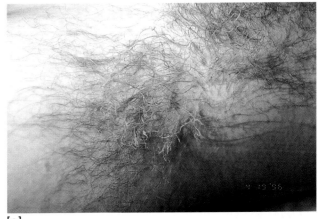

[a]

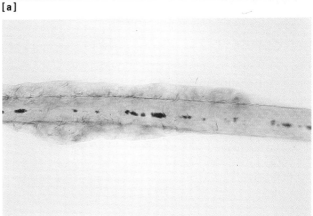

[b]

Fig. 11.11 (a) Trichomychosis axillaris (b) showing the yellow concretions around the hair cuticle.

the hair shampooed daily. Successful treatment with a 6 week course of oral terbinafine has been recently described. Whitfield's ointment can be applied after shampooing to prevent a recurrence. White piedra is resistant to azole antifungals.

Key points

Black nodules occur along the hair shaft in black piedra, while white nodules and fusiform swelling occur in white piedra, which may be accompanied by itching.

11.5 Trichomycosis axillaris and pubis

Definition

Despite the name trichomycosis, this is a superficial bacterial infection. Axillary and sometimes also pubic hairs develop adherent granular nodules.

Epidemiology

Trichomycosis axillaris is seen in all races and climates and in both sexes, but adolescent males are the ones most commonly affected. Axillary hair is a prerequisite for this condition. It is very common and in one study 27% of male university students had this condition.

Aetiology

The nodules consist of masses of predominantly *Corynebacterium tenuis*, but other *Corynebacterium* species may be present and different coloured nodules occur with different *Corynebacteria* species.

Pathogenesis

The bacteria invade and grow within the cuticle and cortex, but the hair shafts are not weakened (Fig. 11.11).

Clinical features and investigation

It is asymptomatic and the first thing noticed by the patient is usually the black, yellow or red staining of their shirt armpits.

Black, yellow or red concretions are visible on the affected hair shafts and these may be hard or soft, nodular or diffuse. The axillary sweat is discoloured. Yellow is the most common colour outside the Tropics.

Investigations

Wood's light examination reveals a dull yellow fluorescence of affected hairs. Other *Corynebacterium* infections may coexist and involvement of the pubic hair, erythrasma and pitted keratolysis should be looked for.

Treatment

Shaving the hair provides a rapid cure as does regular washing, antiperspirant, Whitfield's ointment, clindamycin 1% solution or tetracycline cream.

Key points

Trichomycosis axillaris presents with asymptomatic yellow, red or black concretions of *Corynebacteria* surrounding the axillary hairs. Involvement of the pubic hairs is called trichomycosis pubis.

Chapter 12

Inflammatory dermatoses of the scalp

12.1 Seborrhoea

Definition

Seborrhoea is the term applied to greasy hair. It is due to excessive sebaceous gland secretion.

Aetiology

Seborrhoea begins at puberty when the sebaceous glands enlarge due to gonadal and adrenal androgens. It may also occur in infancy due to the transplacental spread of maternal androgens.

Pathogenesis

Sebaceous gland activity is driven by circulating androgens, while oestrogens lead to decreased activity.

Clinical features

Many patients will also complain of greasy skin and acne, although excessive sebum secretion cannot be objectively demonstrated in all patients. This is because different people have different thresholds for presentation. Greasy hair may be described by men developing androgenetic alopecia, however, this is due to redistribution of sebum among fewer hairs, rather than increased sebum secretion and seborrhoea is not associated *per se* with androgenetic alopecia. Nevertheless, as both conditions are common they frequently coexist.

Pathology

Enlarged sebaceous glands may be demonstrated.

Investigation

Usually none required. Virilism in a woman can usually be excluded clinically.

Associated features

In women the association of seborrhoea, hirsutes, acne, androgenetic alopecia and irregular menses indicate androgen excess that may be pathological and should be further investigated, but seborrhoea alone does not warrant further action.

Prognosis

Gradual improvement over 5–10 years is the norm.

Treatment

Only symptomatic treatment is required. Frequent washing of the hair will remove excess grease and shampoos are specifically marketed for people with oily hair. Selenium disulphide with or without isopropyl alcohol as a vehicle is an effective agent. Tar shampoos are also useful. While oestrogens reduce sebaceous gland activity and the use of oestrogen creams topically is advocated for this condition in some European countries, there seems little need for these potentially problematic preparations.

Key points

Seborrhoea may be a manifestation of virilism in women, but is more often a physiological variant. People with oily hair will empirically establish the type of shampoo and the frequency of application that best controls their seborrhoea.

12.2 Pityriasis capitis and seborrhoeic dermatitis

Definition

Pityriasis capitis means scaly scalp and is popularly known as dandruff (Fig. 12.1). Seborrhoeic dermatitis is an inflammatory dermatitis of the scalp, face, upper chest and back, that is usually itchy.

Pityriasis capitis and seborrhoeic dermatitis are related disorders differentiated on the basis of severity. Pityriasis capitis is the mildest form of seborrhoeic dermatitis of the scalp.

Epidemiology

Pityriasis capitis is an affliction of adolescence, affecting 50% of 20-year-old Caucasoids. It is most prevalent between the ages of 15 and 50. It is rare in the period after infancy and before puberty and tends to become less frequent after 50.

Seborrhoeic dermatitis occurs in infancy, disappears in childhood, returns at puberty and persists into senescence. It has a prevalence of 1–3% of the general population but is much more common among paraplegics and quadriplegics, patients with Parkinson's disease, epilepsy, obesity, chronic alcoholism and people with AIDS.

Aetiology

Both conditions occur in association with increased numbers of pityrosporum yeasts. Whether an allergic reaction to increased pityrosporum numbers causes these conditions is unknown, and these yeasts may simply be proliferating in a favourable environment. A role of pityrosporum yeasts in causing these conditions is suggested by the response to antifungal shampoos. Seborrhoea may or may not be present in the same patient, and consequently appears not to be causative. Seborrhoeic dermatitis may also occur as a reaction to certain drugs (Table 12.1).

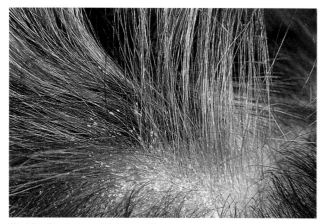

Fig. 12.1 Pityriasis capitis (dandruff).

Table 12.1 Drugs that exacerbate or induce seborrhoeic dermatitis.

Cimetidine
Methyldopa
Chlorpromazine
Isotretinoin
Arsenic
Gold
Bismuth

Pathogenesis

The scales of pityriasis capitis correspond histologically to focal areas of parakeratosis. The parakeratosis overlies areas of hyperproliferative epidermis, where the epidermal transit time is decreased to 3–4 days.

The relationship between infantile and adult forms of seborrhoeic dermatitis is unclear. Longitudinal studies have not demonstrated affected infants to have an increased likelihood of developing seborrhoeic dermatitis in adolescence. Many consider infantile seborrhoeic dermatitis to be a manifestation of atopy, while adult forms are considered by some to be a variant of psoriasis.

Clinical features

Pityriasis capitis is not itchy. It does not produce baldness or damage the hair shafts. Any association with seborrhoea appears to be coincidental as marked pityriasis can occur in the absence of seborrhoea and vice versa. The diagnosis is usually obvious and the most people manage the condition themselves, rarely presenting to their doctor.

On examination of the scalp there are widespread, small, thin, white or greyish, loose scales that fall from the scalp onto the shoulders, where they are particularly noticeable against dark-coloured clothing.

In infants seborrhoeic dermatitis presents with cradle cap (Fig. 12.2), which is soon followed by an erythematous, scaly rash on the glabella, the medial margins of the eyebrows, the central facial region and the retroauricular folds. While the chest and back tend not to be involved, in children, the napkin region is a common site. When the napkin area is involved, discrete secondary psoriasiform lesions may appear in the region.

Infantile seborrhoeic dermatitis is most common in the first 3 months of life and usually regresses within 6 months. In infancy it may also involve the flexures, but this is less common in adults.

In adults, seborrhoeic dermatitis is a chronic relapsing dermatitis, characterized by excessive dandruff, retroauricular scaling, blepharitis and a facial rash that centres around the nasolabial folds. In the scalp, large waxy yellow scales combine with exudates to form crusts, beneath which the scalp is red and moist. Perifollicular erythema and scaling extend to form well demarcated erythematous plaques. Exco-

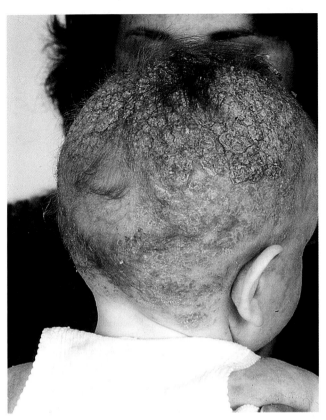

Fig. 12.2 Cradle cap.

riation may produce secondary impetigenization, occasionally with pustulation.

Pathology

The histology most closely resembles psoriasis with the added feature of spongiosis. There is basket-weave hyperkeratosis with focal parakeratosis, hypogranulosis, acanthosis, spongiosis and a superficial perivascular lymphohistiocytic infiltrate. Yeast-like organisms may be seen in the surface keratin.

Investigation

None usually required. Wood's light examination and scalp biopsy are only required in atypical cases or cases resistant to treatment.

Diagnosis

In the scalp the diagnosis of seborrhoeic dermatitis is usually obvious, but the only pitfall is that occasionally histiocytosis X (Letterer–Siwe disease) may occur in the scalp and resemble seborrhoeic dermatitis. The lesions of histiocytosis X tend to be more papular and sometimes haemorrhagic.

The erythematous plaques may resemble psoriasis, but that condition has different scales that are heavy and silvery.

Lichen simplex chronicus over the occiput may also cause confusion, however, the characteristic site, the intensity of the itching and the persistence of the plaque as a solitary lesion often for many years, strongly suggests that diagnosis.

Tinea capitis, especially due to *Trichophyton tonsurans* may very closely mimic seborrhoeic dermatitis and is easily missed if fungal scrapings are not performed in suspected cases.

A potential mimic of seborrhoeic dermatitis on the face is paranasal dermatitis of young women. This is a variant of rosacea that resembles paranasal seborrhoeic dermatitis. It responds to oral tetracyclines, but fluorinated steroids provide only marginal symptomatic relief and rapidly produce perioral dermatitis.

Associated features

Severe and extensive seborrhoeic dermatitis may be a clue to AIDS.

Prognosis

Both pityriasis capitis and seborrhoeic dermatitis are chronic relapsing conditions. Patients should be encouraged to have realistic expectations from treatment. They should understand that treatment is suppressive and the condition is likely to return soon after the treatment is stopped. Ultimately recurrences become less frequent and the condition is less of a problem after the age of 40.

Treatment

Pityriasis capitis can be effectively treated with any of a large number of proprietary agents available over the counter. The problem is that seborrhoeic dermatitis is a recurrent condition and relapses will require retreatment. Thus it is important for the patient to have realistic expectations and to understand that the aim of any treatment is to suppress the scaling at the lowest possible cost and inconvenience to the patient.

Antidandruff shampoos are readily available and effective in all but the most severe cases. Common active ingredients include selenium sulphide, zinc pyrithione and zinc omadine. Shampoos containing tar and ketoconazole are generally reserved for the more severe cases.

True treatment failures (as opposed to unrealistic patient expectations) most commonly result from insufficient usage. Either the hair is not washed frequently enough or the shampoo is not left on the scalp long enough (according to the instructions on the bottle: usually 5–10 minutes) prior to rinsing. Asking the patients to time how long they leave the shampoo on the scalp improves compliance.

Oil of cade BP pomades, coconut oil pomades (Table 12.2), low potency topical steroids and antifungals such as

Table 12.2 Extemporaneous treatments for seborrhoeic dermatitis.

Ung Cocois co (BP)	Coconut oil BP	30%
	Coal tar solution BP	6.25%
	Salicylic acid	4%
	Precipitated sulphur BP	2%
	Emulsifying ointment	up to 100%
Oil of cade ointment (BP)	Cade oil	6%
	Salicylic acid	2%
	Precipitated sulphur BP	3%
	Emulsifying ointment	up to 100%

ketoconazole are all effective suppressers of seborrhoeic dermatitis and are used when shampoos alone have failed.

Key points

Dandruff is very common, but only rarely do people seek medical attention for it. Antidandruff shampoos are readily available and generally effective. The condition is recurrent and treatment will need to be repeated at regular intervals.

Despite its name, sebum secretion is not increased in seborrhoeic dermatitis. It seems likely that the infantile and adolescent forms are two distinct entities bearing the same name. Both are common, itchy, inflammatory dermatoses predominantly affecting the scalp, face and seborrhoeic areas of the trunk. In addition the infantile form often extends to the napkin area.

12.3 Pityriasis amiantacea

Definition

Pityriasis amiantacea is an asbestos-like scale crust that encases and binds down a tuft of hairs. Removal of the scale crust also removes the hairs and leaves behind an erythematous bald patch.

Epidemiology

Pityriasis amiantacea affects females more often than males and most commonly occurs between the ages of 5 and 40 years, with the average age of onset being 25 years.

Aetiology

It most commonly occurs as an idiopathic isolated phenomenon, but it may also appear in association with seborrhoeic dermatitis, eczema, psoriasis or lichen simplex.

Pathogenesis

Hair casts encircle the hair, mat together and form a solid crust. Traction from the scaly crust on the encased hairs releases them from the follicle, producing a localized patch of alopecia when the crust is removed.

Clinical features

Masses of sticky silvery scales, overlapping like roof tiles, adhere to the scalp (Fig. 12.3) and are attached in layers around the hair shafts. Peeling of the scaly plaque removes all the hairs to leave a completely bald patch. The underlying scalp is red and moist, and may show features of the predisposing dermatosis. There is usually only one small patch of pityriasis amiantacea on the scalp, although occasionally a single large patch or multiple smaller ones occur.

Pathology

Biopsy of the underlying skin reveals spongiosis of both the follicular and surface epithelium with parakeratotic scale at the follicular ostia. The parakeratotic scale forms an onion skin layered arrangement around the emerging hair shaft.

Investigation

None usually required.

Diagnosis

Trichophyton rubrum kerion can mimic pityriasis capitis.

Associated features

Usually none.

Prognosis

Often this condition follows a chronic recurring pattern for a few months to a year and then dissapears. Hair loss occurs in the affected area, but it regrows unless there is a complication such as secondary infection.

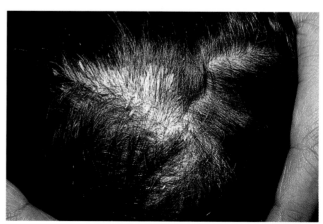

Fig. 12.3 Pityriasis amiantacea.

Treatment

It is important to treat any underlying dermatosis. The pityriasis amiantacea scale can act as a shield preventing active medications reaching their target. The scale should be loosened with salicylic acid (10–30%) in mineral oil, left on the scalp for half an hour before the scale is combed out with a fine tooth comb. Immediately after the scale is removed, daily use for a week of either oil of cade, ung cocois co. BP (British pharmacopea), or a tar and salicylic acid preparation will deal with the underlying inflammation of the skin. These preparations are applied in the evening, left on overnight under a gauze bonnet and rinsed off in the morning with a tar shampoo. Recurrence can be forestalled by regular use of the tar shampoo.

Key points

Pityriasis amiantacea is an asbestos-like scale that mats down a tuft of hair. Removal of the scale leaves behind a patch of alopecia that always regrows. The condition is most commonly an idiopathic isolated disorder, but it may also occur in psoriasis, eczema, seborrhoeic dermatitis and lichen simplex.

12.4 Psoriasis

Definition

Psoriasis is a chronic relapsing, inflammatory papulosquamous dermatosis.

Epidemiology

Psoriasis occurs worldwide affecting at least 2% of the population. Scalp involvement is a prominent feature. Psoriasis may appear at any age, but the age of onset has bimodal peaks in the teens and again in the sixties.

Aetiology

Psoriasis is a polygenic familial disorder that is associated with HLA-Cw6. Triggers that may induce or exacerbate psoriasis include streptococcal pharyngitis and certain drugs (Table 12.3). Stress is commonly blamed.

Pathogenesis

The pathophysiology involves abnormal hyperproliferation of the skin with a rapid cell turnover time in the epidermis (3–4 days). This is probably secondary to activation of the cellular immune system producing a variety of cytokines (especially interleukin-1; IL-1), eicosanoids (especially leukotriene B4; LT-B4) and polyamines. The changes in epidermal cell kinetics, result in alterations in the epidermal cell keratin cytofilament expression, and cellular differentiation.

Table 12.3 Drugs that exacerbate or induce psoriasis.

Lithium
β-blockers
Antimalarials
Aspirin
Nonsteroidal anti-inflammatory agents
Steroid withdrawal

Clinical features

Skin lesions consist of well-demarcated erythematous plaques with a classic silvery scale, that bleeds when scratched off (Auspitz sign). It is usually not very itchy. There may be large plaques, small plaques, guttate (raindrop) lesions or a mixture of all three. Extensor surfaces are predominantly affected, however, flexural involvement also occurs and occasionally the entire skin surface may be erythrodermic. Pustular forms of psoriasis are most common on the palms and soles, but can be generalized and associated with systemic upset. The Koebner phenomenon is the appearance of psoriasis in sites of trauma.

Scalp involvement occurs in about 50% of psoriatics and may be the first and occasionally the only manifestation of the psoriasis. Initially, there may be only patchy or diffuse scaling without any specific features, resembling pityriasis capitis. Pityriasis amiantacea may develop, but more commonly palpable plaques covered with thick scale develop extending just beyond the hair line (Fig. 12.4). Any part of the scalp can be involved and there may be some mild thinning of the hair overlying the plaques.

The scalp lesions frequently irritate or itch, but pruritus is rarely severe. Severe itch is a feature of lichen simplex chronicus, which occurs over the occiput and looks very similar to psoriasis. Seborrhoeic dermatitis may also cause diagnostic difficulty, especially in the absence of skin lesions elsewhere or nail changes. Retroauricular involvement suggests seborrhoeic dermatitis as do fine powdery scales; while thick, large

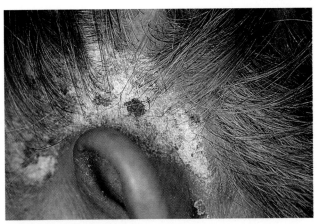

Fig. 12.4 Retroauricular psoriasis.

silvery scales suggest psoriasis. Occasionally it is impossible to differentiate the two conditions until lesions appear elsewhere on the body.

Alopecia is uncommon with plaque psoriasis but well recognized with the erythrodermic and pustular variants. Trichograms from plaques of psoriasis show an increased telogen count, consistent with a 'localized telogen effluvium', and erythrodermic psoriasis may produce a diffuse hair loss due to a generalized telogen effluvium. Pustular psoriasis may result in extensive areas of alopecia. After recovery from a severe episode of pustular psoriasis, Pohl–Pinkus lines may be seen in the hair. Scarring alopecia has been documented in cases of severe long-standing psoriasis of the scalp, but is uncommon.

Pathology

Psoriasis is a dynamic process and the histology of a lesion varies during its evolution and subsequent regression. Well-developed lesions show psoriasiform acanthosis with suprapapillary thinning of the epidermis and oedematous dermal papillae. This leads to the so called squirting papillae. The granular layer of the epidermis is thinned and there is parakeratosis. Occasionally collections of neutrophils in the stratum corneum, known as Munro's microabscesses occur although these are uncommon in the scalp. There is follicular plugging, enlargement of the follicular ostia and follicular parakeratosis. The epidermis may show spongiosis with collections of neutrophils forming spongiotic pustules. In the dermis there is a superficial perivascular mixed cellular infiltrate. Despite the increased epidermal proliferation and reduced transit time, the rate of hair growth is not increased. However, the calibre of hairs from within a plaque is reduced and the cuticles are ruffled.

Investigation

None usually required.

Diagnosis

Pityriasis rubra pilaris is a clinical and histological differential diagnosis of psoriasis. In the scalp this condition produces erythema, fine scaling and diffuse hair loss.

Associated features

Nail changes occur in about 20% and a seronegative arthritis develops in 5% of patients.

Prognosis

Psoriasis has a strong tendency to relapse and often requires ongoing treatment.

Treatment

Mild cases can be managed with tar shampoos alone. Steroid scalp lotions are useful for the itch. Thick scale can act as a barrier to steroid scalp lotions, which work best if the scaling is mild, or has been previously removed by shampooing. The lotion is applied to the scalp after the hair has been parted and left on overnight.

Thick plaques or resistant cases will require a tar pomade (Table 12.4) left on overnight. Ung Cocois co BP (Table 12.2) is a useful pomade and cade oil (Table 12.2), ung pyrogallol co BP (Table 12.4) and dithranol pomades (Table 12.4) are acceptable alternatives. Dithranol should be used cautiously in fair-haired psoriatics as it may stain blond hair mauve, and cause irritation.

Prior application of salicylic acid (10–25%) in mineral oil to the scalp for half an hour to loosen the scale and then combing the hair with a fine tooth comb to remove the scale will enhance the action of the pomades.

To apply the pomade the hair is parted with a comb and the ointment applied down the part. The hair is re-parted a little further along and the pomade reapplied. The part is moved again until the entire scalp has been treated. A shower cap or a Tubifast bandage is applied over the top to protect the pillowcase. Plastic shower caps should never be used in children, who are at risk of suffocation beneath them. The treatment is washed off in the morning with a tar shampoo. Pomades are messy and patients need to be motivated.

Systemic treatments also help scalp psoriasis, but are rarely indicated for scalp psoriasis alone. UVB and PUVA are of little benefit as the scalp is shielded from the light by the hair. Any systemic effect of the PUVA tends to be small and unpredictable.

Key points

The scalp is a site of predilection for psoriasis, which presents with plaques covered in a thick silvery scale. Mild cases respond to shampoos, but treatment for more severe cases is messy and tedious.

Table 12.4 Extemporaneous treatments for psoriasis.

Coal tar pomade	Coal tar solution	6%
	Salicylic acid	2%
	Emulsifying ointment	up to 100%
Dithranol pomade	Dithranol	0.3%
	Salicylic acid	0.3%
	Yellow soft paraffin	4.3%
	Emulsifying ointment	up to 100%
Ung pyrogallol co	Pyrogallol	2.5%
	Salicylic acid	4%
	Phenol	2.5%
	White soft paraffin	up to 100%

12.5 Eczema of the scalp and lichen simplex chronicus

Definition

Atopic eczema is a chronic pruritic, inflammatory dermatitis.

Epidemiology

Eczema affects up to 10% of the population and about 30% of the population are atopic. In 50% of cases it first presents in infancy but may appear at any age.

Aetiology

It is a manifestation of atopy, which is an autosomal dominantly inherited cluster of related disorders; namely eczema, asthma and hayfever. The three do not necessarily occur in the one patient.

Pathogenesis

The pathogenesis is unclear, but an IgE mediated late phase response as well as cell-mediated immunity involving type 2 helper T cells (T_H2) contribute in some way. Type 2 helper T cells secrete interleukin 4, 10 and 13, along with interferon-γ and tumour necrosis factor-β. They also stimulate a B-cell immunoglobin production switch to IgE.

Clinical features

Scalp involvement can occur and presents as an itchy, scaly dermatitis of the scalp. Broken hairs from scratching and rubbing can be seen (Fig. 12.5). Scalp involvement can occur with the simple flexural type of eczema, but it is particularly common in erythrodermic eczema. Telogen effluvium may also occur with erythrodermic eczema and the hair loss may be quite severe.

Lichenification and secondary infection are common complications. Lichenification is the leathery thickening of the skin that occurs in response to repeated scratching and rubbing. Any itchy rash can cause the patient to scratch to gain temporary relief. If the itch returns more severe than ever after a brief intermission and produces renewed scratching, then the patient can fall victim to a repetitive itch–scratch cycle that ultimately produces lichenification. When the original rash is obvious the lichenification is considered secondary, while if the original rash is obscure, the condition is called lichen simplex chronicus.

Pathology

Spongiosis is the histological hallmark of eczema. All other features are variable and nondiagnostic.

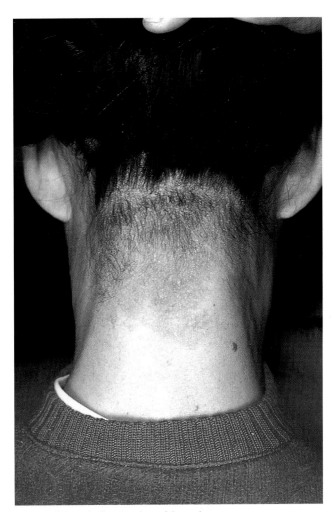

Fig. 12.5 Lichen simplex chronicus of the nuchae.

Investigation

Usually none required.

Diagnosis

In the absence of eczema elsewhere, tinea capitis needs to be excluded. Lichen simplex can mimic psoriasis.

Associated features

Scalp eczema frequently becomes complicated by *Staphylococcus aureus* infection. It may also be involved in Kaposi's varicelliform eruption due to secondary infection of the eczema with herpes simplex virus.

Childhood eczema can be a feature of a number of inherited syndromes, such as the Wiskott–Aldrich syndrome (eczema, thrombocytopenia, impaired immunity with elevated IgE and early death from infection), hyper-IgE syndrome (eczema, recurrent infections, growth failure and raised serum IgE) and hypereosinophilic syndrome (atopic eczema, hypereosinophilia and multisystem involvement). Scalp involvement is common in these conditions.

Prognosis

Eczema is a chronic relapsing condition and the patient should be encouraged to have realistic expectations of the outcome of treatment.

Treatment

Tar shampoos and pomades as well as steroid lotions and creams are used. Oral antibiotics are used for secondary bacterial infection, and oral prednisolone may be required in severe cases.

Key points

Eczema often involves the scalp. It look similar to seborrhoeic dermatitis, but in general it is more itchy, and there is often eczema elsewhere on the body.

12.6 Contact dermatitis

Definition

Contact dermatitis is an eczematous dermatitis, caused by an external agent.

Aetiology and pathogenesis

That external agent may be an irritant or an allergen. Irritants are abrasive substances with the potential to produce a dermatitis in everybody, while allergens will only produce a dermatitis in those people who are sensitized to that substance and who mount an immunological reaction to it whenever it is encountered.

The scalp is generally resistant to irritants because of its rapid epidermal turnover time and the thick epidermis and in particular the thick stratum corneum. The commonest causes of irritation are overuse of bleaching preparations, frequent blow drying and thioglycolates used in permanent waving (which disrupt the disulphide bonds within the hair keratins to allow remodelling of the hair).

Contact dermatitis is common, although the scalp is also relatively resistant to allergens. The initial sensitization may occur on the scalp or at distant sites. The major allergens are hair dyes, bleaches, permanent wave solutions and hair creams (Table 12.5).

Clinical features

The scalp margins tend to be worst affected. Allergy can also occur to hair nets, hat bands or wigs, while an allergy to shampoo is very rare. Contact dermatitis is occasionally induced therapeutically with dinitrochlorobenzene (DNCB)

Table 12.5 Important causes of contact allergic dermatitis of the scalp.

Substance	Allergen
Hair dyes	
Vegetable dyes	Camomile
Metallic dyes	Nickel or chromium
Colour rinses	o-Nitroparaphenylenediamine
Permanent dyes	Phenylenediamine
Hair bleaches	Ammonium persulphate
Permanent wave solutions	Thioglycolates
Hair straighteners	Thioglycolates
Depilatories	Thioglycolates
Men's hair cream	Lanolin, perfume or parabens
Shaving cream	Perfumes
Hair nets	Nylon or elastic
Hat-bands	Leather (chromate) or colophony
Wigs	Adhesives

or diphencypropenone acetate (DCP) in the treatment of alopecia areata (Fig. 12.6); however, these two chemicals are not otherwise encountered.

Contact dermatitis presents with an acute, subacute or chronic eczema that may be localized to the scalp and adjacent areas, or spread to involve other parts of the head and neck. Periorbital oedema may occur and mimic dermatomyositis or angio-oedema.

Investigation

Patch-testing to a battery of known chemical antigens (Table 12.5) will usually diagnose an allergic contact dermatitis, and the patient should be advised to thereafter avoid all proven allergens. Irritant contact dermatitis may not show up on patch testing, but may be obvious on history. A usage test with a suspected irritant may be indicated in difficult cases.

Prognosis

If the allergens can be successfully avoided the prognosis for contact allergic dermatitis is excellent, however many allergens are ubiquitous, making avoidance difficult.

Treatment

The dermatitis is treated with topical steroids. In severe cases oral prednisolone can be used. Irritation of the scalp can be minimized by using a mild shampoo, and avoiding all hairdressing procedures for at least a month following clinical recovery.

Key points

Contact dermatitis of the scalp may present as an acute, subacute or chronic dermatitis of the scalp that sometimes spreads to adjacent areas. A directed history and patch testing can

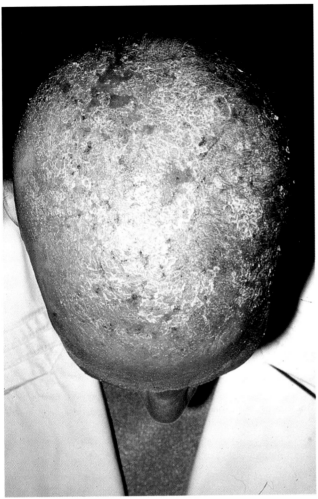

Fig. 12.6 Iatrogenic contact allergic dermatitis from dinitrochlorobenzene (DNCB) in the treatment of alopecia areata. (Courtesy of Dr M. Haskett, Melbourne.)

usually establish the diagnosis. Light testing with a monochromator and a solar simulator can be performed if a photodermatitis is suspected.

12.7 Pruritus and burning of the scalp

Definition

Pruritis means itching.

Epidemiology

An itchy scalp is a common complaint, while a burning scalp is only seen infrequently.

Aetiology

Itch may occur with an obvious pruritic dermatosis or with an apparently normal scalp. A number of conditions which are not traditionally thought of as pruritic dermatoses, such as pityriasis capitis, androgenetic alopecia, lichen plano-

pilaris and psoriasis can also occasionally cause severe pruritus.

Burning of the scalp may be primary and idiopathic or secondary to an inflammatory dermatosis or somatization of a psychiatric disorder such as anxiety or depression.

Pathogenesis

The mechanism of scalp itch is no different to that of itch elsewhere and is mediated by a number of chemicals including histamine, bradykinin, prostaglandins and various neurotransmitters. The pathogenesis of the burning scalp is unknown; however, the role of aberrant expression of substance P in the scalp is being investigated.

Clinical features

Evidence of the underlying dermatosis may be obvious, or the signs may be absent or subtle and only detected after close inspection of the entire scalp. Manifestations of scratching such as broken hair shafts, linear excoriations, prurigo nodules or lichen simplex may also be identified. Broken shafts due to rubbing are most noticeable over the parietal and temporal regions while lichen simplex is seen most frequently in the nuchal area, where it may mimic psoriasis.

Pityriasis capitis and androgenetic alopecia may occasionally produce severe pruritus, but other causes should be excluded before accepting either as the sole cause.

Conditions that can produce itch with few or no objective signs include urticaria, allergic contact dermatitis, endogenous eczema, pityrosporum folliculitis, acne necrotica, dermatitis herpetiformis, and pediculosis. This checklist is incomplete, but serves as a useful starting point for dealing with patients with an itchy scalp and no obvious cause.

The scalp may appear completely normal in allergic contact dermatitis, but there are usually clues in the history. Patch testing can be used to identify an allergen. If avoidance of the allergen cures the itch then it is reasonable to assume that was the cause. Urticaria may also produce very few signs initially, but eventually most people will develop weals elsewhere on the body.

Pustules can be easily missed without a diligent search through the entire scalp. Finding even one or two pustules may enable a diagnosis of pityrosporum folliculitis or acne necrotica to be made. Both these conditions can produce intense focal itching.

If the patient only has a few lice or nits then it is possible to miss this diagnosis. A careful search of the scalp may find some of these creatures and explain a generalized itch. Dermatitis herpetiformis may present on the scalp and produce a severe itch. The only sign may be a few excoriations with or without vesicles.

In the absence of an obvious cause of the itch, and after a thorough examination of the scalp looking for pustules, vesicles and inflammatory plaques, the rest of the skin should be examined for cutaneous disorders such as eczema, psoriasis and dermatitis herpetiformis. Possible contact allergens should be sought in the history and an inquiry should be made into recent stresses coincident with the onset of pruritus. Depression may somatize as scalp itch, in which case it is often described as being present all day and all night. Early morning wakening and loss of appetite may be important clues to the diagnosis.

Frequently no cause is found for the itch, and a diagnosis of idiopathic pruritus capitis is made. The patient is then treated empirically and regularly re-evaluated for a diagnosis that may not have been initially apparent.

Treatment

In the presence of a dermatosis the condition should be treated on its merits. Itch usually responds to tar shampoos, however, steroid scalp lotions may also be required. Sedatives and antidepressant medications are useful for both itch and when there is an associated endogenous depression. Topical capsaicin has been used empirically for scalp pain with varying success.

Key points

Itch commonly accompanies scalp dermatoses, but also occurs with an apparently normal scalp. Contact urticaria, allergic contact dermatitis, stress and depression may be easily overlooked without directed inquiry. An aetiology is not always found. Such cases are called idiopathic pruritus capitis for which empirical treatment of the itch is required.

12.8 Pustular conditions of the scalp

Definition

Follicular pustules on the scalp can occur with or without destruction of the hair follicles and scarring.

Epidemiology

Pustules on the scalp are very common, and almost everybody will develop one or more crops at some time in their life.

Aetiology

Follicular pustules may be infectious or inflammatory. Common infectious organisms include staphylococci bacteria and pityrosporum yeast. Noninfectious inflammatory nondestructive folliculitis can be seen with acne vulgaris, eosinophilic folliculitis and seborrhoeic dermatitis. As the pustules are frequently itchy and excoriated secondary infection may occur.

Destructive folliculitis can be a feature of acne necrotica, folliculitis decalvans and dissecting cellutitis of the scalp.

Clinical features

The first manifestation is an intensely itchy or slightly painful follicular papule that may occur anywhere in the scalp, but is most characteristic on the vertex. These are frequently excoriated before resolving slowly over 1–2 weeks. Lesions may occur singly or in crops.

In acne necrotica the lesions most commonly occur around the frontal hair line. The initial papule becomes a pustule that becomes umbilicated. In acne necrotica it then develops central necrosis and ulceration that eventually crusts over (Fig. 12.7). When the crust is shed it leaves behind a depressed varioliform scar. Patches of cicatricial alopecia may result.

Sometimes there is intense pruritus out of keeping with the objective signs.

Pathology

Histology shows an acute inflammatory infiltrate in the follicular infundibulum and beneath the adjacent stratum corneum. Disruption of the hair follicle produces dermal inflammation. Colonies of bacteria or yeast may be seen in the follicle.

In addition to these changes, in acne necrotica the folliculitis is accompanied by necrosis of the hair follicles and a predominantly lymphocytic perivascular and periappendageal inflammatory infiltrate. Occasionally trichomalacia is seen without scarring, suggesting that the localized hair loss is secondary to scratching.

Investigation

Bacterial cultures may grow staphylococci, while a Gram stain of biopsy tissue may reveal the Gram-positive pleomorphic rods of *Propionibacterium acnes*.

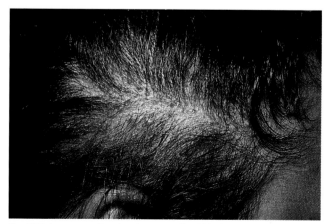

Fig. 12.7 Acne necrotica showing a pustule within the scalp.

Diagnosis

It is not always possible to determine the cause of the pustules clinically and a trial of empirical treatment is useful.

Associated features

Patients may have acne or folliculitis elsewhere.

Prognosis

Untreated, new lesions continue to develop at irregular intervals. The condition runs a long course over many years, although there may be only a small number of active lesions present at any one time.

Treatment

Tetracyclines used as for acne vulgaris will usually induce remission and are often combined with an antiyeast or tar shampoo. Maintenance therapy is usually required with long-term antibiotic therapy and medicated shampoos. Resistant cases may benefit from isotretinoin, which may need to be continued long-term. However, insufficient numbers of patients have been treated with this drug to make firm conclusions about its efficacy.

Key points

Folliculitis presents with an itchy or painful scalp, that is studded with pustules. While most heal spontaneously over 1–2 weeks, some undergo central necrosis and leave behind varioliform scars. Small patches of cicatricial alopecia may result.

12.9 Acne keloidalis nuchae

Definition

Acne keloidalis nuchae is a chronic inflammatory folliculitis of the nape of the neck.

Epidemiology

This condition occurs exclusively in men and most commonly in Negroid men. Most commonly it begins after puberty between the ages of 14 and 25 years.

Aetiology

The cause of the condition is unknown but may relate to short hair styles and in particular using a razor or 'liner' to shape the posterior hairline, with the subsequent development of pseudofolliculitis.

Pathogenesis

Keloids or rather hypertrophic scars develop from the papules and produce a distinctive clinical picture.

Clinical features

Men from all races may be affected by these inflammatory papules that develop diffusely over the nuchal area, just below the hair line (Fig. 12.8). The papules progressively extend towards the occiput and some may grow to be very large. Occasionally linear papules may be seen. Many affected individuals suffer or have previously suffered from acne vulgaris.

Pathology

Histology of early lesions shows a pseudofolliculitis with granulomatous inflammation, foreign body giant cells and naked hair shaft fragments. True keloids are exceptional but scar tissue formation is seen.

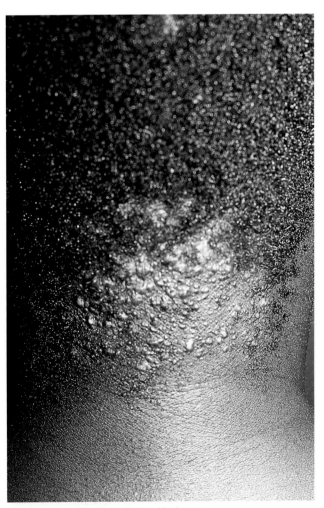

Fig. 12.8 Acne keloidalis nuchae in a black person.

Investigation

Swabs should be taken from pustules or weeping areas. A biopsy may be required, but usually the diagnosis is clinically obvious.

Diagnosis

Cyclosporin A can produce a variant of acne keloidalis nuchae with follicular papules on the vertex of the scalp and in the beard (Fig. 12.9). A biopsy shows an intense neu-

Table 12.6 Scalp involvement in systemic disease

Virilism (hirsutes, androgenetic alopecia)	Androgen secreting ovarian carcinoma Polycystic ovary syndrome Congenital adrenal hyperplasia Cushing's syndrome Prolactinoma Drugs Corticosteroids Anabolic steroids Phenytoin Penicillamine Streptomycin HAIR-AN syndrome Post-menopausal hirsutes
Alopecia areata	Down's syndrome Atopy Thyroiditis Vitiligo Addison's disease Pernicious anaemia Lupus erythematosus Rheumatoid arthritis Scleroderma Ulcerative colitis Diabetes mellitus
Diffuse hair loss	Iron deficiency anaemia Hypothyroidism Hyperthyroidism Chronic renal failure Pregnancy or systemic illness (telogen effluvium) Drugs (see Table 5.2)
Moth-eaten alopecia	Syphilis
Premature canites	Pernicious anaemia Progeria and pangeria
Scarring alopecia	Lupus erythematosus Sarcoidosis Temporal arteritis Scleroderma Dermatomyositis Amyloidosis Follicular mucinosis Mastocytosis
Hair shaft abnormalities	Trichothiodystrophy Menkes' syndrome
Seborrhoeic dermatitis	Acquired immune deficiency syndrome (AIDS)
Scalp hyperpigmentation	Daunorubicin chemotherapy Bleomycin-induced flagellate erythema Minocycline

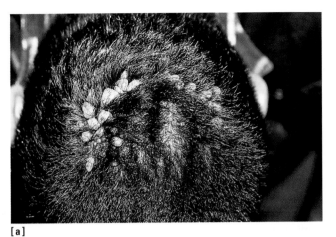
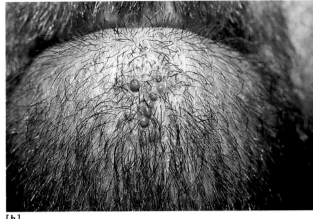

[a]   [b]

Fig. 12.9 Bizarre nodular folliculitis in the (a) scalp and (b) beard areas of a patient receiving cyclosporin A for polymyositis, which resolved when the cyclosporin A was stopped.

trophilic folliculitis without organisms, and culture is negative. Stopping the cyclosporin allows these papules to resolve over 6–8 weeks without scarring. If the cyclosporin is continued the papules enlarge and resemble keloids.

Associated features

Patients commonly have facial acne.

Prognosis

Without treatment the condition follows a chronic progressive course.

Treatment

Acne keloidalis nuchae is a notoriously difficult condition to eradicate. Ideally destruction of the keloids needs to be combined with measures to halt the development of new lesions. Oral antibiotics may reduce the number of new papules that develop, while the hypertrophic scars may respond to liquid nitrogen, (repeated) intralesional triamcinolone injections or carbon dioxide laser ablation. The hypertrophic scarring may recur following treatment.

Key points

Acne keloidalis nuchae presents as grouped papules and keloidal plaques on the nape of the neck of a (Negroid) man.

12.10 Scalp involvement in systemic disease

Systemic disorders frequently lead to abnormalities of hair growth (Table 12.6). The most important of these were discussed in the sections on virilism in hirsutes and androgenetic alopecia and in the section on diffuse hair loss. The relationship of autoimmune disorders to alopecia areata and premature canites has also been addressed in the relevant sections. Systemic diseases that are associated with scarring alopecia were dealt with under that heading in Chapter 8 and include lupus erythematosus, sarcoidosis, giant cell arteritis, dermatomyositis and amyloidosis.

Certain medications may produce hyperpigmentation of the scalp. This is most common with minocycline, and an unusual polycyclic pigmentation of the scalp has been seen with daunorubicin chemotherapy. Bleomycin-induced flagellate erythema may also produce a flagellate hyperpigmentation of the scalp.

Benign and malignant tumours, reticuloses and lymphoproliferative disorders will be considered along with other naevi, tumours and cysts of the scalp in the next chapter.

Chapter 13

Naevi, tumours and cysts of the scalp

13.1 Scalp cysts

The term sebaceous cyst is applied indiscriminately to both epidermoid cyst and pilar cyst. True sebaceous cysts occur in steatocystoma multiplex. The term is confusing and is best abandoned.

Pilar cysts (or tricholemmal cysts) are derived from the external root sheath of the hair follicle (the tricholemma) at the level of the isthmus. Pilar cysts are common on the scalp and present as single or multiple, firm, round nodules. The overlying hair growth may be affected (Fig. 13.1). Cysts can be a nuisance and excision is the easiest treatment. Most pilar cysts can be removed through a keyhole incision.

The cyst contains compactly arranged keratin with occasional foci of calcification, and the wall consists of stratified squamous epithelium without a granular layer. This indicates the keratin is formed by trichohyaline keratinization. Because the cyst arises deep in the hair follicle, and the overlying follicular infundibulum is not dilated, no punctum is seen on the skin and no epidermal connection is seen on histology.

A predisposition to pilar cyst formation is inherited as an autosomal dominant trait. Giant pilar cysts, known as Cock's peculiar tumour may occur on the scalps of older women and are said to resemble squamous cell carcinoma (SCC) (Fig. 13.2). Postauricular pilar cysts may be seen in association with hidradenitis suppuritiva and acne conglobata.

Proliferating tricholemmal cyst is a variant of a pilar cyst. These are solitary lesions and over 90% occur on the scalp. It appears as though a proliferating tricholemmal cyst arises from an ordinary pilar cyst, that grows into a large, elevated lobular mass that may undergo ulceration and resemble an SCC. The cyst lining is acanthotic and shows architectural and cytological atypia. They are well circumscribed and benign. Rarely, true malignant transformation and metastasis may also occur.

Epidermoid cysts are firm and rounded nodules situated in the dermis and attached to the epidermis. They arise from the infundibular portion of the hair follicle. There is usually a diagnostic central punctum. They are common in adult life and adolescence when they may occur as a complication of acne vulgaris. They also occur in Gardener's syndrome associated with fibromas, lipomas and polyposis coli.

The cysts can be subject to episodes of recurrent inflammation. They are found most commonly on the face, neck and trunk, but are not uncommon on the scalp. Lesions on the palms and soles may arise either from the eccrine ducts or from inclusions of epidermis driven into the dermis by puncture wounds. They can be differentiated from pilar cysts histologically by the cyst lining which consists of a stratified squamous epithelium with a stratum granulosum. If a cyst becomes annoying, then it can be surgically removed. The cyst can either be excised or drained with the lining curetted out.

Dermoid cysts are variants of epidermoid cysts that arise from sequestrated epithelial cells along lines of embryonic fusion. Most commonly they occur at the external angle of the eye, but they can also be seen over the cranial suture lines of the scalp. Occasionally dermoid cysts are connected by a stalk that passes through the cranium to a second intracerebral cyst: the so called dumb-bell dermoid. These sinuses may act as a portal of entry allowing infection into the brain if the cyst is traumatized. The bone beneath the cyst may be eroded or absent.

Around 40% of dermoids are present at birth and 60% by the age of 5 years. They enlarge slowly and may get up to 5 cm in size. The overlying skin is usually bald and at birth there may be a surrounding collar of hypertrophic hair which

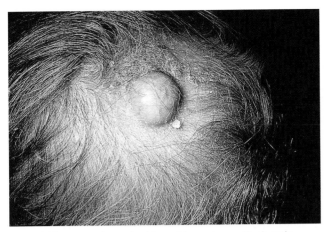

Fig. 13.1 Pilar cyst on the scalp with overlying androgenetic alopecia.

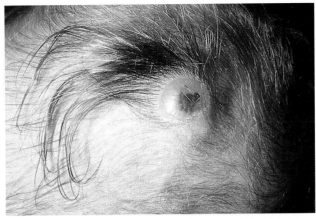

Fig. 13.3 Core of hypertrophic hair surrounding a congenital inclusion dermoid cyst of the scalp. (Courtesy of Dr Charles Darley, Brighton.)

is known as the hair collar sign (Fig. 13.3). Eventually the cysts involute and develop into a tethered bald scar, while the collar of hypertrophic hair blends imperceptibly in with the scalp terminal hairs as they develop.

Dermoids are similar to epidermoid cysts histologically in that the lining of the cyst consists of stratified squamous epithelium with a granular layer, but in addition the dermoid cyst lining gives rise to appendageal structures that bud out from the cyst wall. Dermoid cyst appendages include sebaceous, eccrine and apocrine glands as well as hair follicles.

A number of other conditions may present as congenital bald nodules on the scalp, with or without the collar of hypertrophic hair (Table 13.1), and may be clinically indistinguishable from dermoid cysts. If excision of such a nodule is contemplated for whatever reason then it is imperative that a preoperative assessment is made, looking for intracranial extension of the cyst and erosion of the outer tables of the skull. A CT scan and a plain X-ray of the skull are sufficient for this, but will not exclude a sinus tract penetrating the skull. This should be looked for at the time of the operation and sealed off.

Heterotopic brain tissue is ectopic neural tissue that during embryogenesis has become separated from the rest of the brain. The neural tissue is nonfunctional and the development and intelligence of the child is usually normal.

Eruptive vellus hair cysts are a rare autosomal dominant entity clinically similar to steatocystoma multiplex, and the two conditions may occur concurrently. They arise from the

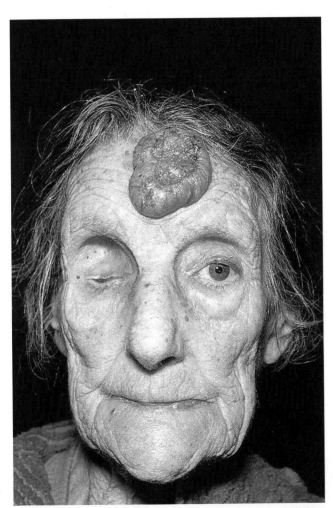

Fig. 13.2 Cock's peculiar tumour.

Table 13.1 Differential diagnosis of childhood scalp lesions with focal alopecia.

Aplasia cutis congenita	Encephalocele
Organoid naevus	Heterotopic brain tissue
Triangular alopecia	Sequestrated meningocele
Cerebriform intradermal naevus	Leptomeningeal cyst
Epidermoid cyst	Osteoma
Inclusion dermoid cyst	Protruding arachnoid granuloma
Dermal sinus tumour	Eosinophilic granuloma
Vascular naevi	Lipoma
Cephalohaematoma deformans	Pilomatrixoma

infundibulum of vellus hairs. Small firm keratotic papules develop on the chest and extremities of adolescents and young adults. Individual lesions may resemble keratosis pilaris, folliculitis or a perforating dermatosis. Histologically thin walled cysts containing numerous vellus hairs are seen to be surrounded by a layer of epidermis without a stratum granulosum. Multiple piloleiomyoma may sometimes look similar and Fox–Fordyce disease is a pruritic condition of the axilla due to sweat retention in apocrine ducts.

13.2 Epidermal naevus

Definition

An epidermal naevus is a circumscribed, congenital, hamartomatous malformation of the epidermis.

Clinical features

Epidermal naevus including linear verrucous epidermal naevi (Fig. 13.4), naevus unius lateris and ichthyosis hysterix; may occur on the scalp and be associated with permanent

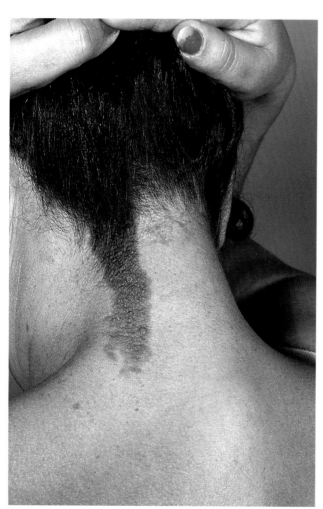

Fig. 13.4 Linear epidermal naevus.

alopecia. Rarely basal cell and SCCs may complicate these. Epidermal naevus syndrome is the association of neurological, ocular and skeletal abnormalities with an epidermal naevus.

Pathology

Histology classically shows hyperkeratosis, papillomatosis, acanthosis with hypergranulosis and basal hyperpigmentation. Many variations of this classic histology are recognized and include epidermolytic hyperkeratosis, porokeratosis-like change, acantholysis, psoriasiform and lichenoid changes.

Treatment

None is usually required. If small, surgical excision may be feasible. They tend to recur after dermabrasion, cryosurgery and carbon dioxide laser ablation.

Key points

Epidermal naevi on the scalp may produce localized permanent alopecia.

13.3 Organoid naevus

Definition

Organoid naevus, which is also known as naevus sebaceous of Jadassohn, is a congenital abnormality of the pilosebaceous glands as well as other adnexal structures.

Epidemiology

It occurs in 0.3% of newborns and seems to be distributed along the lines of Blaschko.

Aetiology

It occurs both as an isolated abnormality and as part of the organoid naevus syndrome associated with vascular, musculoskeletal and central nervous system abnormalities (Schimmelpenning–Feuerstein–Mims syndrome).

Clinical features

An organoid naevus characteristically occurs on the scalp, forehead and face. The appearance of the lesion is sensitive to androgens and alters at puberty. The lesion is usually present at birth as a 1–6 cm, bald, smooth, waxy, slightly yellow plaque (Fig. 13.5). At puberty the lesions enlarge and become verrucous, occasionally grotesquely so. Neoplastic degeneration may occur, most commonly when the patients are in their forties. Common neoplasms include syringocystadenoma papilliferum, basal cell carcinoma and hidradenoma. Rare

acanthosis with papillomatosis. In the dermis there is a reduced number of pilosebaceous units and those that are present are immature and abnormally formed. After puberty the epidermis becomes acanthotic and more papillomatous and the sebaceous glands enlarge. They are seen abnormally high in the dermis, with an increased number of closely set lobules and malformed ducts. Apocrine glands are present in about half and hair follicles are vellus rather than terminal and sparsely distributed. Other tumours, as previously listed, may be seen within the organoid naevus.

Associated features

In the organoid naevus syndrome the sebaceous naevi tend to be more extensive and more numerous. Organoid naevi have also been associated with hypophosphataemic rickets (Sugarman–Reed syndrome), verrucous epidermal naevi, woolly hair naevus, straight hair naevus and dystrophic nails.

Prognosis

The lesions once fully developed remain verrucous throughout life. Tumours may develop within organoid naevi, as mentioned above. While mostly banal in their behaviour, metastasizing tumours have also been reported, albeit rarely.

Treatment

Excision with primary closure is usually recommended around the time of puberty to prevent malignant degeneration. This is often the time when the patients present due to enlargement of the lesion. Once excised, lesions do not recur.

Key points

A smooth, bald, congenital, yellow plaque that enlarges at puberty under the influence of androgens, and which may undergo neoplastic degeneration later in life.

13.4 Skin cancer, melanocytic naevi and melanoma

Solar keratoses

Bald scalps are exposed to the sun and are prone to actinic damage. Solar keratoses are circumscribed, scaly, erythematous lesions, usually less than 1 cm in diameter that occur on sun-exposed sites in older individuals. They frequently occur on the scalp.

Cutaneous horns are relatively common on balding scalps. They are hard, yellowish-brown keratotic excrescences with a height exceeding one-half its greatest diameter. They are most commonly due to solar keratoses, but may also occur with viral warts, epidermal naevi, SCC or seborrhoeic keratosis. Induration of the base of the lesion is a clue to SCC.

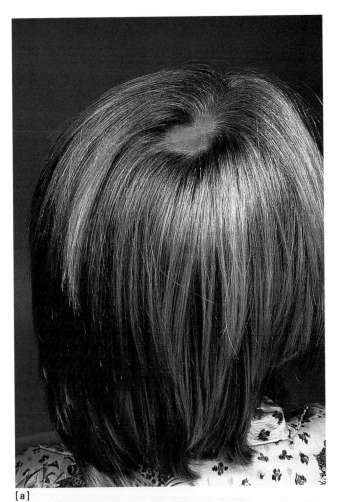

[a]

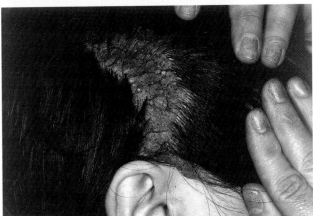

[b]

Fig. 13.5 (a) Organoid naevus in a prepubertal child. (b) Organoid naevus in a postpubertal child.

neoplasms include leiomyoma, syringoma, SCC, keratoacanthoma, porocarcinoma, and other benign appendageal tumours with apocrine or sebaceous differentiation.

Pathology

Histology in prepubertal children shows mild epidermal

Histology of a solar keratosis shows focal parakeratosis with loss of the underlying granular layer. Often there is acanthosis. Basal layer cytological atypia is required for the diagnosis. The atypia usually spares the acrotrichia and the acrosyringia. Solar elastosis is present in the underlying dermis.

Treatment

Solar keratosis can be left alone if asymptomatic, frozen with liquid nitrogen, curetted or treated with 5-fluorouracil cream. Overzealous cryotherapy may be complicated by permanent alopecia. If the lesion is indurated, a biopsy should be performed to exclude SCC. Cutaneous horns are often a nuisance and surgical removal is generally recommended.

Bowen's disease

Bowen's disease is *in situ* SCC. It may occur on any part of the skin. On the scalp it presents most frequently in fair skinned people on bald areas heavily exposed to solar radiation. Sunlight and arsenic ingestion are other known precipitants. Rarely multicentric Bowen's disease occurs on a hairy scalp. Bowen's disease presents as a persistent, asymptomatic, scaly or crusted, well demarcated plaque (or plaques) on a bald scalp. It may resemble psoriasis except that it remains unchanged or enlarges slowly over many years. Invasive SCC develops after a number of years in around 5–10% of cases and can metastasize.

Histologically there is full thickness cytological and architectural epidermal atypia that extends down hair follicles and eccrine ducts. In addition there is an increase in the number of suprabasal mitoses, and atypical mitoses are present. The granular layer is lost and there is overlying parakeratosis and hyperkeratosis. Bowenoid solar keratoses also occur on the scalp and on biopsy show full thickness epidermal atypia, that spares the pilosebaceous units.

Treatment

Cryosurgery with a 30 second single timed spot freeze will cure 98% of Bowen's disease. Because follicular destruction with permanent alopecia would be produced by this dose of liquid nitrogen, excision is more suitable for Bowen's disease occurring on a hairy scalp.

Keratoacanthoma

A keratoacanthoma (KA) is a rapidly evolving skin nodule that is histologically malignant but biologically benign. It occurs predominantly in an elderly balding population in response to solar radiation. It has been suggested that KA arise from hair follicles and that the growth phase corresponds to the anagen phase of hair growth and the involution and apoptosis that accompanies resolution may correspond to catagen. While this hypothesis is attractive, the occurrence of KAs on nonhair bearing sites such as the mucous membranes, palms and soles and the subungual region confounds the theory.

Less than 5% of all KAs occur on the scalp. Their behaviour on the scalp is similar to their behaviour elsewhere on the skin. Classically they enlarge for about 6 weeks, plateau for 6 weeks and involute spontaneously over 6 weeks.

The histology of KA shows a symmetrical exoendophytic lesion in the upper dermis which extends no deeper than the sweat gland coils. A central mass of keratin is surrounded by columns of acanthotic epidermis that form a colarette. The cells show some cytological atypia, but atypical mitoses are not common. The keratinocytes have an eosinophilic cytoplasm and there is a lymphocytic infiltrate at the base of the lesion with scattered neutrophils and eosinophils. Distinction from a well-differentiated SCC can be difficult at times, however, the architecture and cellular morphology usually allow differentiation.

Treatment

On the basis of the clinical and histological features, a prediction of biological behaviour can be made. In the presence of a normal immunological system a KA may be left alone to resolve spontaneously. If however, there is immunodeficiency (e.g. postorgan transplantation) then the lesions tend not to involute and may metastasize, albeit rarely. Such lesions should be removed, as should any lesion that threatens to cause local destruction to the nose or eyelids.

Keratoacanthomas that are still enlarging or which may leave a disfiguring scar after healing, or that are difficult to diagnose clinically with certainty, should also be excised. In practice this encompasses the majority of KAs and only a relatively small percentage are best left to regress spontaneously. A shave biopsy followed by curettage and cautery is usually sufficient. Alternatively an elliptical excision has a slightly lower rate of recurrence. Cryotherapy is less effective and is not recommended for treatment however, radiotherapy may be successful.

Squamous cell carcinoma

Squamous cell carcinoma is the second most common cancer in man and lesions on the scalp are common. They are especially common in organ transplant recipients. Squamous cell carcinoma occurs in sun-damaged, bald scalps, and is usually surrounded by other features of actinic damage such as solar keratoses.

Radiotherapy epilation treatment for ringworm, fashionable in the days before griseofulvin (1950s) has resulted in many cases of SCC after a 20–40 year latency period. Radiotherapy was also used for lupus vulgaris, scalp psoriasis and other benign dermatoses. Scars produced by burns (Marjolin's ulcers) or other chronic sores may also degenerate into SCC.

Squamous cell carcinoma may present in a number of different ways. The development of induration around the base of a solar keratosis or a cutaneous horn suggests SCC. Squamous cell carcinomas may also present as shallow ulcers with a keratinous crust and an elevated, indurated margin (Fig. 13.6). If neglected there may be serious consequences.

Published data suggests that up to 5% of SCCs on the scalp metastasize, predominantly to regional lymph nodes, and up to 10% of lesions recur locally after apparently adequate radiotherapy or standard surgical treatment. Australian experience would suggest that metastasis is less common than this, but this may reflect the greater number of SCCs seen and earlier diagnosis. Mohs' micrographic surgery has a lower rate of local recurrence. Neurotropic spread is indicated by severe pain in the lesion and when present is a sinister feature.

Histology is required to confirm the diagnosis and shows nests of atypical squamous cells arising from the epidermis invading into the dermis. Keratin pearls and individual cell keratinization are common. The cellular differentiation is variable. Finding desmosomes, which manifest as prickles adjoining adjacent cells, is helpful to establish the tumour cell type of a poorly differentiated SCC. Histological variants include spindle cell SCC, adenoid SCC and clear cell SCC.

Treatment

Treatment choices include surgical excision, curettage and electrocautery, radiotherapy and cryosurgery. The treatment chosen will depend on the patient's age, health and preference, the site and size of the SCC, as well as the nature of any previous treatments.

Basal cell carcinoma

Basal cell carcinoma (BCC) is the most common cancer in man and approximately 5% of all BCCs occur on the scalp.

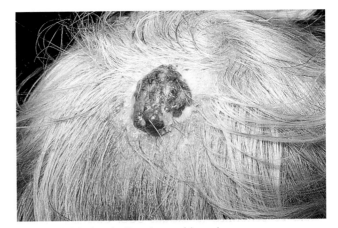
Fig. 13.7 Nodular basal cell carcinoma of the scalp.

Basal cell carcinomas on the scalp usually occur in bald areas (Fig. 13.7) where they are most common in scars. Lesions in hair-bearing skin are often neglected and may be very large at initial presentation (Fig. 13.8). Organoid naevi are predisposed to develop a BCC within them. Radiotherapy for ringworm is another predisposing factor, and the irradiated area is not invariably bald. The incidence is increased two to threefold in organ transplant recipients although this increase is less marked than for SCC.

The clinical appearance does not differ from BCC elsewhere on the skin. The lesions are typically smooth, translucent nodules with superficial telangiectasia, that enlarge very slowly and frequently ulcerate centrally to leave a translucent pearly edge. Basal cell carcinomas may be pigmented, morphoeic, nodular or of the rodent ulcer type. They may achieve great size if neglected. They can recur locally, however metastasis is exceptionally rare, with an estimated incidence of less than one in a million.

Histology reveals a tumour within the dermis that is connected to the epidermis or a hair follicle. The tumour cells are basaloid (dark blue) in colour and there is peripheral palisading and clefting (separation artefact). There is a dermal

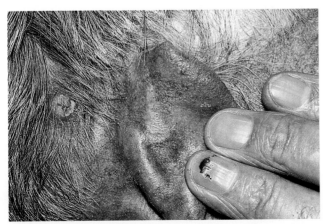
Fig. 13.6 Squamous cell carcinoma occurring behind the left ear.

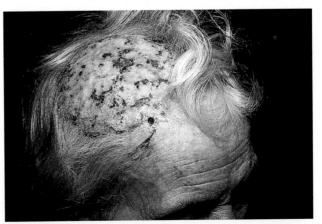
Fig. 13.8 Morphoeic basal cell carcinoma of the scalp.

stromal reaction, which is most marked in morphoeic BCCs. Nerve involvement should be looked for as neurotropic spread predisposes to local recurrence.

Treatment

The diagnosis should be confirmed by biopsy. Treatment options include surgical excision, curettage and electro-cautery, radiotherapy and cryosurgery. The treatment chosen needs to be individualized and will depend on the site and the size of the BCC, as well as the nature of any previous treatments.

Melanocytic naevi and melanoma

Melanocytic naevus is a benign proliferation of melanocytes that may be congenital or acquired. Congenital naevi include Spitz naevi and blue naevi, while acquired naevi may be junctional, compound or intradermal in location. Melanocytic naevi may be precursors to melanoma. Melanomas are a malignant neoplasm of melanocytes with a high metastatic potential. Approximately one in four people diagnosed with melanoma in the United Kingdom will die of metastatic disease. Both benign naevi and melanomas occur on the scalp.

Junctional naevi are flat brown macules. Histology shows a proliferation of melanocytes in nests at the dermoepidermal junction. With time they may evolve into compound naevi.

Compound naevi are dome-shaped brown papules, with nest of melanocytes both at the dermoepidermal junction and also separately within the dermis. The junctional nests produce pigment while the intradermal nests do not. Compound naevi may eventually evolve into intradermal naevi.

Intradermal naevi are flesh-coloured, dome-shaped papules. There are nests of melanocytes within the dermis, but there are no junctional, pigment producing nests. Over time these lesions involute and disappear.

Blue naevi may be macular or papular. They are characterized by a distinctive deep blue colour. Lesions may occur anywhere on the body and are common on the scalp. In one series 17% of cellular blue naevi were found on the scalp. They arise as a result of interrupted migration of embryonic melanocytes from the neural tube to the epidermis. Unlike the dermal melanocytes of acquired naevi, the intradermal melanocytes of blue naevi produce melanin. The colour arises as a result of refraction of light passing through the epidermis, which makes the black pigment appear blue (the Tindall effect). Histologically blue naevi may be either of the common epithelioid cell type or of the spindle cell type. Malignant blue naevus is a very rare complication of blue naevus.

An association between multiple blue naevi and pili annulati occurred in one family, suggesting genetic linkage.

Congenital naevi differ in their morphology and natural history from acquired naevi. Clinically congenital naevi may be small or large (bathing trunk naevi), dark lesions with a verrucous surface. Occasionally the surface is irregularly convoluted and cerebriform. Coarse hairs may grow from within the mole. Histologically they are compound naevi with a periadnexal deeper component. Melanoma may develop in between 1 and 10% of congenital; naevi, usually, but not always, after puberty.

Melanomas in the scalp are uncommon. Out of 4000 invasive melanomas on the University of California, San Francisco (UCSF) database, only 80 were on the scalp. There was a broad range of Breslow thickness of the lesions. They are predominantly superficial spreading, but not uncommonly nodular, in type (Fig. 13.9). Scalp melanomas may arise either *de novo*, within congenital naevi in children and young adults, or within a lentigo maligna in the sun-damaged bald scalp of an elderly person. Often the lesions are well advanced at the time of detection and metastasis is common. The overall survival in the UCSF series was 20%, which is worse than for other body sites, however, there is no evidence that depth for depth, melanomas of the scalp fare worse than elsewhere on the body. The scalp is also the preferred site for desmoplastic melanoma, a rare type of melanoma that is often a nonpigmented nodule (Fig. 13.10), difficult to diagnose both clinically and histologically.

Lentigo maligna or Hutchinson's melanotic freckle is a type of *in situ* melanoma that occurs exclusively on the head and neck. Scalp lesions are common on sun-damaged bald areas. Invasive melanoma is said to occur in 5–10% of lentigo malignas over a period of 20 years.

Treatment

If malignancy can be confidently excluded on clinical grounds, treatment is only required if the naevus is a nuisance to the patient. There is debate over the malignant potential of congenital naevi and whether prophylactic excision of these lesions is justified. Currently the trend is not to excise lesions prophylactically as the small ones carry a negligible risk and excision of the large ones carries significant morbidity.

The treatment of choice for melanoma is unequivocally surgical excision with an adequate margin of surrounding uninvolved skin to prevent local recurrence. A 1 cm margin per 1 mm of Breslow depth is considered appropriate for invasive lesions up to 2 mm deep. *In situ* melanoma can be adequately treated with a 0.5 cm margin. The optimal margins for lesions greater than 1 mm are undergoing constant redefinition. Lesions greater than 3 mm deep have a very poor prognosis and excision margins greater than 1–2 cm do not appear to be justified.

13.5 Vascular naevi and tumours

Pyogenic granuloma

This is a common benign vascular tumour. About 3% of pyo-

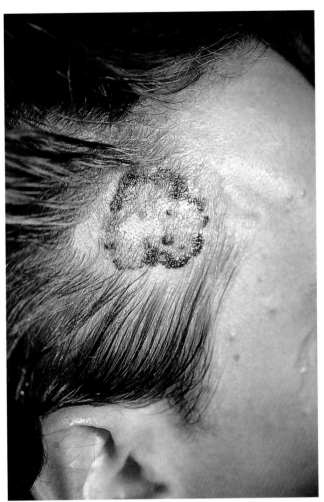

Fig. 13.9 Superficial spreading malignant melanoma of the scalp (level III).

genic granulomas (PG) occur on the scalp. They are bright-red, soft, highly vascular papules or nodules that range in size from 2 to 3 mm to several centimetres. Larger lesions may be pedunculated, mushroom shaped or sessile. The clinical differential diagnosis includes amelanotic melanoma or a Spitz naevus.

Lesions may arise spontaneously or appear following minor trauma such as a scratch from a rose thorn. They enlarge for several weeks and thereafter persist indefinitely unless treated. Pyogenic granulomas are often multiple and may ulcerate and bleed profusely if knocked. Young children often develop PGs on the face, while older children and adults generally develop them on their face, hands, arms and upper chest. The mucous membranes of the mouth and nose can also be affected and lymphangitis is an occasional complication.

Histology shows an epidermal colarette surrounding an upper dermal proliferation of endothelial cells and capillaries, that resembles granulation tissue. Treatment options include cryotherapy, curettage and electrocautery, and surgi-

cal excision. Biopsy tissue should be sent for histology if there is any doubt about the diagnosis. Local recurrences may follow each of these treatment modalities and excision is then advisable for the recurrent lesion.

Salmon patch

Both salmon patches and port wine stains have in the past been called naevus flammeus. However, the two conditions are distinct, hence the term is confusing and best avoided. A salmon patch (or stork bite) is a pink macular area that occurs on the nape of the neck of between 20 and 50% of newborn babies and persists indefinitely throughout life. It is covered by hair and as such is not a cosmetic problem and is usually no more than an incidental finding when the scalp is being examined (Fig. 13.11). A salmon patch may also occur on the forehead or eyelids. Such lesions are much less common than nuchal ones and tend to fade during the first year of life and ultimately disappear.

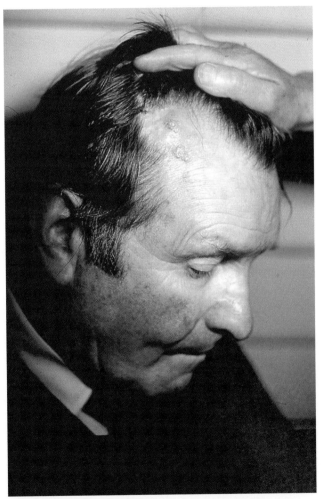

Fig. 13.10 Desmoplastic melanoma occurring in the scalp. These lesions are extremely difficult to diagnose clinically.

Port wine stain

A port wine stain is a developmental vascular malformation present at birth in 0.3% of children. It occurs most commonly on the face and neck, but a significant proportion extend onto the scalp. Single or multiple areas of macular erythema may be present and they are often sharply unilateral or segmental (Fig. 13.12). Unlike salmon patches, with time these lesions persist, darken and develop a raised verrucous surface, sometimes studded with nodular angiomas or pyogenic granulomas.

Histologically there is a dilatation of thin walled vessels in the papillary dermis without an actual increase in the number of vessels or thickening of the vessel walls. In the Sturge–Weber syndrome there is a port wine stain involving the ophthalmic branch of the trigeminal nerve (forehead and upper eyelid), the choroid of the eye and the leptomeninges. Intracranial angiomas predispose to epilepsy.

Various lasers have been developed to treat port wine stains on the face and body. Those on the scalp are generally

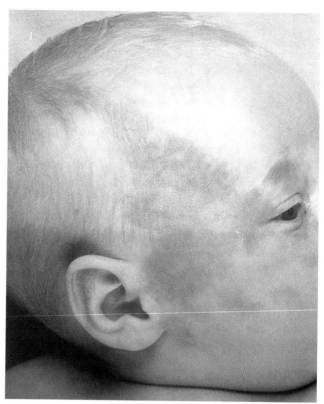

Fig. 13.12 Port wine stain occurring over the face and extending onto the scalp.

covered by hair and require no treatment. The treatment of choice for flat lesions on the face is the 585 nm tunable pulsed yellow dye laser (Candela). The response to treatment is unpredictable, however the majority will improve and many will disappear completely. The great benefit of these lasers is the lack of scarring. Other vascular lasers such as the copper vapour, Nd:YAG and argon have lower response rates and may produce permanent textural changes (scarring) and depigmentation.

Strawberry naevi

These are cavernous haemangiomas that are not usually present at birth. They occur in 5–10% of babies and first appear during the first few weeks of life. They begin as an erythematous macule that becomes papular and rapidly enlarges over a few months to become nodular. At this stage lesions are bright-red, smooth nodules that vary in size from 1 to 25 cm. They frequently ulcerate, but profuse bleeding is rare. Occasionally there is a consumption coagulopathy due to the Kasabach–Merritt syndrome, which has a 40% mortality.

After 3–6 months the lesions stop growing and start to involute spontaneously. In 95% the involution is complete, leaving behind only an atrophic scar. The degree of scarring is variable (Fig. 13.13), but is worst if there has been ulceration or infection of the naevus. The rate of involution is variable

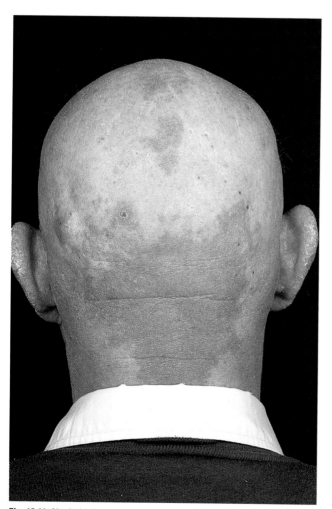

Fig. 13.11 Nuchal salmon patch in a person with total alopecia due to keratosis, ichthyosis, deafness (KID) syndrome.

and 30% will be gone in 4 years, 50% in 5 years and 75% by 7 years. The later the resolution the less likely it is to be complete. When important structures are threatened, or ulceration is developing, intralesional triamcinolone or oral prednisolone (2–4 mg/kg) may be used to hasten resolution. They are most useful during the rapidly growing phase. The candela laser is also useful at the early macular stage, and may abort the lesion.

About 60% of strawberry naevi occur on the head and neck. Twenty per cent of affected children have multiple strawberry naevi. Lesions in the scalp usually resolve without permanent alopecia unless there has been previous ulceration. In a neonate cutaneous extramedullary haemopoesis may mimic multiple strawberry naevi.

Angiosarcoma of the scalp

Idiopathic cutaneous angiosarcoma of the head and neck is a distinct highly malignant neoplasm of blood vessel endothelium that behaves aggressively and often metastasizes to regional lymph nodes, and to the lungs. Local recurrence of the disease is common as the tumour margins are difficult to define. The prognosis of recurrent disease is dismal.

Angiosarcomas commonly present as single or grouped bluish-red nodules on the face and scalp. There may be some thinning of the hair over the tumour nodules, but alopecia is not marked. Less well differentiated tumours present as diffuse indurated plaques or flat infiltrating macules over which there is a cicatricial alopecia. This form is known as the malignant bruise. Nodules may develop from within the areas of macular erythema (Fig. 13.14) and the surface may be verrucous.

The tumours are progressive and extend to involve large areas of the face, neck and scalp. There may be gross oedema of the eyelids and large ulcers may bleed profusely. Involvement of the skull produces erosion of the bone and seeds distant metastases. The average survival from diagnosis is under 2 years.

Histology shows a poorly circumscribed dermal tumour that infiltrates subcutaneous fat. Angiomatous and solid patterns occur within the tumour. In the angiomatous regions a meshwork of anastomosing dilated vessels extends between the collagen bundles. The channels are lined by atypical swollen endothelial cells that are plump and resemble hobnails. The solid areas contain poorly differentiated spindle and epithelioid cells. The histological picture may closely resemble Kaposi's sarcoma. Immunohistochemical stains may be required to distinguish a poorly differentiated angiosarcoma from a spindle cell SCC or amelanotic melanoma.

The prognosis of this condition is poor and the 5 year survival has been estimated at 15%. Surgical excision with a wide margin (2–3 cm) of normal skin is required. Even so local recurrence is common. It has been recommended that once the lesion is excised, closure or grafting should be

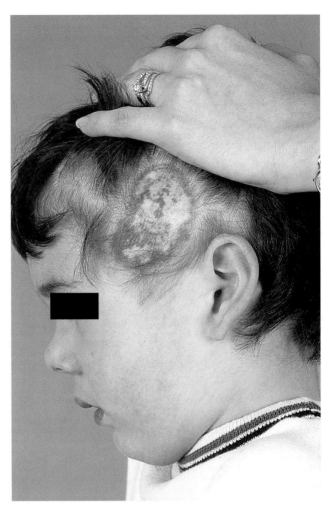

Fig. 13.13 Scarring following resolution of a strawberry naevus in a child. Unusually there was no history of ulceration or infection in this lesion.

delayed for 24–48 hours until a rapid paraffin section can be histologically examined to ensure the margins are clear. A Mohs' type examination of the margins is best. Postoperative radiotherapy should be given as it has been shown to increase the duration of disease-free survival. Large lesions can be treated with interferon α 2b in an attempt to shrink them preoperatively. Massive doses may be required.

13.6 Appendageal tumours

Introduction

A large number of benign appendageal tumours with follicular, sebaceous, apocrine or eccrine differentiation have been described. The more common follicular tumours are pilomatrixoma, trichoepithelioma, trichofolliculoma, tricholemmoma, trichodiscoma, tumour of follicular infundibulum and inverted follicular keratosis. Some have malignant counterpart, but these are very rare.

Sebaceous hyperplasia is common, while benign and malignant tumours arising from sebaceous glands are rare.

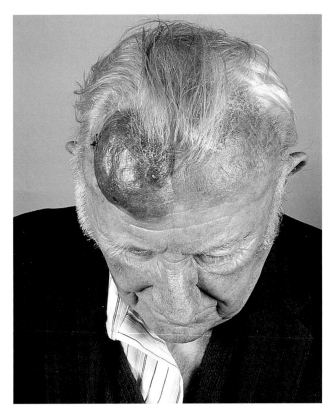

Fig. 13.14 Angiosarcoma of the forehead, with formation of a large nodule on the right side.

The Muir–Torre syndrome is an important autosomal dominant cancer syndrome characterized by the development of multiple sebaceous tumours in association with visceral carcinoma and KAs.

Apocrine derived tumours are rare. Those that affect the scalp are syringocystadenoma papilliferum, apocrine hidrocystoma and tubular apocrine adenoma. Cylindromas are probably eccrine derived.

There are two important considerations in the management of a solitary benign appendage tumour. The first is whether a biopsy is required to rule out malignancy and the second is the cosmetic impact of the lesion, as appendageal tumours are generally asymptomatic. If treatment is required, surgical excision is usually the treatment of choice.

Multiple lesions such as trichoepitheliomas, tricholemmomas, trichodiscomas and fibrofolliculomas may require treatment for cosmetic purposes. Alternatives include excision, curettage, cryosurgery, CO_2 laser ablation or dermabrasion.

Appendageal tumours with follicular differentiation

Trichofolliculoma occurs in adults as a solitary skin-coloured dome-shaped nodule with a central pore. They are usually found on the face but also occur on the scalp or neck. A tuft of fine hairs may be seen emerging from the central punctum. Nodules may coalesce. Histology shows a keratin filled cystic structure in the dermis that is lined by squamous epithelium and in continuity with the skin surface. The cyst is a dilated primary hair follicle from which numerous smaller well differentiated secondary follicles radiate.

Trichoepitheliomas (TEs) first appear at puberty. They may be single or multiple, small (2–8 mm), flesh-coloured, firm nodules that are found mainly on the nose, nasolabial fold, upper lip and cheek. Occasionally lesions may be seen on the scalp or forehead. Multiple lesions can be inherited alone in what is known as epithelioma adenoides cysticum or together with multiple cylindromas (Fig. 13.15) in the autosomal dominant Brooke–Spiegler syndrome. The Rombo syndrome comprises multiple trichoepitheliomas, milia, atrophoderma vermiculata, multiple BCCs, peripheral vasodilatation and cyanosis.

Histology of the TE shows a lobulated basaloid tumour in the upper and mid dermis. The tumour arises from the epidermis and resembles a BCC. The lobules show peripheral palisading, contains numerous horn cysts and are surrounded by a conspicuous connective tissue sheath. The walls of the horn cysts consist of two or three layers of cells with an eosinophilic cytoplasm and large vesicular nuclei. The numerous horn cysts help to distinguish a TE from a BCC, however, some lesions may be equivocal and clinicopathological consultation is required to arrive at the correct diagnosis.

Desmoplastic TE is a variant of TE that clinically and histologically resembles a morphoeic BCC, but has a benign biological behaviour. The lesions are usually solitary, asymptomatic, small, hard annular lesions with a depressed centre and a slightly raised border. They are most common on the face of middle-aged females. Histologically there are narrow strands of tumour cells, numerous horn cysts and a desmoplastic stroma. Horn cysts are not a feature of morphoeic BCCs.

There are a number of clinical presentations of *follicular infundibular tumours*. Solitary lesions present as asymptomatic, smooth or slightly keratotic, elevated papules on the head, neck or upper chest. Multiple lesions may occur on sun-exposed areas of the head and neck of middle-aged men and heal spontaneously leaving discoid lupus-like scars. Alternatively, hundreds of eruptive infundibulomas, 2–15 mm in diameter with complex angular shapes may appear in a mantle distribution over the upper portion of the chest, back or shoulders. Histology shows a plate-like growth of pale staining keratinocytes, running parallel to the skin surface, arising from numerous hair follicles and interconnecting them. There is a peripheral palisade and this benign tumour resembles a superficial BCC.

Inverted follicular keratosis is probably a histological variant of an old wart. It occurs on the face of middle-aged men and women and may be mistaken clinically for a BCC. Histology shows a cutaneous horn composed of ortho- and hyperkeratosis. The base of the horn shows a hyperplastic epidermis

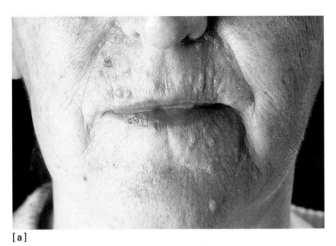
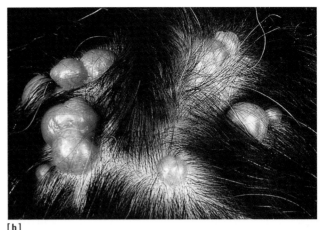

[a]   [b]

Fig. 13.15 (a) Multiple trichoepitheliomas occurring together with multiple cylindromas on the face together with (b) multiple cylindromas on the scalp. (Courtesy of Dr J. Kelly, Melbourne.)

with numerous squamous eddies, but minimal cytological atypia.

Tricholemmomas are benign tumours derived from the outer root sheath (the tricholemma). They occur commonly as solitary tumours, which are small (3–8 mm), asymptomatic, papular lesions usually found on the face. They resemble plane viral warts clinically and old warts histologically, but a virus has not to date been identified from within them.

Multiple lesions can occur as a manifestation of Cowden's syndrome which is an autosomal dominant cancer syndrome consisting of lipomas, neuromas, acral keratoses, palmar pits, acromelanosis, skeletal abnormalities, oral fibromas, fibrocystic disease of the breast, thyroid adenomas, ovarian cysts, gastrointestinal polyps, carcinoma of the breast and thyroid, non-Hodgkin's lymphoma, and SCC of the skin, tongue and cervix.

Histology shows a circumscribed clear cell tumour in the upper dermis, arising from the epidermis or follicular epithelium at several points. The tumour is composed of a number of lobules containing clear (glycogen filled) squamoid cells surrounded by a palisade of columnar cells. The lobules are encircled by a distinct, thick glassy membrane. The overlying epidermis is acanthotic and hyperkeratotic.

Pilomatrixoma, also known as calcifying epithelioma of Malherbe is a benign tumour thought to arise from hair matrix cells, and shows differentiation towards hair cortex. Hence the name pilomatrixoma. It accounts for about 20% of pilar tumours. Clinically it appears as a solitary, hard, dermal nodule up to 3 cm in diameter. Calcification within the lesion is common and may be visible macroscopically in the cut excision specimen. Lesions are found predominantly on the head, neck and arms and usually present in childhood. In one large series 12% were found to occur on the scalp. Pigmented pilomatrixomas, multiple tumours (rarely more than 4), and perforation can all be seen.

Histology shows a circumscribed tumour in the lower dermis and subcutis consisting of lobules within a dense fibrous stroma. There are two cell types. Basophilic (matrix-like) cells are found at the margin of the lobules and transform into eosinophilic shadow (cortex-like) cells in the centre of the lobules. Shadow cells have lost their nuclear staining, but retain distinct cell borders. Calcification occurs in the majority of pilomatrixomas, but true ossification is less common. A foreign body giant cell reaction may surround the lobules, and melanin and haemosiderin are often seen within the tumour.

Recent immunohistochemical studies have shown that the outermost basophilic cells of the tumour lobules express the same cytokeratins as the stem cells of the hair bulge. This implies that calcifying epitheliomas may actually derive from cells more primitive than matrix cells. It has been proposed that bulge cells differentiate into the basophilic cells (corresponding to outer root sheath cells), subsequently into the transitional cells (corresponding to the hair matrix) and finally into shadow cells (corresponding to the hair cortex). Perhaps pilomatrixomas should be renamed pilobulgeomas!

Trichodiscoma is a proliferation of the connective tissue sheath that surrounds the hair follicles. The component of the sheath that gives rise to this tumour is the hair disc or *Haarscheibe*, which is a richly vascularized and innervated mechanoreceptor that contains Merkel cells. The lesions are multiple, asymptomatic, tiny (1–3 mm), flesh-coloured papules. They are most common on the face, but also occur on the trunk and limbs. Histology shows a poorly demarcated dome-shaped, fibrovascular tumour in the papillary dermis, that arises from the side of a hair follicle.

Appendageal tumours with sebaceous differentiation

Sebaceous hyperplasia appears on the face, neck and scalp of elderly people with sun-damaged skin. It presents with small (2–5 mm) yellow umbilicated papules that may be mistaken for an early rodent ulcer. Histology shows lobules of enlarged sebaceous glands surrounding a central hair follicle.

Sebaceous adenomas usually appear on the nose, face or scalp of men over the age of 40 years. They present as slightly keratotic yellow nodules about 0.5 cm in size. Larger ones exist and ulceration and bleeding can occur. Histology shows multiple discrete, incompletely differentiated, sebaceous lobules in the mid to deep dermis, that are irregular in size and shape. The peripheral layer of basaloid cells is separated from the central foamy cells by one or two layers of transitional cells.

Sebaceous carcinoma tends to occur most commonly in the elderly on the eyelids as an aggressive, locally invasive tumour. They arise from the meibomian glands and the glands of Zeis. Sebaceous carcinoma accounts for 3% of all eyelid tumours. They present as solitary, solid or ulcerated, yellow, translucent nodules that enlarge slowly. The upper eyelid is more commonly involved than the lower. Occasionally lesions may masquerade as chalazion or a chronic conjunctivitis. Metastasis is relatively common and the 5 year survival is around 80%. Sebaceous carcinoma may also occur away from the eye, usually on the face and scalp. Histology demonstrates lobules of sebaceous cells in various stages of differentiation, separated by a fibrous stroma and deeply invading the dermis, subcutis and underlying muscle. There are numerous atypical cells and mitoses and there is often focal necrosis. Pagetoid intraepidermal or conjunctival spread occurs in ocular lesions, this makes complete excision difficult.

Sebaceoma or sebaceous epithelioma is a BCC with sebaceous differentiation. Clinically the lesions is a solitary yellow nodule on the face. It may occur as a part of the Muir–Torre syndrome or arise within an organoid naevus. Histology shows a basaloid tumour arising from the epidermis with a random admixture of sebaceous cells. The basaloid cells outnumber the sebaceous cells, as compared to a sebaceous carcinoma where the sebaceous cells are in the majority.

Appendageal tumours with apocrine differentiation

Apocrine hidrocystoma is a cystic dilatation of the apocrine secretory duct that presents as a small (less than 10 mm), solitary, well-defined, dome-shaped, translucent nodule with a blue hue. They occur most commonly on the outer canthus of the eye and the penis, but can also be found on the scalp, ear, chest or shoulders. Multilobulated lesions can also occur. Histology shows one or several large cystic spaces lined by a row of secretory epithelium that shows decapitation secretion. Papillary projections can delve into the cystic spaces.

Syringocystadenoma papilliferum is an exuberant proliferating lesion that is most commonly seen on the scalp and is accompanied by alopecia. It may appear at birth as a solitary translucent or pigmented papule with a blue hue, or as several papules in a linear arrangement following Blaschko's lines. Extensive verrucous plaques may develop at puberty when the congenital lesions enlarge and become papillomatous and crusted with androgen stimulation. About one-third of syringocystadenoma papilliferum appear later in life in association with an organoid naevus.

Histology shows epidermal papillomatosis, and beneath this a cystic invagination extends downwards into the dermis. Numerous papillary projections extend into the

Table 13.2 Classification of hair follicle tumours (after Weedon).

Hamartomas and tumours of the hair germ	Hair follicle naevus
	Trichofolliculoma
	Trichoadenoma
	Trichoepithelioma
	Desmoplastic trichoepithelioma
	Trichoblastoma
	Generalized hair follicle hamartoma
	Basal cell hamartoma with follicular differentiation
	Linear unilateral basal cell naevus with comedones
Infundibular tumours	Follicular infundibular tumour
	Dilated pore of Winer
	Pilar sheath acanthoma
	Inverted follicular keratosis
External root sheath tumours	Tricholemmoma (Cowden's syndrome)
	Tricholemmal carcinoma
	Basal cell carcinoma (some)
Hair matrix tumours	Pilomatrixoma
	Pilomatrix carcinoma
Tumours of follicular mesenchyme	Trichodiscoma
	Fibrofolliculoma

lumen of the cystic invagination. The cyst is lined by a double layer of columnar cells showing decapitation secretion and the underlying stroma contains abundant plasma cells.

Tubular apocrine adenoma is a very rare tumour that occurs most commonly in the scalp or the axilla. It presents as a dermal nodule which gradually enlarges and may grow as big as 7 cm in diameter. Histology shows a poorly circumscribed dermal tumour connected to the epidermis. The tumour is composed of lobular masses that contain a central tubular structure. The tubular lumen is lined by a double layer of cells, the inner columnar cell layer shows decapitation secretion, while the outer consists of myoepithelial cells. A malignant counterpart of this condition also exists.

Appendageal tumours with eccrine differentiation (Table 13.3)

Cylindromas are dome-shaped nodules that mainly occur on the scalp and forehead of middle-aged women. They arise from the intradermal coiled duct region of the eccrine gland. Cylindromas may be single or multiple (turban tumours), bald, smooth, firm, pink, pedunculated slow-growing tumours that reach up to 5 cm in size. Occasionally tumours are painful and in some families they occur as an autosomal dominant trait with variable penetrance. They can be inherited in conjunction with multiple trichoepitheliomas (Fig. 13.15), parotid adenomas and eccrine spiradenomas. Long-standing lesions may become locally aggressive or occasionally undergo malignant transformation, however, metastasis is very rare.

On histology the low-power appearance of these tumours is characteristic. Isolated islands of basaloid cells are surrounded by thick PAS-positive hyaline basement membrane, and fit together like the pieces of a jigsaw puzzle. The islands contain palisading small, dark cells at the periphery and centrally there are larger cells with pale vesicular nuclei. Small duct-like structures may be present in the centre of the lobules. Malignant degeneration is characterized by loss of the PAS-positive basement membrane and very large cellular islands almost completely composed of the larger pale cells.

Chondroid syringomas are solitary, slow growing, firm intradermal or subcutaneous nodules, between 0.5 and 3 cm in diameter. They occur most commonly on the head and neck of the elderly, but can also be seen on the trunk.

Histologically two types of chondroid syringoma are recognized:

1 chondroid syringoma, with small, tubular lumina, that shows a circumscribed dermal tumour containing numerous small islands of epithelial cells and duct-like structures in a myxoid, chondroid and fibrous stroma;

2 the more common chondroid syringoma with tubular branching lumina. This contains larger tubular structures as well as more solid islands of epithelial cells within the dense stroma.

Table 13.3 Classification of eccrine tumours (after Weedon).

Benign	Malignant
Eccrine hamartomas	Microcystic adnexal carcinoma
Eccrine hidrocystoma	Eccrine carcinoma
Papillary eccrine adenoma	Adenoid cystic carcinoma
Aggressive digital papillary adenoma	Mucinous eccrine carcinoma
Chondroid syringoma	Malignant chondroid syringoma
Syringoma	Malignant cylindroma
Cylindroma	Malignant eccrine spiradenoma
Eccrine spiradenoma	Malignant eccrine poroma
Eccrine poroma	Hidradenocarcinoma
Dermal duct tumour	Eccrine ductal adenocarcinoma
Hidroacanthoma simplex	Other sweat duct carcinomas
Syringoacanthoma	
Syringofibroadenoma	
Hidradenoma (acrospiroma)	

Eccrine spiradenoma presents as a solitary grey-pink nodule on the head and neck, trunk or, less commonly, the extremities. They occur in adults and are often painful. Giant forms, linear lesions and multiple lesions have been described, as has their occurrence in association with cylindroma. Histology shows one or more well demarcated basophilic nodules in the dermis and subcutis surrounded by a thin fibrous capsule. The lobules are composed of two cell types admixed together and arranged in cords, and some contain duct-like structures. Large, pale cells are predominantly located in the centre of the lobules and outnumber the small basaloid cells found towards the periphery.

Primary cutaneous adenocystic carcinoma is a very rare tumour with a predilection for the scalp and chest. Both local recurrence and metastasis are common. Histologically it closely resembles adenoid cystic carcinoma of the salivary gland. The tumour is composed of islands and cords of basaloid cells that contain tubular structures within. There is abundant sialomucin in the tubular structures and diffusely in the lobules. These tumours should be differentiated from metastasis either from a salivary adenoid cystic carcinoma or a large intestinal mucinous adenocarcinoma.

Mucinous eccrine carcinoma is a slow growing tumour that usually occurs on the face, scalp, axilla or trunk of an older individual. The morphology is of a painless, red-brown nodule, 0.5–1 cm in diameter that tends to recur locally and metastasizes early. Histology shows the tumour is divided into a number of compartments. In each compartment islands of epithelial tumour cells float in a sea of mucin and are connected by fine fibrovascular septae.

13.7 Other primary tumours of the scalp

Neurofibromas are a benign neoplasm of Schwann cells arising from peripheral nerves. They may be solitary or multiple. Multiple neurofibromas occur as part of the autosomal dominant genodermatosis, von Recklinghausen's disease, which occurs in 1 in 3000 births.

The commonest manifestations of von Recklinghausen's disease on the scalp is neurofibromas, which may be single or multiple and appear during the second or third decade. They appear as soft flesh-coloured nodules with or without overlying alopecia. Some are very large. Plexiform neuromas may also occur on the scalp. Malignant change is rare and usually occurs in deeper structures. Surgical excision of a troublesome neurofibroma is generally simple, but may result in anaesthesia in the skin supplied by the excised nerve.

Dermatofibrosarcoma protuberans (DFP) is a rare tumour of fibroblasts that often begins in early adult life. The most common site for DFP is the trunk, but up to 10% occur on the head or neck (Fig. 13.16). Lesions look like a scar, but there is no history of preceding trauma or surgery. On palpation there is a firm dermal plaque. On the scalp DFP may directly invade the skull and brain. Histology resembles a dermatofibroma (DF) with spindle cells in a storiform pattern extending from the papillary dermis into the subcutis. Ulceration of the epidermis, invasion of the subcutis and the relatively numerous mitoses help to differentiate DF from DFP.

Atypical fibroxanthoma (AFX) is a low-grade malignant tumour that only occasionally metastasizes. Clinically they are raised nodular lesions that occur in elderly sun-damaged skin. The head and neck are most commonly sites. Nodules may have been present for many years at the time of diagnosis, but rarely grow larger than 2 cm. Atypical fibroxanthoma often ulcerates (Fig. 13.17). Histology shows a highly cellular dermal infiltrate that abuts the epidermis above and extends deeply into the subcutaneous fat below. The infiltrate comprises spindle-shaped fibroblasts, pleomorphic histiocytes with a ground glass cytoplasm, and giant cells that are strikingly atypical. Atypical mitoses are common.

Histiocytosis X is an umbrella term that incorporates three different, but related conditions characterised by a proliferation of Langerhans cells. The three clinical forms are Letterer–Siwe disease, Hand–Schuller–Christian disease and eosinophilic granuloma. In addition there are transitional cases with overlapping features.

Letterer–Siwe disease tends to occur during the first year of life and is most often associated with extensive and often fatal visceral involvement. The most common features are fever, malaise, anaemia, thrombocytopenia, hepatosplenomegaly, lymphadenopathy, and pulmonary lesions. Cutaneous lesions occur in 80%, and the most common manifestation is an eruption in the scalp consisting of numerous indurated, waxy, yellow-brown papules covered with scale and crusting. At first sight it resembles seborrhoeic dermatitis or bacterial folliculitis, however the child is obviously sick. The papules appear in crops and also occur on the trunk, face, neck and buttocks. The flexures are involved and there is often an intertrigo. Associated thrombocytopenia may make the papules haemorrhagic.

Hand–Schuller–Christian disease occurs in older children and comprises the classic triad of diabetes insipitus, exoph-

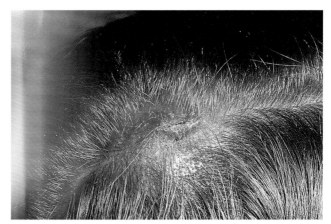

Fig. 13.16 Dermatofibrosarcoma protuberans (DFXP) presenting as an ulcerated patch of cicatricial alopecia. The lesion was very firm to palpation.

thalmos and multiple pathological fractures due to osteolytic lesions. Skin lesions occur in around 30% and are occasionally the presenting complaint. Infiltrated plaques with ulceration in the flexures, yellow papular xanthomas and lesions identical to those of Letterer–Siwe disease may occur.

Eosinophilic granuloma is a chronic localized disease that tends mainly to affect bone. The skin is only occasionally involved and the lesions may resemble the waxy papules of Letterer–Siwe or the ulcerating plaques of Hand–Schuller–Christian disease.

The histology of the scalp lesions tends to show an upper dermal band-like infiltrate with exocytosis of the cells into the epidermis. The epidermis may be ulcerated. The infiltrate is composed of large rounded cells with an abundant eosinophilic cytoplasm and an eccentric kidney shaped nucleus. There is nuclear pleomorphism and atypia. There are occasional foam cells in the infiltrate and a few multinucleate giant cells in those lesions that clinically show transition to the infiltrated plaques.

The prognosis depends on the extent of systemic organ

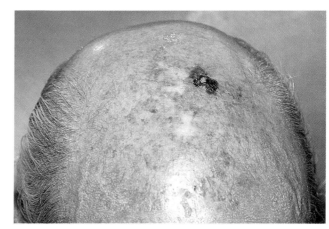

Fig. 13.17 Atypical fibroxanthoma (AFX) presenting as a haemorrhagic nodule on the scalp. (Courtesy of Dr H. Rothstein, Melbourne.)

involvement. Patients with single organ involvement have a good prognosis and often require no treatment or only limited measures. For the skin, topical nitrogen mustard, PUVA therapy or intralesional steroids can be used. If vital structures or bones are compromised low-dose radiotherapy can be given. In multisystem disease the advice and care of a paediatric oncologist is required. Prednisolone (2 mg/kg), vinblastine, methotrexate, 6-mercaptopurine, etoposide, cyclosporin A and interferon α have all been reported as useful.

Benign cephalic histiocytosis is a rare 'non-X' histiocytosis that first appears late in infancy and spontaneously resolves without scarring in childhood at around 9 years of age. Multiple 2–5 mm asymptomatic erythematous macules, papules, nodules and plaques develop on the cheeks, forehead, earlobes and neck. Scalp lesions may also occur. With time the lesions darken and new ones appear on the trunk and arms. In contrast to histiocytosis X, systemic involvement does not occur. Histology shows an infiltrate of histiocytes in the superficial and mid-dermis that is well circumscribed. The cells are S100 and CD1 negative and no Birbeck granules are seen on electron microscopy, allowing the lesions to be

distinguished from histiocytosis X. There are no Touton giant cells or foamy macrophages to suggest juvenile xanthogranuloma.

Lymphomas not uncommonly occur on the scalp. Mycosis fungoides (MF) is the most common of the cutaneous lymphomas. It is a lymphoma of T helper lymphocytes that are epidermotrophic. In the initial stages MF is confined to the skin, but in later phases there is lymph node and internal organ involvement. The skin lesions begin as macules (patch stage MF) and progress first to plaques and later into tumours (Fig. 13.18). All stages of MF may be seen on the scalp, as may the rare variant called follicular mycosis fungoides. This condition produces total alopecia and follicular papules that may clinically resemble lichen planopilaris (Fig. 13.19). Overall the prognosis of MF is good with the majority of patients surviving many years with minimal inconvenience from their disease.

Treatment of MF is palliative and not curative. First line therapy consists of potent topical steroids for a localized patch, or whole body PUVA if the patches are generalized. Topical nitrogen mustard (diluted 10 ml mustine in 50 ml of water and applied with a cotton ball) is also an effective palliative treatment that may actually cure a minority of patients. Tumours generally require radiotherapy. This can be done using superficial X-ray therapy to the tumour or with total body electron beam therapy.

Follicular mucinosis (p. 124) presents with widespread follicular accentuation and alopecia. It may be seen at any stage during the MF, but is more typical of advanced disease. Occasionally follicular mucinosis will precede other manifestations of MF. Histology is important in these cases to differentiate the benign form of follicular mucinosis from the MF-associated form.

Sézary syndrome is an erythrodermic leukaemic variant of mycosis fungoides. It is associated with diffuse hair loss or a total alopecia (Fig. 13.20). The nails may be dystrophic and resemble psoriatic nails. Sézary syndrome tends to be resistant to conventional MF treatments, but may respond to extracorporeal phototherapy. This condition has a high mortality, and death often occurs suddenly after several years.

Cutaneous B cell lymphoma may be primary in the skin or develop during the course of a nodal lymphoma. They can occur on the scalp as a solitary, firm, purple nodule, or a plaque up to several centimetres in diameter (Fig. 13.21). Grouped lesions may occasionally occur. Histology shows a dense mononuclear cell infiltrate involving the mid and deep dermis. There is usually a Grenz zone of normal dermis between the tumour and the epidermis. Lymphocyte marker studies are required to confirm the diagnosis.

Cutaneous Hodgkin's disease is a rare entity. It occurs as a late manifestation of Hodgkin's disease in 0.5% of affected patients. Firm erythematous nodules, that are sometimes ulcerated may occasionally occur on the scalp as the initial presentation of Hodgkin's. The diagnosis should be

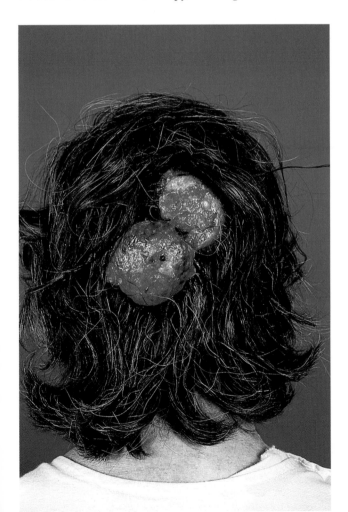

Fig. 13.18 Two large nodules of mycosis fungoides (MF) with overlying alopecia.

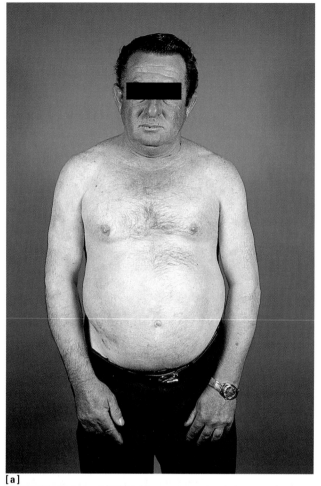

[a]

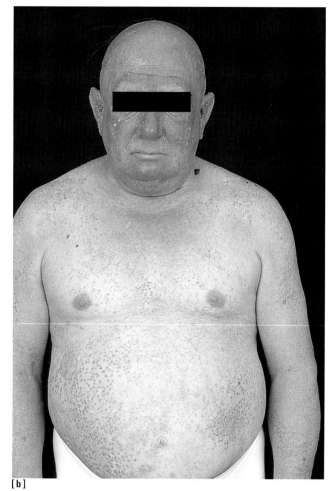

[b]

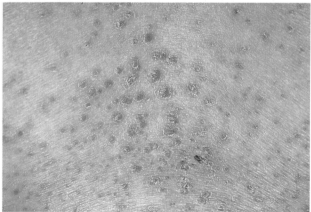

[c]

Fig. 13.19 Follicular mycosis fungoides, (a) on initial presentation and (b) 2 years later. (c) The follicular papules shown in greater detail.

confirmed by biopsy. Cutaneous lesions can be treated by either radiotherapy or chemotherapy.

Leukaemia cutis may involve the scalp and produce multiple plum coloured nodules or an erythematous plaque. It is usually associated with a poor prognosis (Fig. 13.22)

Merkel cell carcinoma is an exceptionally rare neuroendocrine carcinoma of the epidermis. It presents as a rapidly enlarging flesh-coloured nodule or tumour that may ulcerate (Fig. 13.23). It has a very high metastatic potential and while many treatments produce a temporary remission this is invariably short lived. Surgical excision of the primary tumour is the treatment of choice and radiotherapy or single agent chemotherapy with etoposide is useful for palliation of disseminated disease. Scalp lesions produce alopecia.

13.8 Metastatic carcinoma of the scalp

Definition

Metastasis to the scalp may present with nodules or alopecia neoplastica.

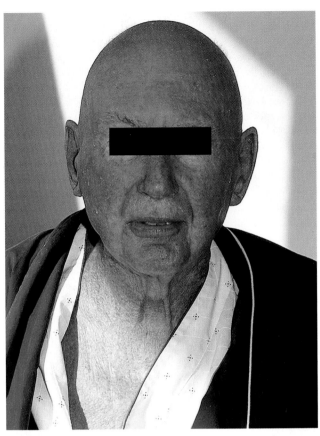

Fig. 13.20 Sézary syndrome.

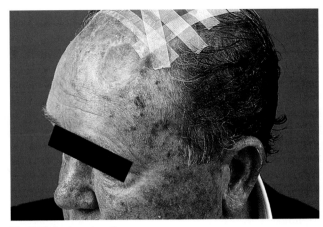

Fig. 13.22 Leukaemia cutis.

Epidemiology

Cutaneous metastasis occurs in 2–4% of patients with internal carcinoma.

Aetiology

The most common malignancies to metastasize to the scalp are breast, bronchus and renal. Others include melanoma,

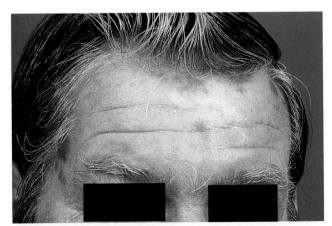

Fig. 13.21 B cell lymphoma producing an erythematous plaque along the scalp margin, and extending into the scalp.

stomach, colon, rectum, ovary and prostate. Rarely a scalp metastasis arrives from a pancreas, liver, uterus or bone primary malignancy. Meningiomas may also involve the scalp either through direct extension, through an operative defect or by metastasis.

Pathogenesis

A visceral carcinoma may directly invade overlying skin or metastasize to skin via lymphatic or bloodstream embolic dissemination. The scalp is a site of predilection, possibly because of its abundant blood supply.

Clinical features

A cutaneous metastasis to the scalp may be the initial presentation of an internal malignancy. More commonly patients have known metastatic disease. Single or multiple, firm, nontender nodules that rapidly enlarge (Fig. 13.24) are the commonest presentation. Alternatively a cicatricial alopecia (Fig. 13.25) with scleroderma-like plaques (known as alopecia neoplastica) may occur. Rarely multiple nodules may simulate turban tumours. Recently alopecia neoplastica without alopecia has been described. In this case a metastasis to the scalp did not produce clinically obvious alopecia (Fig. 13.26).

Histology may mirror that of the primary tumour or the cells may be too anaplastic for identification. In general oat cell carcinoma of the bronchus, malignant carcinoid, testicular orchidoblastoma, malignant teratoma, gastric signet ring carcinoma and metastatic clear cell renal carcinoma can be identified. Immunohistochemical techniques facilitate identification of the primary when the metastasis presents before the primary tumour is detected. The characteristic histology is of a dermal tumour nodule separated from the epidermis by a broad Grenz zone. The cells may invade the adjacent dermis in single file.

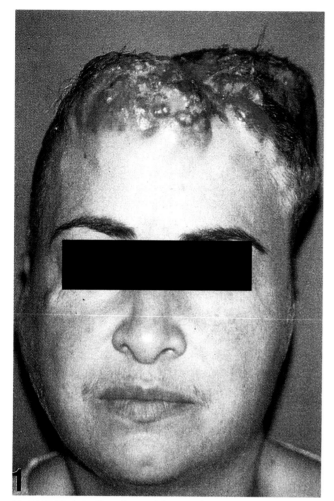

Fig. 13.23 Merkel cell carcinoma of the scalp. (Courtesy of Dr Francesco Ferrau *et al.*, Cantania, Italy and the *Journal of the American Academy of Dermatology* (1994) **31**, 271.)

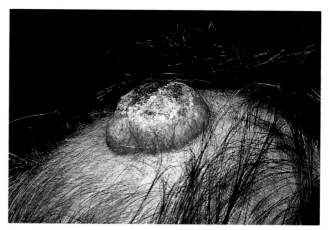

Fig. 13.24 Cutaneous metastasis from unknown primary cancer.

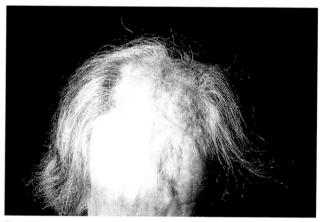

Fig. 13.25 Alopecia neoplastica due to metastasis from carcinoma of the breast.

A meningioma is an extremely rare tumour that presents as a solitary, soft or rubbery nodule, usually in the midline of the occiput. The overlying skin is usually thickened but may be atrophic. Meningiomas enlarge slowly over a number of years and may reach 10 cm in size. The diagnosis is suggested by the site and requires histological confirmation. Treatment is by excision.

Rarely tumours such as osteogenic sarcoma (Fig. 13.27) can involve the skin by direct extension from underlying bone or soft tissue.

Pathology

The histology may mirror that of the primary tumour or be undifferentiated.

Investigation

A scalp biopsy is required. Investigations pertaining to the primary tumour and other distant metastases are required.

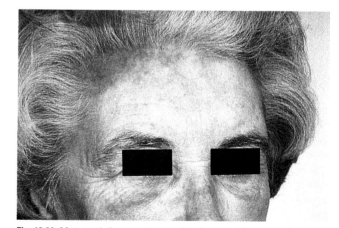

Fig. 13.26 Metastasis from carcinoma of the breast, without associated alopecia.

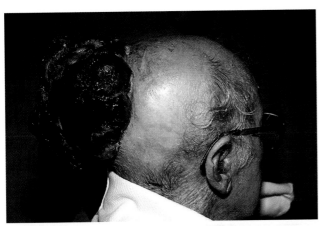

Fig. 13.27 Osteogenic sarcoma of the scalp with associated cicatricial alopecia.

Treatment

Every attempt should be made to treat the primary lesion. If this is not possible then the prognosis is poor. Hypernephromas are notorious for presenting with a solitary scalp metastasis at a stage when excision of the primary and the metastasis is possible and often associated with prolonged survival.

Key points

Scalp metastases frequently present as either single or multiple firm nontender bald nodules; or evolving patches of scleroderma-like cicatricial alopecia. It may be the initial presentation of an internal malignancy.

Index